Stepping into Emotionally Focused Therapy

This accessible, practical, and thoroughly updated second edition introduces and presents how emotionally focused therapy can be used effectively across all three modalities, couple, family, and individual therapy, with clients from a diversity of backgrounds.

Responding to critical updates in the field, this second edition once again follows Emily, an EFT therapist, to demonstrate how EFT can be used in practice. With updated references, research, and terminology throughout, this new edition reflects recent theoretical and practical updates by refocusing the model toward therapist interventions, such as the "EFT Tango," rather than the client change events, making it more accessible for readers to learn. It addresses the current need to integrate explicit socio-cultural sensitivity into EFT by including diverse case studies, explicit discussion of how the model can be applied with a diversity of clients, and how EFT therapists can integrate cultural sensitivity and attunement across multiple and diverse identities, such as race, gender, sexual orientation, disabilities, neurotypicality, class, and religion. It can also be used alongside a practical new workbook, *Workouts for Stepping into Emotionally Focused Therapy*, providing therapists with all the tools needed to confidently integrate this approach into their practice.

This book is an essential read for all marriage and family therapists in practice and in training as well as counselors who are looking to use EFT with couples, families, and individuals.

Lorrie L. Brubacher, MEd, Director of the Carolina Center for EFT, adjunct at UNCG, Greensboro, NC, has authored many EFT training videos, articles, and chapters. She trains in EFT internationally.

"This second edition is a thorough and much needed work that engages therapists in compelling new ways to personally explore how to apply the amazing growth in the EFT model. The focus on clinical interventions in the moves of the EFT Tango is, like the first edition, presented in a concrete, readily-digestible manner. Brubacher breaks new ground with an informative journey of the three modalities of EFT, combining much needed integration of culture & racial trauma."

Paul T. Guillory, PhD, Associate Professor UC Berkeley, EFT Trainer, author of
Emotionally Focused Therapy with African American Couples: Love Heals

"Lorrie Brubacher's *Stepping into Emotionally Focused Therapy* is the perfect introductory book for those who want to learn about and begin to practice EFT. Brilliantly organized around the experience of a beginning EFT therapist, Brubacher builds a clear understanding of all the essential aspects of this approach, including not only how to conceptualize and intervene, but also how to experience the powerful emotions involved. Updated and expanded to include all of the latest developments in EFT, including its adaptation to individual and family treatment modalities, and filled with evocative clinical vignettes, this book is a great resource for anyone who wants to learn more about the practice of EFT today."

Jay Lebow, PhD, ABPP, Family Institute at Northwestern University, Evanston, Illinois

"This second edition of *Stepping into Emotionally Focused Therapy* is an essential reading for all trainees and qualified practitioners who want to use the wisdom of emotionally focused therapy (EFT) ideas and techniques in their clinical work. The book has cleverly integrated all the latest advances in attachment theory and research and in the practice of EFT in an accessible and immediately useable format. It offers all the information newcomers need to integrate EFT within their clinical work, but also provides an up-to-date account of the cutting-edge expansion of EFT to individual and family therapies. The volume reads quickly and effortlessly because of the engaging author's clinical examples and insights. I enjoyed reading this informative and fascinating book. I consider it as a must-read for mental health practitioners who are looking for a compassionate and transformative approach, like EFT, to help their clients in unlocking the puzzle of their core wishes and unmet needs, healing old wounds, and moving them toward personal growth, satisfactory close relationships, and a meaningful life."

Mario Mikulincer, Professor of Psychology, Founding Dean, Baruch Ivcher School of
Psychology, Reichman University, Israel, co-author of *Attachment Theory Applied* (2023);
Attachment Theory Expanded (2023); *Attachment in Adulthood* (2018)

"This second edition of *Stepping into Emotionally Focused Therapy* is fantastic! Brubacher captures the many innovations in EFT over the last decade in simple, clear terms. For those who want to access the power of EFT with individuals, couples, and families, this is a great resource!"

Scott R. Woolley, PhD, Distinguished Professor, Couple and Family Therapy, California
School of Professional Psychology, Alliant International University, San Diego, California

Stepping into Emotionally Focused Therapy

Key Ingredients of Change

Second Edition

Lorrie L. Brubacher

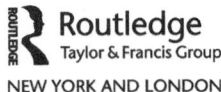
Routledge
Taylor & Francis Group

NEW YORK AND LONDON

Designed cover image: brytta © Getty Images

Second edition published 2025
by Routledge
605 Third Avenue, New York, NY 10158

and by Routledge
4 Park Square, Milton Park, Abingdon, Oxon, OX14 4RN

Routledge is an imprint of the Taylor & Francis Group, an informa business

© 2025 Lorrie L. Brubacher

First edition published by Routledge 2018

Library of Congress Cataloging-in-Publication Data
Names: Brubacher, Lorrie L., author.
Title: Stepping into emotionally focused therapy: key ingredients of change /
Lorrie L. Brubacher. Other titles: Stepping into emotionally focused couple therapy
Description: Second edition. | New York, NY: Routledge, 2024. |
Earlier edition published in 2018 as: Stepping into emotionally focused couple therapy. |
Includes bibliographical references and index. |
Identifiers: LCCN 2024004472 (print) |
LCCN 2024004473 (ebook) | ISBN 9781032151342 (hardback) |
ISBN 9781032151335 (paperback) | ISBN 9781003242673 (ebook)
Subjects: LCSH: Emotion-focused therapy. | Couples therapy. | Family psychotherapy. | Psychotherapy.
Classification: LCC RC489.F62 B78 2024 (print) |
LCC RC489.F62 (ebook) | DDC 616.89/1562–dc23/eng/20240327
LC record available at https://lccn.loc.gov/2024004472
LC ebook record available at https://lccn.loc.gov/2024004473

ISBN: 978-1-032-15134-2 (hbk)
ISBN: 978-1-032-15133-5 (pbk)
ISBN: 978-1-003-24267-3 (ebk)

DOI: 10.4324/9781003242673

Typeset in Times New Roman
by codeMantra

Support Material

Additional material, including chapter summaries and exercises, can be accessed online. Please go to www.routledge.com/9781032151335 and click on the link that says Support Material. A link to the supplementary material will appear.

Dedicated

to my mother, Alice Brubacher (1921–2020), a many-faceted crystal of love: artistry, precision, empathy, connection, self-doubt, persistence, humility, tenacity, and hope. May you live on in every act of kindness and rest in peace with your beloved family

and

to Sue Johnson (1947–2024), whose creative genius brings attachment to the forefront of individual, couple, and family psychotherapy, continuing to revolutionize the field, making therapy a process of love. May this book help to carry on your legacy of love in our profession!

Contents

About the Author

Lorrie Brubacher, MEd, LMFT, RMFT is the Founding Director of the Carolina Center for EFT. Certified with the International Centre for Excellence in EFT (ICEEFT) as a therapist, supervisor, and trainer, she has worked in private practice in individual, couple, and family therapy since 1989, and has private practices in North Carolina, USA, and Manitoba, Canada. She has an adjunct appointment at UNC Greensboro and has previously been an instructor at the University of Manitoba, University of British Columbia, and University of Winnipeg. She publishes and presents internationally on EFT, having taught Emotionally Focused Couple Therapy (EFCT) and Emotionally Focused Individual Therapy (EFIT) since 2009. Lorrie has co-authored six chapters with Dr. Sue Johnson, the originator of EFT, a chapter with Dr. Ting Liu on online EFT, is published in the *Encyclopedia of Couple and Family Therapy, in the Journal of Marriage and Family Therapy, in Person Centered and Experiential Psychotherapies*, and, with Dr. Stephanie Wiebe, on Process Research to Practice in the *Journal of Family Psychotherapy*. She serves on the editorial board for the international *EFT Community News* and is a contributing author to *Becoming an Emotionally Focused Therapist: The Workbook* (2022). She is co-developer, with Dr. Lillian Buchanan (2014) of the first EFT interactive video training program, accessible at www.attachmentinjuryrepair.com. She has many EFCT and EFIT training videos available at https://steppingintoeft.com/. The first edition of this book (2018) is in nine languages, with more translations in progress. As a companion to this book, she has authored *Workouts for Stepping into Emotionally Focused Therapy: Exercises to Strengthen Your Practice*. See more at www.lbrubacher.com, www.carolinaeft.com, and www.eftandme.com.

Foreword

This second edition of *Stepping into Emotionally Focused Therapy* is a wonderful resource to all Emotionally Focused Therapists across the spectrum from novice to highly experienced therapists and as personable and accessible as the first edition. The focus extends beyond what therapists need to do, by helping them walk into the experience of engaging the power of emotion and shaping interpersonal encounters to create change. As in the first edition, the reader is provided with an experiential sense of what it is like for a therapist to integrate the mindset and skills of EFT, by means of the personal experiences, clinical choice points, and ongoing reflections, uncertainties, and triumphs of the fictitious EFT therapist, Emily, who is growing in her practice of EFT.

Brubacher integrates the theoretical and practical advances in EFT that have occurred since her first edition, embracing the expansion of the EFT model from couple intervention, to a general psychotherapeutic model with relevance to three modalities: couple, individual, and family therapies. In this edition, the reader has an opportunity to learn alongside Emily as she experiments and develops her skills in both *Emotionally Focused Couple Therapy* (EFCT) and *Emotionally Focused Individual Therapy* (EFIT), and as she considers dipping her toe into *Emotionally Focused Family Therapy* (EFFT). This book is a practical testament to how EFT offers a clear model of change across modalities.

Lorrie also engages the reader in exploring how EFT works sensitively with racial, contextual, and intersectionality differences. The addition of cultural awareness and skills woven into the case examples is sure to be a valuable resource to readers.

Last, but not least, this text brings life to how an EFT therapist attunes to and connects with clients across the five moves of the EFT macro-intervention, the *EFT Tango*. The therapist moves and micro-interventions are broken down into practical, easy-to-follow clinical examples of EFCT and EFIT, illustrating how these therapist moves facilitate client progress through the change events that lead to significant and lasting shifts in models of self and other and in emotional balance and integration.

This book and its companion workbook, *Workouts for Stepping into Emotionally Focused Therapy: Exercises to Strengthen Your Practice*, provide a wonderful compliment to my recent books (*Attachment Theory in Practice: Emotionally Focused Therapy with Individuals, Couples and Families*, 2019; *The Practice of Emotionally Focused Couple Therapy* (3rd ed.), 2020; and with L. Campbell, *A Primer for Emotionally Focused Individual Therapy*, 2022). You are sure to enjoy Lorrie Brubacher's *Stepping into Emotionally Focused Therapy: Key Ingredients of Change* and will emerge as a more confident and competent EFT therapist after reading it.

S. Johnson

Preface

Why a Second Edition of *Stepping into Emotionally Focused Therapy*?

Trainees had been asking me since 2012 to write a book on emotionally focused individual therapy (EFIT) and after the publication of the first edition of *Stepping into Emotionally Focused Couple Therapy* (2018) and its translation into seven languages, readers have been asking for an accompanying workbook. This volume, including couple and individual therapies, is a response to both requests while also integrating the recent expansions in EFT with regard to theory, practice, and diversity. I am committed to retain what readers value in the first edition: accessibility, clarity, structure, and the musings and challenges of a fictional therapist, Emily, as she steps into the EFT model with her couples and individuals. A readily accessible companion workbook, *Workouts for Stepping into Emotionally Focused Therapy: Exercises to Strengthen Your Practice*, accompanies this second edition.

Since the publication of the first edition, EFT has undergone theoretical and practical advances (Johnson, 2019; Johnson, 2020; Johnson & Campbell, 2022) supported by new research and literature on topics, including EFT and sex (Johnson et al., 2018; Wiebe et al., 2019), EFT and violence (Slootmaeckers & Migerode, 2018, 2020), EFT and emotional and physical health (Greenman & Johnson, 2022), and EFT and cultural sensitivity (Allan et al., 2022; Guillory, 2022; Nightingale et al., 2019). Racist and culturally violent events have shaken me to the core and heightened my sense of urgency to explicitly name how EFT can be informed by racial sensitivity and multicultural concerns (Day-Vines et al., 2020; Guillory, 2022; Hardy, 2022, 2023; McGoldrick & Hardy, 2019).

The most significant theoretical advance since the first edition is that EFT has shifted from being presented primarily as a couple therapy model to a general psychotherapeutic model with relevance to three modalities: couple, individual, and family therapies (Johnson, 2019). This leads me to include parallel tracks of couple and individual therapies in a second edition, to update the terminology to reflect shifts that the expanded applications of the model to individual therapy have created, and to invite my colleagues Furrow and Palmer to write a guest chapter on Emotionally Focused Family Therapy (EFFT), to help Emily explore what it would mean to add EFFT to her practice going forward.

There is a new focus in current EFT literature and training on the specific interventions and moves made by the therapist practicing EFT (Johnson, 2019, 2020). The *EFT Tango* (described in Chapter 2 of the first edition) is a macro-sequence of EFT interventions, that practitioners find to be more accessible and easier to apply in practice than to focus on directing clients through steps and stages of change. The essence of EFT practice and the steps and stages of client change have not altered. *In practice*, to shape change events, EFT therapists repeat the five moves of the *EFT Tango* one or several times throughout each session and many times through each step of client change. In this second edition, I identify the *EFT Tango* in case examples that illustrate how the therapist's *tango moves* facilitate clients to take the nine steps and three stages toward lasting change.

Through online training experiences during the pandemic, I had the amazing privilege of connecting with trainees across the globe – from North Carolina to Hawaii, Iran, Malaysia, Greece, Africa, Brazil, Hong Kong, China, Mexico, Italy, Egypt, Romania, New Zealand, Australia, Ukraine, Romania, Canada, Israel, Russia, and more! Given my growing awareness of how the centrality of middle-class, heterosexual, whiteness can perpetuate experiences of invisibility and otherness for clients and therapists alike (Chan & Howard, 2020; Hardy, 2022, 2023; McGoldrick & Hardy, 2019), I sought out conversations and consultations with EFT colleagues around the world to explore how this edition can embrace more racial and cultural diversity. These conversations and my ongoing EFT practice keep me continually in awe of the core of EFT – the power of "empathic listening as an iterative relational process" (K. Arnold, 2014, p. 365) in which emotional restructuring and the healing potential of human connection are released! Like the first edition, this revision is an invitation for you, the reader, to receive support and encouragement to make EFT your *way of being*, as you engage with *Emily* seeking to do the same.

Acknowledgments

It is impossible to acknowledge everyone who has influenced and supported this second edition, written during difficult times of political unrest and the global pandemic. While retreating from social settings during the pandemic, my world did not shrink. It opened up in a new way with increasing online trainings and connections. To all the international colleagues I have connected with over the past seven years, since the first edition, thank you for the impacts you have had and continue to have on my perspective of humanity and psychotherapy. Everyone I connected with as colleagues, trainees, supervisees, and clients has shaped me and my writing. Thank you!

Thank you to Sue Johnson for nudging me to write the first edition and writing the forward to this second edition.

One of my greatest encouragements to keep writing has been the extensive efforts of so many colleagues to translate the first edition and to write forewords to these translations. I treasure my affectionate meeting with SungDeok Park, EFT Trainer and co-translator of the Korean translation, my warm connections with EFT supervisor, Ioanna Koukou and EFT trainer Kyriaki Polychroni, responsible for the Greek translation, the book launching for the Norwegian translation, replete with a steppingintoeft.com training video, and the enthusiastic responses for translations in EFT communities in Denmark, the Netherlands, Germany, Ukraine, Iran, and Russia. Others, waiting for this second edition to translate, have also inspired me.

Paul Guillory, Feion Villodas, Mary Hinson, Tanisha James, and Ting Liu, each in your own way, have been influential diversity consultants to me while I was writing this second edition. Thank you for your support and challenges as I have sought to explicitly integrate racial and cultural sensitivity into EFT. Thank you for challenging me to listen more deeply and to risk more curiosity. My blind spots with respect to diversity and racial-cultural trauma are ongoing learning edges for me.

Special gratitude goes to EFT trainers James L. Furrow, PhD, Couples and Family Therapy Program, Seattle University, Seattle, Washington, and Gail Palmer, MSW, co-director of the International Centre for Excellence in EFT (ICEEFT) for accepting my invitation to contribute the chapter, Emotionally Focused Family Therapy (EFFT): Stepping into EFT with Families. I am thrilled with how they joined the journey with Emily, the fictional therapist learning EFCT and EFIT throughout the book, as she ponders how to respond to a couple that has returned for family therapy. Thank you for successfully embracing the challenge of portraying the essence of EFFT in such a concrete and digestible way that Emily and the readers are left with the confidence that they can successfully extend their EFT practice to include families.

Thank you to all the members of the Carolina Center for EFT for your dedication to EFT, specifically Tanisha James, Mary Hinson, and Jenna McGown for all you do to keep the center thriving! And thank you to Maria Wood, James McCracken, Steve Wampler, and countless others for all you do to expand the center's support of EFT. Jenna McGown, my Carolina officemate, and Carolina EFT support from the earliest days of EFT at UNCG, thank you for always being there!

To UNCG graduate students and faculty, who are continuing to spread EFT in the world, thank you for the ways you support my work and give me encouragement to keep writing. While there are too many to mention by name, I hold many of you consciously in my heart and want to give specific thanks to Drs. Craig Cashwell, Scott Young, and Christian Chan. And thank you to Kelly Wester and Mitzi Lorenz for supporting my ongoing connection to UNCG.

Very specific to the labor pains of birthing this book, thank you to all who held my hand and breathed with me! I could not have done this without you! To my many colleagues and friends, thank you for all the chapter drafts you read, feedback you shared, and encouragement you gave me during the extended delivery of this book: Janet Bergsgaard, an accessible cheerleader, competent editor, and Canada-office partner; Dan Perlman, with brilliant, ever-ready responses to my queries; Ali Barbosa and Dimitrij Samoilow, EFT trainers, always encouraging and collaborating; Amanda Giordano, for your expertise and suggestions on the addictions chapter; Caroline Gasparetto, EFT supervisor, for your steady support and excellent touches to keep me grounded as I moved back and forth between this book and its companion book, *Workouts for Stepping into EFT*. And, strong and steady, Jackie Evans, a friend and editor par excellence; you are amazing at detecting nuances requiring clarity! To each of you, I am endlessly grateful!

To my loved ones, Shannon Friesen, Josh Friesen, Sandy Brubacher, Colette Minion, Bev Fehr, and Brian Kowalchuk, thank you for being who you are and bringing joy, stability, and laughter into my world. Last and most importantly, thank you to my dear husband, Dan Perlman, my accessible and responsive source of support and encouragement. Your love sustains me as a partner, a parent, a friend, and an author! Thank you!

Epigraph from *The Practice of Emotionally Focused Couple Therapy: Creating Connection*, (3rd ed.) by Susan M. Johnson. Copyright © 2020 by Routledge. Used with permission of Taylor & Francis Group LLC- Books; permission conveyed through Copyright Clearance Center, Inc.
Figure 7.4 Intersecting Axes of Privilege, Domination, and Oppression from Therapeutic Utility of Discussing Therapist/Client Intersectionality in Treatment: When and How? by M. E. PettyJohn, C-F Tseng & A. J. Blow in *Family Process, 59*(2). Used with permission of John Wiley & Sons – Books; permission conveyed through Copyright Clearance Center, Inc.

Chapter 8

Epigraph from Emotionally focused couple therapy by Susan M. Johnson. In A. S. Gurman, J. L. Lebow & D. K. Snyder (Eds.), *Clinical handbook of couple therapy* (pp. 97–128). Copyright © 2015 by Guilford. Used with permission of Guilford Publications, Inc.; permission conveyed through Copyright Clearance Center, Inc.

Chapter 9

Epigraph from *The Practice of Emotionally Focused Couple Therapy: Creating Connection*, (3rd ed.) by Susan M. Johnson. Copyright © 2020 by Routledge. Used with permission of Taylor & Francis Group LLC- Books; permission conveyed through Copyright Clearance Center, Inc.

Chapter 10

Epigraph Excerpt(s) from *A General Theory of Love* by Thomas Lewis, M.D., Fari Amini, M.D., & Richard Lannon, M.D., copyright © 2000 by T. Lewis, F. Amini, & R. Lannon. Used by permission of Random House, an imprint and division of Penguin Random House LLC. All rights reserved.

Chapter 11

Epigraph from *Attachment Theory in Practice: Emotionally Focused Therapy (EFT) with Individuals, Couples and Families* by Susan M. Johnson. Copyright © 2019 by Guilford. Used with permission of Guilford Publications, Inc.; permission conveyed through Copyright Clearance Center, Inc.

Chapter 12

Epigraph from *Inuksuit: Silent Messengers of the Arctic* by N. Hallendy. Copyright © 2001 by Douglas & McIntyre. Used with permission of Douglas and McIntyre, Inc.

Chapter 15

Epigraph from In the Realm of Hungry Ghosts: Close Encounters with Addiction by Gabor Maté, American edition published by North Atlantic Books in cooperation with Penguin Random House Canada, copyright © 2010 by Gabor Maté. Reprinted by permission of publisher.

Chapter 17

Epigraph from The Making & Breaking of Affectional Bonds, by John Bowlby. Copyright © 1979 by Taylor & Francis. Used with permission of Taylor & Francis Informa UK Ltd – Books; permission conveyed through Copyright Clearance Center, Inc.

Chapter 18

Epigraph from *All About Love* by bell hooks. Copyright © 2000 by Gloria Watkins. Used by permission of HarperCollins Publishers.

Introduction

Why an Introductory Book on Emotionally Focused Therapy?

Whether you are a new or a well-seasoned clinician learning EFT or an EFT therapist seeking an EFT refresher, I am writing this book to provide you with a panoramic view of EFT chock-full of practical nuggets, encouragement, and culturally sensitive, attachment-based inspiration. I hope to offer you an easy-to read, emotionally evocative experience that conveys the technical and artistic aspects of Johnson's (2004, 2020) EFT model of change, relevant across modalities of individual, couple, and family therapies (Johnson, 2019). I want to enhance your therapy practice and deepen your attunement to the interactive present-moment processes *within* yourself, *within* your clients, and *between* each participant on this therapeutic journey, while also sensitizing you to the impact of the dominant social context of power, prejudice, and oppression on the persons embarking on this journey. The journey of change through EFT is a journey of transformative bonding events that have the power to shift internal working models of self and other. At the same time, we need to be aware that reshaping attachment security may not serve to make the external environment any safer for clients who do not have the privileges of a dominant white, heteronormative society. In this endeavor, I offer you a model whose primary focus across all modalities is to work with the active process of emotion to foster the social connectedness that restores emotional balance and protects against the mental and physical health risks of social isolation (Greenman & Johnson, 2022) and socio-cultural inequities (Mikulincer & Shaver, 2021) with particular sensitivity to intersectionality and oppression (Crenshaw et al., 1995; Guillory, 2022; Nightingale et al., 2019; PettyJohn et al., 2020).

This edition continues to introduce EFT through the experience of Emily, a therapist learning EFT. Emily is a fictional white, cisgender, heterosexual female therapist newly stepping into the practice of EFT, keen on being racially and culturally sensitive. In *Workouts for Stepping into Emotionally Focused Therapy: Exercises to Strengthen Your Practice*, written to accompany this second edition, Emily's responses are included as a benchmark from which the reader can compare their responses and consider whether there is anything in Emily's responses that they may want to integrate into their EFT style. The first edition of this book focused almost entirely on Emily's couple therapy, with only one chapter detailing her discovery of how smoothly EFT could be extended from couples to individuals. This second edition offers parallel tracks of her exploration of EFT with couples (EFCT) and with individuals (EFIT) as two complimentary modalities of the same therapy model. After following her journey, with couples and individuals, readers will have the opportunity to witness her ventures into Emotionally Focused Family Therapy (EFFT) in a chapter by guest authors J. Furrow and G. Palmer.

How This Book Can Enrich Your Therapy Practice

First, by exploring the attachment theory of love, you are provided with a unifying theoretical foundation for formulating clients' problems and the endpoint of successful treatment, and for operationalizing therapeutic interventions shown to help clients reach those outcomes. Second, attachment theory offers a map of the terrain that clients step through to move from distress to secure bonds and full engagement with life. Having access to this map helps you locate where your clients are in their change process. Third, by immersing in the experiential roots of EFT, your therapy can become more infused with moment-to-moment engagement with clients. This active engagement with clients increases their depth of in-session experience, a factor proven to be associated with therapeutic change. Lastly, the attachment theoretical definition of love as a safe and secure attachment bond has some very important cultural, systemic implications. This book will hopefully broaden your capacity as an EFT therapist to be more attuned to racial and intersectional trauma and the impacts of the larger socio-cultural context as well as increase your awareness of times you cannot assume to understand and need, humbly and with empathic curiosity, to invite clients to share as much of their story as they are willing to share.

A Theory of Love and Its Implications for Therapy

EFT is the only model of therapy that is based on a clearly delineated and empirically validated theory of adult love. The definition of adult love as a secure attachment bond (Johnson, 2019) puts the quality of people's sense of emotional connectedness to significant others in the forefront as both etiology and source of recovery from anxiety, depression, post-trauma reactions, and relational distress. It provides guidance to questions EFT therapists ask themselves, such as, "What is happening in emotional distress?" "Where am I headed with this couple?" "How do we get to a better place?" "What emotional processes and repetitive patterns are driving a couple's distress or an individual clients' depression and anxiety?"

A clearly articulated theory of adult love equips a therapist with a precise picture of well-functioning adult love, emotion regulation, and emotional balance. It provides a map of how to help distressed clients arrive at a safe destination. The map of therapeutic change leads clients to secure attachment bonds that provide the optimum sources of emotion regulation, vitality, and resilience. A theory of adult love keeps a therapist from getting lost in a jungle of conflict, distance, distress, depression, and anxiety. By promoting the innate mammalian need for safe and secure connection, attachment theory provides a therapist with a clear destination for therapy. It also creates a distinct formulation of the core issue in relational and mental distress. Extending beyond surface disagreements and disappointments, unmet needs for secure connection are seen to be at the heart of relational distress, anxiety, depression, and persistent trauma reactions (Barlow et al., 2018; Bowlby, 1980). Attachment theory of adult love provides a therapist with a pragmatic, reliable guide to help a couple to reach a destination of love at its best or an individual to move from despair to hope, resilience, and emotional fitness.

The attachment theoretical view of trauma, love, and emotion regulation holds that human beings are innately wired to survive and to thrive in a context of meaningful emotional connections (Bowlby, 1980; Thompson et al., 2021). It also maintains that predictable behaviors of *separation distress* – protest, clinging, despair, detachment – arise when relationships do not offer this security. This orientation releases a therapist from the pressure to problem solve and remediate symptoms of depression, anxiety, or relationship conflict. Instead, it offers a map for change that guides the collaborative therapist-client team to stabilize habitual emotion regulation patterns (*How are we shaping our world?/How am I shaping my world?*) and to restructure attachment views of self as lovable, worthy, and competent, and of some others as trustworthy and reliable (*How we can reshape our world/How I can reshape my world*).

The EFT Map of Client Change

The science of romantic relationships, as portrayed in attachment theory and research, provides a reliable map for transforming relationships dominated by unexpressed attachment emotions and needs. Correspondingly, the attachment view of personality, health, and emotion regulation disorders (Bowlby, 1973, 1980, 1982; Johnson, 2019) provides a reliable map for shaping interpersonal corrective emotional experiences that reshape individuals' depression, anxiety, and post-trauma reactions into emotional balance and full engagement with life. This book provides case examples of how a clinician frames and normalizes some of the most difficult and daunting couple interactions and individual emotional disorders with an attachment lens. The attachment view of *separation distress* reactions provides therapists with a solid foundation to de-pathologize and make sense out of what may, at first glance, appear to be crazy-making, irrational behaviors playing out in front of them in session. The attachment view also provides therapists with a hopeful reframe and map of how to respond to what may feel like overwhelming, hopeless presenting problems.

The nine steps in three stages of client change in the empirically validated model of EFT remain the core of the clients' process and provide a map to locate where a client is in the journey of change. Current EFT literature and training, however, are focusing on a more accessible way for therapists to learn *how* to practice EFT and help clients step through the EFT steps and stages of change (Beasley & Ager, 2019; Johnson et al., 1999). Johnson (2015) created a streamlined, practical macro-intervention known as The *EFT Tango.* This macro-intervention simplifies the *how* of EFT into five basic therapeutic moves for guiding clients through the EFT steps and stages of change. The parsimonious, macro-sequence of five specific *moves* integrates the micro-interventions of empathic reflections, evocative questions, validation, empathic conjectures, tracking sequences of interactions, reframing, and shaping, processing, and integrating corrective emotional experiences, into a flexibly attuned, yet very systematic way of practicing EFT.

The interventions in the EFT Tango make it possible for therapists to focus on a repeating series of moves with different pacing and varied degrees of intensity depending upon where in the change process the client is. With the Tango moves, client change events recede into the background and precise attunement to clients' emotional interpersonal dance and internal processing moves into the foreground. The EFT Tango provides therapists with a flexible set of tools for moments when client stages of change take nonlinear turns. Moreover, the moves of the Tango are a consistently reliable guide with flexibility, supportive of EFT deliberately expanding to welcome more racial and cultural diversity (Nightingale et al., 2019).

The Experiential Roots of EFT

Research on the processes of EFT that make it effective points to the salience of present-moment experience (Brubacher & Wiebe, 2019; Greenman & Johnson, 2013). Changing attachment security is based on corrective emotional experiences, not on insight, explanations, or problem solving. "An event must be lived in a moment of presentness" writes Stern (2004, p. xiii). EFT therapists do not attempt to determine causes and origins of problems. They engage empathically in present-moment process, helping clients to notice stuck points, rigid patterns, and the primary, core underlying emotions driving those patterns as the pathway to reshape secure interpersonal connections. To create lasting change in EFT, clients need "an experience, not an explanation" (Ehrenwald, 1976, p. 392).

EFT can change your perception of what is happening in client distress and "alter your vision of what is happening in a psychotherapy session" (Stern, 2004, p. xiii). After their initial struggle to shift away from trying to *fix clients' presenting problems* to following a *process model*, new EFT therapists are frequently enthused. They find it liberating to replace problem solving with acknowledging and stabilizing negative patterns, reprocessing the underlying emotions driving these patterns, and shifting typical patterns into ones that foster safe and secure bonds. Therapists are energized to discover that they can accept individual and relational distress as normative and not something they must fix or explain. When they empathically understand clients' presenting problems as best attempts to manage attachment panic at disconnection, therapists can help clients identify coping patterns of anxious escalation or avoidant numbing that have become rigid and ineffective. Stabilizing automatic, reactive patterns gives clients enough emotional balance to access core, unexpressed, underlying emotions, which contain motivations and meanings that are used to shape new strategies for interpersonal connection and reshape a sense of self and other.

Cultural Attunement to Racial and Intersectional Trauma

Based in attachment theory, EFT requires the therapist first and foremost to be a secure attachment figure who, like a fully attuned, responsive, and engaged parent, creates a safe context of unconditional acceptance and empathic understanding for therapeutic exploration. The imperatives for creating this secure attachment space in a racially humble and culturally sensitive manner are that the therapist be genuinely willing to disclose their own social location and positions of power and privilege (Jones, 2016). The therapist must also be empathically curious and courageous to initiate conversations about intersectional or racial trauma and to invite exploration about experiences of marginalization (Allan et al., 2022; Hardy, 2023; PettyJohn et al., 2020).

New to this edition will be conversations about Emily's attempts to integrate racial, ethnic, and cultural (REC) sensitivity into the EFT process. The prominence that EFT gives to empathic curiosity, increasing specificity of client's experience, lingering in the present moment, and therapist humility and genuineness, makes it well suited for broaching these contextual issues. When the terms "*race*" and "REC" are used, it is with the awareness that the term *race* is a discriminatory term, created by whites to justify enslavement and marginalization based on the color of skin; however, race "continues to be an organizing principle … [dictating] … every stage of the human lifecycle" (Hardy, 2023, p. 5) and thus *race matters* (Guillory, 2022; West, 2017).

Key Ingredients of Change

The *experiential manner* in which the key ingredients of change are implemented is an integral part of what makes them effective. The three significant client change events: (1) Stage 1 Stabilization/De-escalation; (2) Stage 2 Engagement; and (3) Stage 2 Softening are deliberately shaped in session, through collaborative, alive-in-the-moment, relational experiences. Three key ingredients (or tasks) on the route toward these transformative change events are creating and maintaining a therapeutic alliance, assembling and deepening emotional experience, and restructuring ways of engaging through interpersonal dialogues. These elements of change in EFT are distilled in the acronym TEA for Therapeutic task alliance, Emotional depth, and Affiliative interactions (Brubacher & Wiebe, 2019).

Transcripts and videos demonstrating EFT's key ingredients in couple and individual therapies are available at www.SteppingintoEFT.com in English and with subtitles in a range of languages.

Overview of the Book

In *Stepping into Emotionally Focused Therapy: Key Ingredients of Change*, I provide guidance with which to gradually learn EFT, one step at a time. I offer a concise introduction to EFT (Johnson, 2019, 2020) with practical handles for working successfully with couples, individuals, and families with this empirically validated model of therapy (Beasley & Ager, 2019; Greenman & Johnson, 2013; Wiebe & Johnson, 2016). Readers of the first edition have confirmed that the tools in this book are equally relevant for new clinicians or graduate students wanting to integrate EFT into their practice, for seasoned therapists seeking to shift paradigms or curiously dip a toe into EFT waters, and for EFT therapists wanting to deepen or broaden their EFT skills.

A therapist new to EFT will learn (1) a new paradigm of adult love and relational needs, (2) a new view of emotional distress and emotion regulation, (3) a map of sequential client change events, (4) a flow of five basic therapist moves that integrate experiential and systemic interventions, all oriented toward attachment emotions as the target and agent of change, and (5) awareness of ones' own social location and relationship to power, prejudice, and oppression, and skills to initiate conversations about the impacts of minority stress and privilege.

Despite being a short-term therapy, the experiential nature of EFT requires slow, repetitive, moment-to-moment engagement and attunement. Therapists can become discouraged as they encounter challenges with various complexities in applying the EFT model. They need a gradual yet focused, accepting, alive experience of stepping into a new paradigm. One of the dramatic shifts, however, that therapists report following EFT training is a more empathic, collaborative stance toward themself as a therapist and toward clients (Conrad, 2015; Koren et al., 2022; Rodríguez-González et al., 2019; Sandberg & Knestel, 2011).

Whether or not you decide to make the paradigm shift to this attachment-orientated model, you can enhance your current practice by learning about the EFT elements that studies have identified are key to creating lasting change (Brubacher & Wiebe, 2019; Greenman & Johnson, 2013, 2022). My intention in this book is to support clinicians to gradually integrate elements of EFT into their work and to experience how to collaboratively guide clients through a contextually relevant, attachment-based, humanistic, experiential change process. I intend to help clinicians from different therapeutic orientations to discover how the EFT processes leading to change are qualitatively and practically different from seemingly similar interventions in other approaches.

Chapter Structure

To meet the need for stepping slowly and mindfully into this model, I introduce the EFT model in Chapter 1 and describe the therapist interventions and key ingredients for change in Chapters 2–4. I outline the attachment perspective of adult love in Chapter 5 and in Chapter 6, detail how emotion is both the target and agent of change. I structure Chapters 7–11 according to the EFT steps of client change. These central chapters illustrate the process of change with a series of three questions noted below. In Chapters 12–14, I help you to integrate and consolidate the key ingredients of change by summarizing markers to locate where clients are on the EFT map of change. I show how Emily explores her own "felt sensing" to follow these markers. Then in Chapters 15–17, we examine EFT in special circumstances – working with addictive behaviors, resolving relationship-specific *attachment injuries*, and, finally, extending the model to working with families. Chapter 18 closes with suggestions for you to plan your next steps with EFT.

The responses to the questions in Chapters 7–11 illustrate clients' movement through the steps and stages of EFT change with couple and individual case examples that include multiple cultural identities. Each of these chapters addresses the following questions:

1. **What do EFT therapists SEE and HEAR?** How does attachment, as a theory of adult love and cultural attunement, guide a clinician to identify what they see and hear in clients' distress?
2. **What do EFT therapists and clients DO?** I describe therapist interventions used in the five moves of the EFT Tango to reflect present process, assemble and deepen emotional experience, shape engaged encounters, process these encounters, and finally, integrate corrective emotional experiences. Since EFT is a collaborative process, I also include client processes through each stage of change.
3. *HOW* **do EFT therapists move with clients through the change process?** Since EFT is both an art and a science, I discuss the attuned, fluid manner in which therapists engage with clients to guide this process.

Online Support Material: There is online support material to accompany many of the chapters. Interactive exercises, succinct summaries, text boxes with tips and guidelines serve as useful tools; several detailed case examples with transcript and more are available (routledge.com/9781032151335).

Terminology Updates

Changes in terminology in this second edition reflect how the EFT language has expanded to more accurately describe a model of psychotherapy, relevant across modalities of couples, families, and individuals. For example, with the moves of the EFT Tango, *encounter* replaces the earlier term *enactment* to refer to a therapist-choreographed dialogue between individuals in the therapy room, such as between partners or family members, between the client and the therapist, or with an *imaginal other* or between two aspects of self. Another shift is a greater use of the term *stabilization* to describe the first change event, initially described as *de-escalation*. The term *patterns* will be used somewhat interchangeably but more prominently than *cycles*. I also primarily use the pronoun *they* to convey greater gender inclusivity. Terminology referring to the active process of emotion is also updated. Since Johnson (2019), the terms for *primary* and *secondary* emotions have been revised into simpler and more practical terms. Now an emotional response which quickly goes underground and is rapidly replaced by a self-protective reactive emotion and action is referred to as a *core emotion* instead of as a *primary* emotion, and a reactive emotional response is referred to as *reactive* instead of as *secondary* emotion.

Hopes for the Reader

It is my hope that reading this book will enrich your therapy practice by integrating EFT one step at a time into your *way of being* with clients. In so doing, you can embark on a lifetime discovery of the art and science of moving with clients from distress to meaningful connection, emotional resilience, and flexibility. You will engage with each individual and couple client in transformative change processes toward the essential ingredient for survival and thriving among all mammals: *effective dependency* (Bowlby, 1988), or as later scholars have called it, *optimal dependence* (Feeney et al., 2015). You can also expect to become more compassionate and intimate in your personal relationships (Conrad, 2015; Rodríguez-González et al., 2019; Sandberg & Knestel, 2011) and as readers of the first edition attest, more confident and competent in your practice of EFT.

EFT therapists are continually learning from practicing EFT. Inspired by an interview with long-time songwriter Paul Simon, an EFT therapist described how Simon continues to learn from the *practice of his craft*. "Just thinking about how you, over decades, learn a sense of what words to stay away from, what words to go to, how rhythm could be used, how melody… You just learn from your craft" (Ogner, 2015). Dr. Sue Johnson replied, saying, "This is what I love about my work – it captures exactly how I feel in my practice. I find myself seeing a new couple or individual, and muttering to myself, 'fascinating,' and, 'now what?' Loving the process is what keeps me passionate here."

If this model proves to be a good fit for you, you may be reassured to know that therapist passion and allegiance for a model are found to be a strong determinant of therapy outcomes (Blow et al., 2007). May your journey through this book be an inspiring adventure.

Part I

Key Ingredients of Change on the EFT Roadmap

1 Stepping into Emotionally Focused Therapy (EFT)

In this chapter, you will meet Emily, a therapist newly learning Emotionally Focused Therapy (EFT). Her reflections and challenges with practicing EFT permeate the book. Her reflections are sprinkled through the brief history of the development of EFT, after which the EFT model of the client change process and the research validating EFT as an evidence-based approach are reviewed. Scenarios of Emily's clients reappear throughout Chapters 7–11, evoking a real-life sense of being an EFT therapist. Emily will become your companion as an EFT learner.

Clients presented here are composites of different clients with identifying characteristics altered. You may well recognize similarities with some of your clients and, no doubt, will identify with some of Emily's challenges and reflections.

On a Tuesday morning with autumn leaves swirling on the path between her steps, Emily walks toward her office, anticipating her first session of the day with Jessica and Wayne. Emily enjoys working with this couple, caught in a classic pursue/demand–withdraw/defend attachment dance. Jessica reactively pursues and pushes for responses from Wayne, and Wayne reflexively withdraws and defends. In her work with this biracial couple, Emily continues to be humbly curious about how her whiteness may be interfering with her empathic attunement with Jessica whose father is white and whose mother is from Argentina, and with Wayne who is black, with an Ethiopian heritage. "Am I fully attending? Is my whiteness interfering with my attunement to their relational and contextual experience? Am I understanding their experience as they need me to understand it?" she asks herself.

As much as she dislikes acknowledging it, Emily is also aware of feeling some dread about meeting with her second couple, Phil and Julie. Underneath their very calm exteriors and rather positive presentation of their relationship, Emily picks up hints of fragility in Julie, particularly as she references her discovery of Phil's extensive use of pornography in the past and her tempered admiration for his current sobriety. She senses self-sufficiency and a volatile protectiveness in Phil, who attributes his sobriety to investing in 12-step groups for alcohol, narcotic, and pornography addiction. Certainly, with this couple – brave Caucasian childhood trauma survivors – it is a challenge for Emily to retain a de-pathologizing, attachment frame. While feeling some pulls to pathologize Phil, she strives to respectfully and collaboratively explore their relationship distress as an attachment dynamic of emotion regulation. She recalls the attachment theoretical frame for substance use and other additive processes as attachment disorders and as *best-attempt strategies* to provide relief from negative emotions (Barlow, 2002; Flores, 2004).

Emily's heart flutters as she anticipates with the usual excitement and trepidation, the new couple she has scheduled later that day. It is typical for her to feel nervous excitement before meeting new couples and she also feels an added layer of pressure to be grounded and well attuned with transparency and curious empathy to this lesbian, Asian/American cisfemale couple.

DOI: 10.4324/9781003242673-2

Her thoughts skim lightly over recent interactions with two individual clients she will be seeing that day as well: A young immigrant cisgender woman named Sahra with whom she has met for several sessions; and a cisgender male named Max, in his late forties who self-identifies as neurodiverse. Sahra is struggling with loneliness, anxiety, and depression. Emily reminds herself to slow her pace with Sahra, whose ready access to tears and rapid story telling can be mesmerizing. Emily is discovering that she needs to slow the process so they can both be attuned to Sahra's present moment experience. She needs to tread the fine line between connecting with Sahra's depth of experience, while containing her emotion so that it does not become overwhelming and lead Sahra to shut down and disconnect. Emily also aches for Max when she thinks of what he has survived – childhood sexual abuse, scenes of death, time in jail, family losses, and now the end of his marriage. She hopes she can adequately engage him in therapy, as he rather methodically seeks to come to terms with the traumas he has survived and to spend less energy attempting to block them from consciousness.

As a young therapist passionately devoted to her profession, Emily frequently finds herself amidst intensely charged emotional turmoil between romantic partners. At times, the extreme emotions surrounding their staunchly pronounced differences can pull her off-balance emotionally. She feels a pressure to help them solve seemingly irreconcilable conflicts, and to dissolve the palpable tension that arises as they discuss issues that range from extended families, childrearing, time spent at work, a lack of sexual intimacy, racial or homophobic discrimination, or a recently discovered affair. Secrets, rage, indifference, disgust, accusations, and her own failed attempts to intervene, whirl around her like a swarm of bees. Then, like a cool refreshing breeze wafting through an open window, Emily draws a reframe from attachment theory for this emotionally distressing drama playing out before her. As she looks through the attachment lens, Emily begins to detect melodies of longings for secure connection and acceptance. Beneath a couple's battle over the recent family vacation gone wrong, she hears one partner's plea for respite from complaints and demands, and the other partner's protest for engagement and closeness. In the moment one partner dismisses their partner's experience of prejudice, Emily hears a loud call for acceptance and validation of their lived experience of racial trauma.

Recently stepping into EFT, Emily feels some degree of relief with the de-pathologizing framework that this model provides for her couple and individual therapy. The various dramas of romantic love in distress and individuals' depression, anxiety, and trauma reactions which at first all looked like problems for her to solve are beginning to take a new form. EFT is giving her a different view of both couples' and individuals' problems, providing a perspective that the real problem is the recurring pattern of self-protective emotional responses to threatening signals. She admits, somewhat sheepishly to herself, that the communication techniques and problem-solving skills she taught her clients in the past, while effective in her office, routinely slipped out the window when emotions ran high at home. While slowly integrating the theory and science of attachment and beginning to see emotion as a *perception-feeling-meaning-action process*, she feels like she is getting a new lease on life and on her work! "My job is no longer to fix and teach and change clients!" Emily repeats to herself:

> I no longer have to find the solution to their problems. I do not need to help partners fight more politely, nor teach individuals skills for self-compassion. All I need to do to begin the process of change is attune and listen to their *emotional music.*

In her work with couples, Emily is discovering that change begins when she helps each partner to participate in identifying the predictable sequence of dance steps they take when one partner's hurt or fear is conveyed as an angry protest or an abrupt disappearance. Emily calms down with the recognition that these predictable steps form the *dance* or repetitive pattern unfolding before her eyes. "I need to trust myself to be fully present to the emotional music and the dance of interaction – that is my most important offering!"

Emily knows that after couple clients have disentangled their cycle of repetitive interactions, they will explore together, the softer, more vulnerable emotions, fears, and good intentions that have gone underground and been buried under reactive emotions and behaviors. She realizes that reactive, protective emotions and behaviors become so automatic that they are almost imperceptible. It takes time before a couple moves to the next part of the work but Emily reminds herself that when they do, their more vulnerable feelings and longings will be uncovered and explored like newly discovered treasures. Previously unacknowledged, unexpressed emotions, when accessed and experienced, become alchemist's gold from which partners can transform previously imprisoning patterns of distancing/suppressing and hyperactivating/complaining into positive cycles of increasing safety, connection, and joy.

"I don't know how to do all this yet," Emily realizes, but she sits more calmly and hopefully with each couple, recognizing that the tension before her is the normal attachment distress of two people who are important to one another. She is learning to trust that her empathically attuned presence and validating understanding of each unique attachment drama is the first and hugely important step out of oppressive disconnection. She takes comfort in Bowlby's essential message to caregivers of infants that they do not need to be perfect; they just need to be *present* (Karen, 1994).

While enthusiastically following EFT for her couple therapy, she is delighted to see how EFT's refreshingly de-pathologizing attachment approach extends smoothly to her individual clients who are struggling with depression, anxiety, suicidal despair, grief, interpersonal conflicts, and post-traumatic stress. Recalling the words of Lewis et al. (2000, p. 169), "Love is not only an end for therapy; it is also the means by which every end is reached," Emily is overjoyed to embrace this model that can also make her individual therapy an experience of love and transformational change. In a Facebook message to her new Ugandan friend, Akiiki, whom she met online in an EFIT training group, she excitedly writes:

> Since EFT can shape secure bonds that have tremendous benefits for relational, emotional, and physical health, we can use EFT to support our individual clients too. Trauma-survivors, individuals suffering in emotional isolation, clients who have no *significant other* relationships in their lives can all benefit from this transformative model. We must help each other to master it.

Emily is thrilled that the revolution, which Johnson initiated with her therapeutic applications of the science of love to romantic relationships (2013), applies to her work with individuals, including those who have no secure relational bases. Liberation from the typical pressure she has felt to help individuals flooded with anxiety or flattened by depression and lethargy is offered to her from the attachment theoretical frame. Attachment theory frames emotional disorders as rigid stuck patterns for dealing with threatening, foreign, and unacceptable emotions (Barlow et al., 2018; Bowlby, 1988). It is revolutionary in individual therapy, not to pathologize individuals suffering from emotional disorders but to collaborate with them on identifying their stuck patterns of emotion regulation. Emily is passionate about the nonjudgmental nature of this model that validates the appropriateness of different strategies at different times and prioritizes flexibility over maintaining that there is one correct way to regulate emotions. She has emblazoned in her heart Bowlby's de-pathologizing words, "clinical conditions are best understood as disordered versions of what is otherwise a healthy response" (1980, p. 245). What may be useful in one context will not be helpful as a rigid strategy. Emily is discovering that change begins to happen as she helps her clients discover, with empathic curiosity and acceptance, the imprisoning patterns that are blocking them from their deepest longings for connection and support.

Initially, her client Max's depression and anxiety looked like a problem she needed to fix. Now it is taking the shape of a recurring pattern they can identify together: A threatening cue of others' laughter triggers his reflexive action tendency to self-isolate which, in turn, heightens his perceived threat of being taunted. Assembling his emotion in this pattern provides the foundation for case formulation, treatment planning, goal setting, and the first change event of stabilization.

The Tripartite Origins of EFT

EFT began with Johnson and Greenberg (1985, 1988) observing their couples in therapy to identify the effective therapeutic moves and the client processes that lead couples from distress to relationship satisfaction and trust. While observing their recorded therapy sessions, they were admittedly biased toward an experiential approach of empathic reflections of emotional experience, non-pathologizing acceptance, and the power of therapist congruence and moment-to-moment engagement in the relationship (Perls, 1969; Rogers, 1961, 1980). Given that they were tracking interactions between partners and observing the context of partners' impact on one another, they realized that it was necessary to add a systemic orientation to the general experiential perspective. Systems theory (Bertalanffy, 1968) is epitomized in family therapy by Minuchin and other structural family therapists (Minuchin & Fishman, 1981). In both systems theory and experiential approaches, problems are seen in terms of process, rather than as being inherent in the person.

It wasn't long before Johnson noticed recurrent themes in couples' stories – fears of loss and abandonment, loneliness, loss of connection, broken trust, fears of rejection, and a sense of failure. She recognized that these themes pointed couple therapy in a new direction. No longer did intimate relationships appear to be rational bargains or co-habiting arrangements to be negotiated. She recognized that, in fact, they were *emotional bonds*, replete with the same intense longings, needs, and thrills, as the bonds between parents and infants. What a remarkable and revolutionary discovery this was! In fact, Johnson's creative and compassionate genius was one of the initial steps of *cracking the code for love* in the field of psychotherapy (Burgess Moser et al., 2015).

The therapeutic model of EFT was developed and first tested in the early 1980s in the context of couple therapy (Johnson & Greenberg, 1985, 1988). Unique to this model was a clearly delineated theoretical integration of experiential (Perls, 1969; Rogers, 1961) and systemic traditions (Minuchin & Fishman, 1981), focusing simultaneously on intrapsychic and interpersonal experiences. No other psychotherapeutic approach had previously synthesized these two traditions. Emotion was featured as both target and agent of change in creating corrective emotional experiences that repaired distressed couple relationships. Johnson's (2004) addition of the attachment orientation (Bowlby, 1973, 1979, 1980, 1982) resulted in EFT becoming the only empirically validated couple therapy based on a theory of adult love. Adding the attachment base to EFT strengthened and streamlined the tasks of transforming distressed couple relationships into safe and secure emotional bonds.

Emily smiles, recalling the metaphor of integration she has heard: Rogers, Minuchin, and Bowlby, sitting together over a cup of tea to discuss what it is that makes psychotherapy effective. When we listen in to their conversation, we can recognize the exquisite integration of Johnson's model of EFT. Carl Rogers, with his experiential focus, is emphasizing empathic attending and responding to how people organize and process their internal emotional experience. He addresses the values of attending moment-to-moment to clients' in-session process and of focusing on people's innate capacity to grow when they are understood and accepted in a genuine relationship. Rogers highlights that the task of the therapist is not to fix but to join with clients and walk into painful experience with them, and to help them process that experience more fully. He says, "We are *process consultants* – not problem solvers or insight givers. We are validators of each person's internal emotional experience." Rogers' focus on reshaping internal experience features emotion as the target and agent of change in psychotherapy.

Salvador Minuchin, with his systemic approach, is accentuating the impact of the system, pointing out that the patterns of interaction that people engage in take on a life of their own and become self-reinforcing. The problem, he says, is not in the individual but in the system – in the reinforcing patterns of interaction in which people are caught. Change, from a systemic point of view, begins with change in the leading elements of the system. Rogers reiterates that emotion is indeed the leading element in the system, while Minuchin focuses more on elements of the interpersonal context as the leading element.

John Bowlby, with the attachment perspective, interrupts to say, "Friends, you are essentially talking about the same thing. You are talking about the power of human connection – safe and secure interpersonal bonds – and how we are all shaped through our interactions and emotional connections with others." When we understand the attachment needs for safe and secure interpersonal connection, the experiential emphasis on internal processing and the systemic focus on interpersonal exploration are inextricably intertwined.

Emily imagines Bowlby whispering into Sue Johnson and Les Greenberg's ears about *disconnection* as the essential problem in couple distress and individual emotional disorders. She visualizes them painting the path away from distress, isolation, and loneliness, toward emotional balance and secure bonds of interpersonal connection. Attachment science points a clear path to secure connection by processing the core emotions driving negative patterns and then shaping interpersonal, emotionally infused dialogues to reshape patterns of interaction into *broaden-and-build cycles* (Mikulincer & Shaver, 2021, 2023a). Connection is the heart of the matter.

Attending to Intersectionality

A powerfully effective model of therapy was created in this tripartite integration (Beasley & Ager, 2019; Johnson, 2020) and in the 2020s, there arose a loud cry (Allan et al., 2022; Guillory, 2022; Nightingale et al., 2019) for the systemic elements of EFT to include more explicit attention to socio-cultural context and intersectionality of client and therapist systems (Hill et al., 2020). Intersectionality, first defined by Crenshaw et al. (1995), refers to multiple social identities and positions such as race, gender, sexual orientation, age, and neurodiversity, creating varied experiences of power and oppression. When intersectionality becomes part of EFT, it makes explicit the need to attend to contextual traumas and impacts of marginalization that may have been far too often overlooked. As *process consultants*, EFT therapists do not get derailed by content and problem solving, but they do invite discussion of the contextual impact of socio-cultural marginalization and trauma. EFT therapists seek to attune to how lived experiences of minority stress are undeniably part of clients' ongoing emotional experiencing (Day-Vines et al., 2018, 2020). As one client said, "The stresses of being a Black, neurodiverse woman in America are complex and ongoing."

Eager to place socio-cultural diversity more prominently in the EFT model, some EFT educators (Seiff-Haron & Calamur, 2022) suggest inviting other leaders and storytellers to the metaphorical Rogers-Minuchin-Bowlby tea party that Johnson has suggested symbolizes the integrative essence of EFT. Much could be learned from those experiencing anti-black, anti-Asian, anti-Hispanic, anti-LGBTQIA+ threats, and from those experiencing neurodiverse, socio-economic, religious, and other types of marginalization. This EFT tea party guest list could include figures such as African American authors James Baldwin, Toni Morrison, bell hooks, politicians, and spiritual leaders Martin Luther King, John Lewis, Desmond Tutu, Nelson Mandela, Thich Nhat Hanh, and Temple

Grandin from the neurodiverse community, and labor leaders, trans and civil rights activists, Indigenous leaders across the globe, and many more.

Another way to imagine this *tea-party-turned-international-conference* is that EFT is essentially a model that invites dialogue between people from many races, genders, and classes. In our therapeutic conversations with each couple or individual, we invite stories and lived experiences where race, class, neurodiversity, and gender may be in the forefront. We engage in empathic attunement, open to enter the world of each client's lived experience. Their context and story are theirs' to share – as much or as little of it as they wish. We cannot presume to understand what is not shared. At the same time, elements of each client's lived experience may well be something they have never yet put into words or *known* with a clear *felt-sense*. As we listen, and in relationship therapy also help partners to listen to each other, we are engaging in a collaborative, evolving experience of honoring stories shared in a new way.

Cultural, contextual considerations are part of all three elements integrated in EFT, as befits a model based on science. Berscheid (1999) asserted that a science of interpersonal relationships "requires transcendence of psychologists' traditional individualistic orientation, as well as more research on the impact of affect on cognition and research on the impact of relationships' exterior environments on their interior dynamics" (p. 260).

1. *Attachment theory* relinquishes an individualistic orientation, claiming that survival depends on connection with others. Racial-cultural consciousness in EFT broadens the attachment context to include significant impacts that may otherwise be overlooked.
2. *Experiential* therapy holds that emotion shapes meaning and has precedence in driving behaviors (Tronick, 1989). Racial-cultural threats can ignite rapidly unfolding emotional-survival processes. These threats and coping responses may be entirely missed in EFT without specifically invited conversations.
3. *Relational/Systemic* therapies focus on the intertwined impact which internal and external environments have on one another. Paying attention to and inviting exploration of the impacts of racial and cultural contexts expands EFT's systemic focus. As a systems theorist, Bowlby focused on how *we do as we've been done to*, with the inner rings of emotional processing triggering and maintaining the outer rings of interpersonal patterns. The third ring of socio-cultural context (Figure 1.1) symbolizes clients' lived experience and the EFT therapist's humble readiness to engage and respond to contextual issues.

One Attachment-based Model with Couple, Individual, and Family Modalities

EFT has made a significant impact on the conceptualization of relationship distress and repair and has expanded the empirical base for placing emotion and emotional connection in the forefront as the agent of change. By extending attachment theory as a map for treating couples, individuals, and families, EFT is reshaping the entire field of psychotherapy. As the only couple therapy based on an empirically validated theory of adult love, it is also recognized as successfully treating the most common presenting problems in individual therapy – anxiety, depression, existential crises, relationship problems (Greenman & Johnson, 2022; Johnson, 2019) – and restoring connection and promoting resilience in families (Furrow et al., 2019).

While validating the existence of multiple attachment figures (Magnavita & Anchin, 2014; Mesman et al., 2016; Mikulincer & Shaver, 2023b), attachment dyads remain the fulcrum of the EFT model, whether working with couples, individuals, or diverse forms of families. Despite the ways attachment theory has evolved in response to culture (Fern, 2020; Gillath & Ai, 2021; Keller, 2021, 2022; Shaver et al., 2016; Thompson et al., 2021) and the increasingly diverse family structures in contemporary society (Bird, 2019; Brill & Kenny, 2016), the bold conjectures of attachment theory have not been refuted (Mesman et al., 2016). Survival depends on having others upon whom to rely. "All of us, from the cradle to the grave, are happiest when life is organized as a series of excursions, long or short, from the secure base provided by our attachment figure(s)" (Bowlby, 1988, p. 62).

The practice of emotionally focused couple therapy (EFCT) is the best preparation for mastering this relational model because it compels therapists to master the challenges of working with an attachment dyad in the therapy room. These two people invariably have differing perspectives that need to be validated without invalidating the other; safety needs to be created in the face of hostility and vulnerability; the two people in the therapy room are at once the greatest trigger for attachment fears and reactivity, as well as the best resource for each other. Throughout the book, the original modality of EFCT will frequently be mentioned before emotionally focused individual therapy (EFIT), as Emily, along with you, the reader, seeks to integrate EFT as a model across modalities of couples, individuals, and eventually, the unique nuances to keep in mind, with families.

EFT integrates attachment theory with systemic and humanistic-experiential approaches in a pragmatic manner that respects clients' innate ability to change and grow, and that views health, dysfunction, and growth from the perspective of surviving and thriving in relationships. In Emily's quest to apply EFT to individual therapy, her heart skips a beat as she realizes that the *ear of empathic attunement* is at the core of all successful EFT therapy. To Emily, EAR (Box 1.3) represents three key ingredients of shaping secure bonds and restructuring attachment orientations: (a) follow **emotion**, with attunement to its cultural nuances; (b) focus on **attachment** and contextual threats for safety; and (c) **reshape** strategies for engaging through interpersonal dialogues while respecting relational/contextual resources and experiences of oppression.

Follow Emotion and Its Patterns

Emily values how EFT relieves her of the need to solve problems, and instead, directs her to begin with tracking the repetitive and automatic patterns of emotional *perception-feeling-meaning-action* reactions when a person experiences threat. EFT Tango Move 1 Reflecting Present Moment Process, rather than trying to fix most content problems, engages all parties in a collaborative effort toward stabilizing negative patterns and discovering the underlying vulnerable emotions, which are then reliable guides toward change. Emily, feeling renewed energy for her upcoming individual therapy sessions, says to herself:

> I don't have to know solutions to my individual clients' presenting problems. There are actually no solutions to some of their tragic circumstances. I can begin, however, with helping my individual clients to identify the patterns of emotion regulation in which they are stuck — their best attempts to cope with adverse events. Then I can help them discover their underlying core emotions and listen to the messages of needs and the motivation embedded in those emotions.

She also recalls that *emotion is contextual*, marking the interface between the individual and the outside world (Knudson-Martin et al., 2015). Socio-cultural context shapes emotional experience and expression. Thus, following emotion means being fully curious to learn how each client is impacted by their socio-cultural context.

Focus on Attachment

Emily values the attachment perspective that humans are bonding mammals wired for interpersonal dependency in a physically and emotionally safe and secure attachment context. She

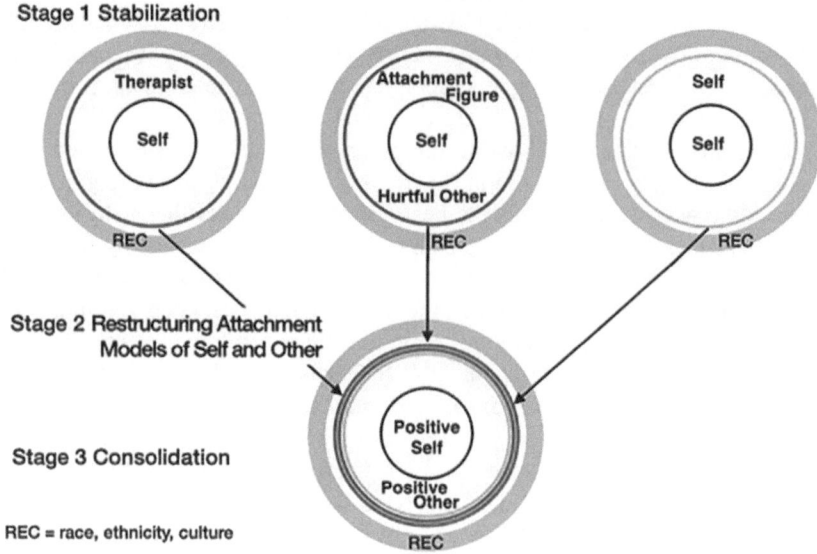

Figure 1.1 EFIT Change Process.

appreciates how attachment theory normalizes anxious and avoidant behaviors as best attempts to find "effective dependency" (Bowlby, 1988). She values how an attachment orientation can reframe *making mountains out of molehills* and *numbing out and disappearing* as common, understandable separation distress responses. Emotion-regulating moves of hyperactivating or deactivating – pushing and demanding, shutting down, turning away, and turning against – are all reframed as best attempts to cope with the primal panic of emotional isolation. Emily thinks:

> Reframing presenting problems as problems of emotion regulation makes sense with individuals as well as couples. Given that we are wired to depend on having a reliable, safe haven and secure base in the world, individuals without secure attachment figures to rely on during stressful times are particularly vulnerable to becoming habitually caught in patterns of hyperactivating or de-activating attachment needs for support and comfort.

Emily is discovering how distress and perception of threat are lessened when clients experience proximity to a trusted other (Johnson et al., 2013). She recognizes this dynamic of soothing threat with interpersonal connection in both her couple and individual sessions. At the same time, she is expanding her focus on attachment to include empathic curiosity to the larger ring of the sociocultural context and possible minority stress which her clients may be experiencing (Jordan, 2018) (see Figure 1.1).

Reshape Strategies for Engaging

Emily has esteem for the EFT Stage 2 change events of reshaping interpersonal bonds to restructure attachment security. She loves witnessing partners becoming each other's primary source of emotion regulation. As she savors the joy of having helped couples move from fierce independence and exasperated dissatisfaction to vulnerable confessions of need, dependency, and trust, she feels herself faltering. "Can this transformative part of EFT take place with individuals? Are there any relationship partners in individual therapy? Can I facilitate transformative dialogues in session?" Then, the puzzle begins to fit together. With emerging clarity, she says to herself:

> The attachment perspective focuses upon dyadic relationships and there are three basic relational contexts in therapy with my individual clients: The client's relationship with me; the relationships they have with others in their life, however supportive or hurtful those relationships might be; and, the mental representations of relationships with attachment figures from the past often blend into conflictual inner relationships between parts of self.

Emily repeats to herself, "Follow Emotion (and the dynamic interface between self and system), focus on Attachment (and threats of socio-cultural context), and Reshape strategies (for engaging with life)." EAR – The Ear of empathic attunement (Brubacher, 2020) captures the essence of EFT. It also readily fits with the acronym CARE for tuning in to context, attachment, relationship, and emotion (Furrow et al., 2022; Johnson & Campbell, 2022).

The EFT Map of Steps and Stages of Client Change

An EFT therapist uses a macro-sequence of interventions to guide clients through a three-stage process of change: stabilization, restructuring, and consolidation. Stages of client change and therapist interventions are standard across all modalities of EFT. (See Steps and Stages of Client Change, Boxes 1.1 and 1.2.) Details of the macro-intervention, known as the *EFT Tango* and the series of micro-skills making up the EFT Tango, are described in Chapters 2–4. Before examining the interventions EFT therapists use, I present the stages of clients' change process.

Stage 1 Stabilization

Building and maintaining an alliance is the first and most important task of this stage. An EFT therapist carefully and empathically listens to understand the client's story. In couple therapy, this includes careful attunement to each partner's description of how they experience the relationship. The alliance is built with an attuned, empathic, accepting stance, where the therapist genuinely believes that people do what they do for very good reasons and that there is no *bad guy* in the room except for *the cycle or repetitive pattern of interaction*. EFT therapists frame a couple's presenting problem as the pattern or cycle, tracking and normalizing their distressed interactions with an attachment perspective; an individual's default coping pattern for regulating emotion and relating to others is framed as legitimate and understandable, in fact, as a helpful strategy at one point in time – though now likely seen as the circular causality of the problem.

The EFT Stage 1 change event of *de-escalation/stabilization* occurs when clients recognize the *circular causality* of their distress: They recognize *the problem is the pattern*. Stabilization "is called de-escalation or stabilization in EFT for couples, for the obvious reason that to create stability it is necessary to de-escalate negative interactional patterns" (Johnson, 2019, p. 84). Partners in EFCT recognize that the real problem creating their relationship distress is the increasingly negative interactive feedback loop in which they are both stuck. Their automatic strategy for engaging with their own emotion and with others has become an increasingly rigid, repetitive pattern of protection from their core, underlying, unacceptable emotions – core existential fears of abandonment and rejection, sometimes also expressed as fears of irrelevance and annihilation.

Box 1.1   Steps and Stages of Client Change, Emotionally Focused Couple Therapy (EFCT)

Stage 1: De-escalation Change Event/Stabilization of Negative Cycle or Repetitive Pattern

Step 1. Form alliance with therapist; collaboratively assess *core attachment struggle*, including impact of cultural and racial stress; identify compatible agendas and goals.

Step 2. Identify the automatic reactive cycle (triggers, actions, meanings) and typical positions of pursuit and withdrawal.

Step 3. Access underlying unexpressed, unmet attachment longings, and core attachment fears that are driving the cycle.

Step 4. Recognize the problem to be a negative cycle/a rigid repetitive pattern of interaction and best attempts to meet needs. *Delineating the pattern disempowers it from dominating the relationship.*

Stage 2: Restructuring the Bond – Engagement Change Event

Step 5. More withdrawn partner accesses underlying emotions, disowned needs, aspects of self: Distill – Deepen – Disclose.

Step 6. More pursuing partner begins to accept this new view of partner; the dance expands.

Step 7. More withdrawn partner steps close to partner, expressing needs and wants; asking for needs to be met to feel safe to stay engaged in relationship. New interactions between partners: Withdrawer risks stepping close, asserting needs and wants; pursuer responds; withdrawer receives the response, marking the first antidote bonding event: Reach – Respond – Receive.

Stage 2: Restructuring the Bond – Softening Change Event

Step 5. More pursuing partner accesses underlying emotions, disowned needs, aspects of self: Distill – Deepen – Disclose.

Step 6. Newly engaged partner accepts new view of partner; further expand the dance.

Step 7. More pursuing partner owning attachment fears and needs, risks reaching from a vulnerable place of engaged fear to ask for needs to be met to feel safely connected. New interactions between partners: Pursuer risks reaching; engaged withdrawer responds; pursuer receives the response. This second antidote bonding event of Reach – Respond – Receive redefines the security between partners.

Stage 3: Consolidation

Step 8. Partners integrate the new secure bond with old problems. New solutions to pragmatic issues emerge. They safely solve problems and cope with differences.

Step 9. Partners consolidate new responsive positions and cycles and tell stories of problems and repair. Create resiliency story of past distress and current bond. Create future love story and rituals to keep love alive.

Box 1.2   Steps and Stages of Client Change, Emotionally Focused Individual Therapy (EFIT)

Stage 1: Stabilization

Step 1. Form alliance with therapist; together assess the core attachment and emotion regulation struggle, including impact of cultural and racial stress; identify goals for therapy.

Step 2. Identify ineffective, repetitive patterns of affect regulation, working models of self and other, and patterns of interaction with others and within self that prime distress, depression, and anxiety.

Step 3. Access core frightening, and/or unfamiliar and unacceptable emotion; gain coherence and deepen.

Step 4. Recognize the problem as the negative dramas with key others, triggering vulnerabilities and unmet needs. Recognize that constricted ways of addressing these needs, in turn, trigger and confirm negative dramas. *Delineating the pattern disempowers it from remaining the rigid default strategy for regulating emotion, relating to self and others, and responding to life's challenges.*

Stage 2: Restructuring Safety, Working Models of Self and Other

Step 5. Distill and deepen core fears, vulnerabilities/insecurities, existential dilemmas. Disclose to imaginal other, to therapist or between parts of self. Distill – Deepen – Disclose.

Step 6. Process real or imagined response to disclosure – the response may be accepting and warm or dismissive or hostile – regardless, the dance expands.

Step 7. Express increasingly congruent, assertive, vulnerable, core emotions and needs, creating corrective emotional experiences of reaching, responding, and receiving. Process and integrate coherent, secure models of self and other. The first Stage 2 change event may be followed by more corrective emotional experiences – expressions of fears and needs and antidote bonding events of *engagement* and *softenings* across relationships.

Stage 3: Consolidation

Step 8. Explore new solutions to past problems with newly shaped views of self and other, engaging in accessible, responsive, and engaged ways with safe others.

Step 9. Consolidate new *broaden-and-build* cycles to engage with life.

Adapted from Johnson (August, 2019, p. 30).

At this point, each partner recognizes and takes ownership for how they get automatically pulled into this dance and for how their reactive behaviors trigger the other into a self-protective mode of reactivity. This negative, self-reinforcing cycle is nicknamed the Demon Dialogue in *Hold Me Tight* (Johnson, 2008). EFIT clients in the stabilization change event recognize their habitual, self-reinforcing patterns as the problem, have gained enough emotional balance that they are able to explore the frightening, unacceptable emotions that are driving their pattern, and are ready to move into corrective emotional experiences whereby they can explore new ways to engage with their experience, with others, and with self.

Stabilization signifies that clients have an emerging sense of how they get thrown off-balance emotionally and what triggers them to experience a sense of threat from another. EFCT clients have a growing appreciation for their partner's specific vulnerabilities and how their own self-protective behaviors threaten their partner's sense of being loved, accepted, wanted, or supported. EFIT clients recognize the real problem is not them but their repetitive pattern which dominates their life as their best attempt to avoid underlying fears, anguish, or despair. It could be a rigid, ineffective pattern such as anxious, disappointing pursuit of others in times of vulnerability, or the pattern may be habitual avoidance, minimizing relationships, and turning to hurtful behaviors in moments of need.

Stage 2 Restructuring: Engagement and Softening

In Stage 2, the therapeutic focus is on deepening and expanding core attachment emotions to create new ways of reaching and responding that reshape attachment bonds into ones of security and connection. In EFCT, each partner, in turn, accesses the longings and needs embedded in the newly expanded core emotions that drive the negative cycle. Each partner takes a monumental risk to reach to their partner and ask for these previously unexpressed attachment needs to be met. These events consist of very intentionally structured dialogues known as *engaged encounters,* forming two change events that actually *restructure* the attachment bond.

The Stage 2 change events have traditionally been called Withdrawer Re-engagement and Blamer Softening (Bradley & Furrow, 2004, 2007; Johnson, 2020; Lee et al., 2017). For several reasons, including illustrating their relevance across modalities of EFT, they are referred to in this book as simply Engagement and Softening change events. "Re-engagement" implies that the down-regulating client has previously been engaged with their own emotional experience and brought themself fully and assertively into the relationship and over time has slipped away. Given that many avoidant clients have relied upon avoidant strategies and self-protective emotional distancing for much of their lives, it feels more accurate to refer to the first Stage 2 change event as *engagement or withdrawer engagement* (as in Johnson, 2004, p. 21; 2020, p. 24), rather than *withdrawer re-engagement.* For many clients, the kind of emotional engagement they are helped to take in Stage 2 is a totally new experience of connection with self and other – a new experience of engaging with the inner and outer rings of experience that Bowlby described. *Engagement* as a change event occurs in EFIT as well as EFCT. Johnson (2019) confirms that stages of client change and therapist interventions are standard across modalities of EFT. Thus, naming the change event as *engagement* fits more generically across modalities. The second Stage 2 change event is referred to simply as a *softening* (see Johnson, 2020, pp. 179, 181; Johnson & Campbell, 2022, p. 90), since the adjective *blamer* carries a pathologizing tone, while attachment theory validates both strategies of avoidance and anxiety as being adaptive at times (Bowlby, 1980).

Engagement precedes a softening. In EFCT, the previously more withdrawn partner – who, in the negative cycle, has been holding back and turning away – takes the risk of stepping forward to ask for attachment needs to be met. These are typically requests for acceptance and assurance that they are really wanted and needed, and requests for the partner to ease up with their demands and criticism. For someone who has been holding back, avoiding conflict, and defending themself against escalating demands, it is indeed a big risk to make these congruent, assertive requests. It is also typically a new experience to access longings for emotional connection since closeness and dependency had become associated with the other partner's demands and dissatisfaction. Asking for what they need to fully step into the relationship and experience safe connection is the change event of *engagement.*

In EFCT, a *softening* change event follows. The previously anxious, demanding partner now risks, from a vulnerable, congruent position, to express fears of abandonment and unworthiness, and asks for comfort and assurance. Studies show that these softening events predict change in relationship satisfaction and in relationship-specific attachment security, and that these changes endure over time (Johnson et al., 2015).

In EFIT, the Stage 2 change events have similar corrective emotional impacts. In the *engagement* change event, the individual client engages more deeply with their core fears and needs that have been unattended to by self and others. Underlying grief and loss, unacknowledged fears of being unlovable, insignificant, and unwanted, terrors of being rejected and abandoned are fully engaged and clearly expressed in encounters. The encounters can be with the therapist, with imaginal significant others, or between two internal parts, such as a harsh internal judge and a cowering fragile self. Assertive expressions of needs, requests for acceptance and support, and integration of affiliative responses complete the corrective emotional experience of the *engagement* change event. *Softening* change events follow from deeper engagement with emotional experiencing. They can involve risks taken in vulnerable encounters with a therapist, with an imaginal other, or between two parts of self, one part softening, embracing, and being embraced by a now engaged, formerly disregarded part of self.

Stage 3 Consolidation

In Stage 3 of EFT, positive cycles of bonding are consolidated and integrated. In couple therapy, partners and the therapist reflect on the evolving positive *broaden-and-build cycles* (Mikulincer & Shaver, 2023a) and co-create stories of resilience – how they moved from distress to security and how these changes project into their future life together. Once partners have found the path to a deeply satisfying sense of felt security, they are likely to stay on this path of secure connection (Mikulincer & Shaver, 2015). In individual therapy, shifts in view of self and other are summarized, heightened, and celebrated. New cycles of emotion regulation, of reaching to others for support, and of building relationships and activities which affirm a positive sense of self and others are celebrated and heighted across relational contexts.

Relational Contexts in the Change Process of EFIT

The top row of circles in Figure 1.1 represents the inner and outer rings of an individual's system. Self is embedded in and shaped by several relational contexts. These include the client's relationship with the therapist; the client's present-day relationships in their outer and inner worlds, which can include relationships with attachment figures, present and past, and supportive and hurtful others; and the client's relationships between two parts of self. Bowlby (1973) claimed that the inner and outer rings of a system complement and maintain each other in a homeostatic way. The third concentric ring, surrounding self and other, represents the impacts of the racial, ethnic, cultural (REC) context, where *cultural* includes diversity in gender, sexual orientation, differing (dis)abilities, neurodiversity, spiritual/religious orientations and more.

Therapeutic change in EFIT begins, as in Stage 1 with couples, with alliance building, assessment, and tracking of ineffective patterns and repetitive processes for regulating emotion across these varied relational contexts represented in the top of Figure 1.1. The automatic negative patterns for regulating emotion are identified as either hyperactivating attachment needs and pushing self and others for more gratifying responses, or deactivating and suppressing attachment needs and displaying self-reliance. After identifying the habitual patterns, core emotions that are typically unexpressed, outside of awareness, or perceived as dangerous and unacceptable, are accessed, assembled and attended to as valuable sources of energy and information. Stage 1 clarity is stabilizing and affirming of client's worth.

Assembling and attending to the newly accessed core emotion leads into Stage 2 corrective emotional reprocessing experiences. The middle of Figure 1.1 conveys a coming together of relational processes and patterns as clients are helped to restructure in Stage 2. Clients' corrective emotional experiences may be directed to the therapist; to imaginal significant others in their past or present life, including hurtful or supportive others, frequently attachment figures; and between dyadic parts of the self. The change events create transformational shifts, opening clients to new ways of interacting and expanding their sense of self. By accessing positive intentions in previously conflicted internal parts and by creating secure attachment bonds with others in the present or from the past, or accessing confidence and clarity to dismiss hurtful others, individual clients shift to positive internal working models of self as lovable, worthy and competent, and of select others as reliable and trustworthy.

The corrective emotional experiences of Stage 2 converge into a secure base with newly shaped views of self and other, as shown in the bottom of Figure 1.1. In Stage 3 consolidation, clients are supported to integrate new-found interpersonal and intrapsychic resources across a series of problems, to heighten and build secure relationships with others and within the self, continuing the new *broaden-and-build* cycles they have initiated.

Research Base of EFT

Outcome studies on EFCT provide empirical validation that this approach to couple therapy is effective and that the results are lasting. It is an evidence-based therapy. Spengler et al. (2022) conducted a meta-analysis with 300 couples. Their findings validate support for EFT as an evidence-based therapy for couples experiencing significant relationship distress, with 70% symptom free at the end of therapy and gains stable up to two years posttreatment. They also found greater therapist fidelity to the model to be associated with stronger gains for the couple. These findings are consistent with earlier meta-analyses (Beasley & Ager, 2019; Johnson et al., 1999) showing EFT to demonstrate a larger effect size than any other couple therapy. Additionally, there are excellent results on EFT follow-up, showing little relapse, with some studies showing significant numbers of couples *continuing to improve after therapy ends* (Wiebe & Johnson, 2016). Individual changes in attachment security over the course of couple therapy (Burgess Moser et al., 2015) remained changed in the direction of secure attachment at follow-up (Wiebe & Johnson, 2016). Given that insecure attachment strategies are associated with depression, anxiety, and suicidal ideation, it is significant that EFT is now validated to go beyond creating relationship satisfaction, to changing attachment orientations. See Mikulincer and Shaver (2023a) for a recent summary of research on the effectiveness of EFT.

fMRI brain scans show that the capacity for EFT to create secure attachment bonds is also changing individuals' responses to threat (Johnson et al., 2013), and is changing attachment orientations from insecure to secure (Burgess Moser et al., 2015; Wiebe et al., 2019). There are many benefits of secure attachment (Johnson et al., 2015; Mikulincer & Shaver, 2015), including the capacity to retain emotional balance during times of stress and threat, to seek and receive care and support in ways that constantly renew attachment bonds, and to implicitly access the powerful mental and physical health benefits of social connections (Feeney & Collins, 2014; Greenman & Johnson, 2022).

EFT meets the standards to classify as an evidence-based couple therapy treatment (Snyder et al., 2006). To be *evidence-based*, a therapy needs to have a specific model of treatment with clearly defined outcomes, there needs to be a measure of therapist fidelity, the problem needs to be clearly identified, the context of treatment needs to be clearly identified, and there need to be valid outcome measures. EFT has all this.

A therapist seeking an effective couple therapy needs to be wary of approaches which may claim to be based on solid research. They could be *evidence informed,* in that they are based upon one or more evidence-based models yet have not been rigorously tested or may contain a series of individual techniques from separate models yet lack a coherent model of practice (Sexton et al., 2011). Alternately, an approach may have a clearly defined model yet lack sufficient outcome research that represents long-term effectiveness of a clearly defined goal of couple therapy. Sexton et al. (2011) contrasted *evidence-based treatments,* such as EFT, with treatments that show promising preliminary research results yet are limited in methodological rigor or lack replication studies. Authors described three categories of evidence-based treatments, with EFT being in the highest category of "evidence-based and ready for dissemination and transportation within diverse community settings" (p. 377).

Research on EFIT as a separate modality is in its infancy with the first study currently underway across three sites, examining variables such as depression, anxiety, and post-trauma symptoms. Data is currently being analyzed (Wiebe at al., in preparation). In spite of EFIT not having the extensive research base that EFCT has to date, EFT therapists are encouraged by several factors. First, much of what is measured in EFCT is actually change *within individuals*. EFT is shown to be effective to significantly alleviate depression and symptoms of PTSD (Ganz et al., 2022; Greenman & Johnson, 2013; Wiebe & Johnson, 2016; Wittenborn et al., 2019), in addition to alleviating relationship distress and significantly improving relationship satisfaction with lasting benefits. Changes in individual orientations toward more attachment security are found to be stable at three-year follow-up (Burgess Moser et al., 2015). Second, EFT therapists use the same interventions to move clients through the same basic process of change across all modalities of couple, individual, and family therapy. Given the empirical validation of the couple modality of EFT, Mikulincer and Shaver (2023a) suggest we have good reason to be optimistic about the EFIT outcome research findings. This is enough for Emily, whose moving experiences of change in her couple and individual clients confirm that working with the same evidence-based model across modalities is indeed the most authentic and effective way for her to work.

Applicable over Different Clinical Populations

EFT is widely used across differing cultural contexts (Greenman et al., 2009; Johnson & Brubacher, 2016), and with a diversity of spiritual, religious, sexual and gender orientations, as well as differing forms of families and socio-economic conditions. With the racial reckoning movement in North America in the early 2020s, however, there is a marked emphasis upon the need for EFT therapists to expand their cultural awareness, humility, and competency to elicit and process racial and cultural content. There has been a burgeoning of literature about applying EFT across cultures and races, illustrating how to explicitly include impacts of REC in therapy (Allan et al., 2022; Guillory, 2022; Nightingale et al., 2019). Whether the buffering effects of attachment security can mitigate against others' racist and discriminatory behavior is yet to be seen (Mikulincer & Shaver, 2021), but there is some evidence that secure connection to one's own ethnic group seems to buffer impacts of racism. This suggests that security created in culturally sensitive therapy may add to resilience and effective coping for those hurting from colonialism, slavery, and other forms of discrimination.

A discussion of the usefulness of EFT across modalities of individuals, couples, and families to enhance experiences of social connectedness that are shown to contribute to mental and physical health can be found in Greenman and Johnson (2022) and Johnson (2019, 2020). EFT is validated as an effective treatment for many previously identified individual disorders, such as depression and post-traumatic stress, and is shown to be a promising treatment for couples facing the stress of chronic illness. Studies have validated the effectiveness of EFT for couples facing depression (Alder et al., 2019). Preliminary research on EFT's efficacy in improving sexual relationships and on a model for addressing sexual concerns in EFT has been conducted (Johnson et al., 2018; Wiebe & Johnson, 2016; Wiebe et al., 2019). EFT therapists also report successfully working with couples struggling with violence (Slootmaeckers & Migerode, 2018, p. 220), addictive processes (Landau-North et al., 2011), and physical health (Greenman & Johnson, 2022). There is also data on lasting outcomes for key issues such as the forgiveness of injuries (Wiebe & Johnson, 2016; Zuccarini et al., 2013), discussed in Chapter 16.

EFT is also backed by more process research than any other couple therapy. The therapeutic tools I present in this book are those found in the nine process research studies of EFCT (Greenman & Johnson, 2013) that have carefully examined the actual change processes in therapy and have validated the key ingredients of change for creating secure connections. It is expected that these same processes will predict success in individual and family therapy modalities (Johnson, 2019; Mikulincer & Shaver, 2023a).

EFT Self-help and Psycho-education Programs

EFT continues to expand in areas such as scientifically based self-help books (Johnson, 2008, 2013, 2022; Johnson & Sanderfer, 2016) and video programs, including psycho-educational programs for couples and families for the general public, with effectiveness research validating the psycho-educational-group-based version of EFT (Conradi et al., 2017; Kennedy et al., 2018; Morgis et al., 2019; Wiebe & Johnson, 2016; Wong et al., 2017). Thus, it is shown that EFT works in the real-world, not only in the therapy room. A new EFIT self-help program is being piloted as this goes to print (T. Y. Wong, personal communication, July, 2023).

EFT Training

Therapists worldwide are gravitating toward EFT training and finding EFT to be applicable to their differing contexts. This is not surprising, given the cross-cultural support for the core tenets of attachment theory, and the findings of attachment processes across cultures (Mesman et al., 2016; see also Liu & Wittenborn, 2011; Thompson et al., 2021). Studies of the effectiveness of EFT training in Spanish-speaking counties (Rodríguez-González et al., 2019) and in Hungary (Koren et al., 2022), illustrate EFT's applicability in those cultures. EFT literature and materials have been translated into 34 languages and are expanding, including the first edition of this book into more than seven languages. This is certainly making EFT accessible to practitioners across the globe with trainings occurring in over 40 countries.

In addition to the summary provided above, a summary of the EFT research and list of publications and commentaries can be found at http://www.iceeft.com/index.php/eft-research.

Introducing Five EFT Cases

Three couples in a typical clinical day for EFT therapist, Emily, represent the most common negative patterns of interaction in which distressed couples get stuck. First, we explore three couples and then two individuals with whom Emily is working.

Emily remembers that before she learned to view romantic love through an attachment lens, she became overwhelmed with some of the volatility, hostility, silent distancing, and rationalizations that partners would evoke in one another. She cringes to recall how often she wondered if there would be much hope for couples like these to repair their relationships. Now that she can see each of the following couples' different stories of relationship distress through an attachment lens, the chaos begins to have order. The attachment view of what is happening makes it possible for Emily to validate and normalize the seemingly excessive over- and under-reactions of partners to one another. She has confidence in her mantra, "In attachment, even the most bizarre behaviors all make sense. I just need to attune and understand."

The attachment perspective that all forms of clinging, protesting, blaming, and turning away are normal, universal, survival responses when a significant other is unavailable, sheds clarity and acceptance on the complex stories that unfold within her office. Metaphors from the self-help book, *Hold Me Tight* (Johnson, 2008), for the negative cycles of attachment behaviors regularly come to her mind: *Protest Polka, Freeze and Flee,* and *Find the Bad Guy.* As Emily attunes through the attachment channel and engages in collaborative exploration with each couple and individual client, hostility, pain, silence, and despair are normalized. With this perspective, she experiences and conveys a sense of hope for each couple and each individual, and for the collaborative work ahead of them.

Jessica and Wayne: Protesting Nonchalance (Protest Polka)

Jessica, a large and very beautiful young woman, noticeably lighter-skinned than her husband Wayne, bursts into tears repeatedly during their sessions with Emily. Much of the time, Jessica is exasperated with Wayne's apparent nonchalance and seeming unwillingness to move "even an inch to show he cares." Except for the constant shaking of his left foot crossed over his right, he does look rather motionless and blank. Every now and then, he turns to Emily and gently protests that Jessica is being far too hard on him or expects more than anyone could accomplish. But mostly, he shrugs his shoulders and sighs, "What can you do? I get it wrong and she turtles or fires up. I never know what to expect." This routinely triggers either an outpouring of exasperation from Jessica or silent sobs as she buries her face in her hands, her beautiful, dark curls falling in layers, revealing nothing but whimpers.

Slightly mesmerized by Jessica's beauty, Emily finds herself also distracted by Wayne's remarkable lack of response in his self-contained, handsome, black body with his attractive dreadlocks. Jessica's complaints range from despair over Wayne's lack of willingness to help with household chores, to being marginally involved with their three children, two pre-school daughters and an eight-year-old son, to "never taking time to talk with me or even notice me!" Jessica is a publicist for the one of the city's largest arts organizations, while Wayne work for a computer business in a mid-sized office and is heavily involved in social justice work in their racist, predominantly white community.

A clear pattern of interaction emerges from the first session: The louder and more dramatic efforts Jessica makes to get Wayne's attention and response, the more stoic, nonchalant, and disengaged he becomes. The quieter, more distant, and utterly nonresponsive Wayne becomes, the louder, more frantic, and exasperated Jessica gets, until Wayne finally throws up his hands, sighing in a tone of exclamation, "How can anyone be expected to measure up here!"

Emily's attachment-informed view of romantic love helps her to recognize the strong, albeit tattered, attachment bond between Wayne and Jessica, and to sense the powerful attachment panic (Panksepp et al., 2014) that is driving this escalating behavioral pattern. Emily can hear Jessica's fear of abandonment beneath her desperate anger at failing to get an engaged response from Wayne. Embedded in Wayne's surface nonchalance and eventual dismissal of Jessica's demands, Emily hears his panic at Jessica's expressed disappointments and determination to get him to change.

Phil and Julie: Protecting Selves in a Withdraw/Withdraw Cycle (Freeze and Flee)

Phil and Julie seem the quintessential opposite of Jessica and Wayne. Phil chatters on endlessly about how good things are between them and speaks with pride about the great progress he has made. Julie, appearing very timid, admits to finding it difficult to talk, but agrees she is very proud of him for being willing to join his "sex addiction group," and is extremely grateful to him for how hard he is working at his sobriety. Phil constantly jumps in to explain how he and Julie both feel that, in some ways, her discovery of his porn obsession was the best thing that has happened for them. In fact, their unified story of having come back together after several episodes of Phil's disappearances from the marriage into a series of addictive episodes involving alcohol and pornography prompts Emily to express curiosity about what they are hoping to achieve in couple therapy.

Phil describes having amnesia from before the age of 18 and is terrified of remembering what may have happened. "We are just here to strengthen our marriage," Phil states, "and to improve the intimacy." Julie admits she cannot tolerate any physical contact with Phil at this time and needs help to decide if they can repair their distance, or whether they need to part ways.

Julie speaks proudly of "Phil's progress," and both protect each other from having to discuss what they refer to as "horrific childhoods." In spite of their shared celebration of how they have weathered this shattering discovery of his secret life, the therapist detects subtle hints that Julie's discovery of Phil's pornography use has shaken her to the core, but that she prefers not to touch that at the moment.

This couple is definitely a challenge for Emily, who attempts to follow hints of distress from two highly intellectualizing partners who back away from any simple reflection she makes. She notes that, time and again, they seem to gloss over any hints of distress or to suddenly be flooded and speechless when she refers to their distress. Emily struggles to engage them in their emotional process without overwhelming them or rupturing their tentative alliance.

Although Phil is ready to speak at any moment and seems to prefer to talk than to let Julie respond, the pattern of interaction which Emily is noticing between Phil and Julie appears to be a withdraw/withdraw cycle. Phil tends to withdraw from Julie rather than turn to her for support. Historically he withdrew to his alcohol and pornography habits, and now he turns to his 12-step groups, his movies and novels, and his intellectualizing. Julie openly admits she is holding back. She finds it hard to get words to pass her lips. She wrings her hands and expresses fears and uncertainties about the future of this relationship. Although every now and then when Phil opens slightly to say, for example, "I get how hard it is for her to talk. We both feel that way," she sighs a big smile and says, "That is why I married you! You get me!" Emily can feel how important they are to each other and gradually begins to sense the underlying emotions – longings to feel safe with each other and fears about getting hurt if they get too close.

Sophie and Ella: Caught in Attack /Attack Sequences (Find the Bad Guy)

Sophie and Ella, a lesbian, cisfemale couple, begin their first therapy session in a highly escalated state. "The problem is her close-knit Asian family!" shrieks Sophie, "Everyone is more important than me!" "The problem is her impossible, unending, ridiculous demands," sighs Ella, "I just can't do it anymore. I am getting ill from the stress – nothing is ever enough for her!" Before long, she too is raising her voice! Sophie is the more anxious and pursuing partner while Ella is more avoidant and withdrawn.

Emily has difficulty maintaining control of the session; however, she knows that in order to create safety in the room, she must be in charge of the process. To contain the volatility and to regulate the emotion, she stays very close to each partner's experience with brief, simple empathic reflections, and takes charge of whom she allows to speak at a time. When Ella jumps in to interrupt Sophie, Emily gently looks Ella in the eyes and reaches her hand toward her while saying in a soothing tone, "Ella, I know it is hard to hear this right now, but can we let Sophie finish – and then I'll hear from you?" She continues to soothe Ella with her outstretched hand and by occasionally turning her face toward her as she listens to Sophie describe her view that the problems in their relationship are really all the fault of Ella's family. Then in an attempt to validate and soothe Sophie while at the same time protect Ella from the sting of Sophie's words, Emily says, "Sophie, you are almost frantic here, aren't you? And you don't have any other way of describing the anguish and frenzy you feel between you and Ella, except to take shots at her family. Am I getting it?" Calmed a little by hearing that the therapist hears her frenzy, Sophie sighs, "Yeah, I guess I am pretty frantic." Emily checks, "Frantic for more of Ella?" "Of course!" states Sophie. When the therapist turns to hear from Ella, she invites Ella to disclose what it was like to hear that under Sophie's frustration with her and her family, she is actually frantic to have *more of her*. By linking their responses to the immediate moment experience, Emily knows she can both maintain more control of the session, thereby keeping it safer, and also keep each partner focused on their present moment interactions.

Their rapid attack/attack sequences leave Emily unclear about who is pursuing for contact and who is fighting back in defense before withdrawing. As she attunes closely to each partner's experience, she hears Sophie as an anxious, lonely partner demanding to be loved, triggering exhaustion and a sense of failure in Ella, a more avoidant partner who is longing to please, to feel accepted, and to be loved. She begins to sense Sophie's demands as a kind of "fighting to matter to Ella." Likewise, Ella's fighting back seems like a kind of defense against annihilation or rejection of who she really is – a fear that she will be remade into the person Sophie would prefer her to be.

At the end of this first session, there is a glimmer of hope in the room. There is agreement that the real enemy threatening their relationship is the *Find the Bad Guy (fighting for survival)* pattern in which they are caught. Ella feels a willingness to return to therapy when hearing Sophie acknowledge, "I do blast you and put all the blame on you and your family when I feel alone. I get so frustrated that I don't seem to matter to you." Hope flickers for Sophie when she hears Ella express, "It is true, most of the time I am frustrated and fed up that you are so disappointed in me. I just want us to be good together." The first session over, Emily is proud to have created enough safety to contain their volatility and thrilled that, together, they are beginning to name the core relationship problem as the repetitive cycle that evolves in the face of different cultural and family values, in particular, the threat that Sophie experiences from Ella's close family ties.

Sahra: Anxious, Depressed, Fearful Avoidant Strategies

Sahra, born to a Ukrainian mother and Somalian father, identifies as an Afro-Ukrainian immigrant to the United States. She is a medical student and a single parent of a two-year-old daughter. She has a self-protective pattern of fluctuating between anxiety and numbing, frequently using what in attachment terms is called a *fearful avoidant strategy*. This strategy has helped her survive numerous traumatic events, but she is getting weary of the highs and lows of overwhelming anxiety and the lethargy of depression. She longs to "feel or to have a good cry," yet finds herself flitting from one troubling story to another, as though she is "telling someone else's story."

In her early childhood, she had a close relationship with her mother and was heartbroken at six years old when her mother began medical school and would be away for most of the week, returning only for the weekends. She remembers burying herself into her mother's sweet-perfumed fur coat, hugging her goodbye, feeling like her world was crumbling each time her mother left, and that all was right with the world again every time she returned home. When Sahra was eight years old and her brother was ten, her father unexpectedly left the family and returned to Somalia. Sahra has not had any contact with him since then. She recalls vividly how devastated her mother was when he disappeared, and how she dropped out of medical school and turned to her orthodox faith for comfort.

Sahra's fearful avoidant strategy has helped her survive numerous traumatic events, including childhood sexual abuse and her father's harshness and abandonment, as well as incidents of blatant racism and what Jana and Baran (2020) term *subtle acts of exclusion* due to her dark skin, which was much darker than her mother's. Despite the racial and cultural differences between them, Emily is pleased to hear Sahra comment on how safe she feels working with her.

Max: Driven by Fear, Grief, and Avoidance

Max, a cisgender, white male, nearing his fifties, works as a meteorologist and is grieving the loss of his romantic relationship. Having spent his childhood in Spain and moving back to his home country of the United States as a young teen, Max felt he didn't belong in either culture. To meet his need to belong, he says, he got involved with a group of friends who engaged in the dangerous, illegal sport of street-racing. In his late teens, Max was badly injured in a street-racing crash that tragically took the life of his friend and resulted in Max, the driver of the vehicle, going to jail for criminal negligence causing death. Sustaining physical damage to his face and his back and traumatized by his time in jail, Max defines himself as a full-blown alcoholic by age 24, unable to hold a job and drinking daily.

Decades later, while in the vulnerable throes of separating from his long-time partner, Max enters therapy to face the impacts of trauma which are feeling pervasive and disruptive now that he is on his own. In addition to the trauma of being in jail and subject to hostile others who did not have his best interests in mind, he lives with the weight of responsibility for his friend's death, haunted by a terror of consciously remembering what his friend's body looked like at the scene of the accident. Additionally, he struggles with memories of other trauma and experiences of death.

He distances from his traumatic memories as much as possible and struggles to regulate what he calls "over-the-top" emotional reactions and outbursts. Max self-identifies as neurodivergent with Aspergers and ADHD. He describes having had previous diagnoses and treatments for depression and anxiety. He longs to become more aware of his emotional experience and to safely face traumatic memories that he has tried to block for most of his life. His identification on the autistic spectrum and the challenge in his youth of leaving the country he called home left him feeling he didn't belong in any culture. He struggles with an ongoing, sense of what he calls "cognitive dissonance."

Emily finds herself wanting to sidestep his intellectualizing and move closer to his experience to get a felt sense of what he means by *cognitive dissonance*. She appreciates that his capacity to distance from his emotions is a well-honed survival strategy that has gotten him through various traumatic experiences. She also suspects that his autistic spectrum characteristics and his facial damage from his motor vehicle accident accentuate his matter-of-fact manner. Working online, she is frequently surprised when, beneath his almost stoic exterior he pulls out a handkerchief to wipe his tears, or identifies, without hesitation and in response to her evocative invitations, the tension or relief he feels in his chest and bodily core.

Buckle your seat belt! You are about to embark on a journey with Emily through the EFT change process with these five clinical cases and more! Summaries of the key EFT ingredients of change and the five cases introduced in this chapter are in Chapter 1 Support Material (routledge. com/9781032151335).

Box 1.3   The EFT EAR of Attunement

The EAR of attuned listening (Brubacher, 2020) is an acronym with a focus similar to attuning with CARE (context, attachment, relationship, emotion; Furrow et al., 2022). The EAR of attunement helps us keep in mind that *context* is everywhere – in emotion, in attachment, and in relationships through which we restructure attachment by shaping engaged encounters. We need to constantly attune to impacts of context. It is the air we breathe.

E - signifies attuning to the *emotional process* as it unfolds in the present moment in session and to the ways that culture impacts a client's emotional experience and expression. Emotion is contextual – a continual loop of self and system in interaction. Attuning to emotion requires a therapist to be constantly tuning in to how the client is regulating their emotion, what are the contextual impacts on how they are engaging with their emotion, and what is the optimum level of engagement for this particular client in this moment. That is, what is the depth of emergent emotional experiencing that is increasingly active, vivid, immediate, shifting or resolving? Clients are most open to change when their emotion is engaged in an alive, deep manner, yet within manageable depths, where they remain able to think and feel clearly, without freezing or becoming overwhelmed.

A - signifies attuning to the *attachment dynamics* and strategies clients develop for responding to threat. Attuning to attachment means attuning to the degree of coherence in a client's narrative and making room for clients to tell their stories in a way that shows respect for their context. Contextually, threats may be racial, ethnic, cultural, or interpersonal. Attuning to clients' perceived threats and strategies for responding to lack of safety entails attuning to historical and current dangers that clients are facing. Attuning to attachment includes attuning to whom clients can turn to for support - historically and in the present. Who are the key attachment figures populating our clients' worlds? How do they see themselves in the eyes of their key attachment figures? What pivotal events have shattered their trust and sense of safety or have bolstered their sense of trust and positive views of self, other, and the world? What are the clients' attachment strategies and patterns for coping and regulating emotion?

R - signifies *Restructuring or Reshaping, Respecting Racial-socio-cultural experience, and drawing on Relational Resources*. Engaged interpersonal encounters are the crux of change in EFT and the apex of the EFT tango. Attuning to the relational aspects of clients' lives, including experiences of exclusion and marginalization to reshape, through encounters, is how we restructure attachment, view of self, view of other, and create a safer world.

2   Key Ingredients of Change

Therapeutic Tasks and the EFT Macro-Intervention

The ideal therapist is, first of all, empathic. (Rogers, 1980, p. 146)

The two most general clinical implications of attachment science are that *harnessing the power of emotion within* the client is the most potent way to promote change… and that *change is inherently interpersonal* in nature, sculpted by the emotional messages that occur in dialogue with another. (Johnson, 2019, p. 25, italics added for emphasis)

The key ingredients of change on the EFT roadmap are presented in this chapter. I discuss tasks and therapist interventions that facilitate clients to move through the EFT steps and stages of change. Given the relational nature of EFT and its origins in couple therapy, I continue to lead with the couple modality, followed by EFIT applications. After describing the three main tasks of EFT, the five basic moves of the macro-intervention, the EFT Tango, are described.

The therapist's foremost task is to build a trusting alliance – an engaged, responsive relationship of safety and empathic understanding – emblematic of the safe-haven, secure-base relationship provided by a secure attachment figure (Bowlby, 1988). Creating and maintaining a therapeutic alliance remain salient throughout all EFT steps and stages of client change. The other two basic tasks on the EFT roadmap are assembling and deepening emotional experience, and shaping *affiliative encounters* where newly formulated emotion is expressed in interpersonal dialogues. Engaging in these three tasks is possible with deliberate, empathic, and artful use of the empirically validated EFT interventions (Greenman & Johnson, 2013, 2022; Johnson, 2019, 2020) described in this and the following two chapters.

Key Ingredients for Operationalizing the Three Basic Tasks of EFT

Emily uses the acronym TEA to monitor and foster the three tasks or process factors, found to be central to success in EFT (Brubacher & Wiebe, 2019; Furrow et al., 2022; Johnson, 2019): "T" represents the therapeutic alliance and in particular, the task aspect of that alliance; "E" represents depth of emotional experiencing; "A" represents affiliative sharing through therapist choreographed engaged encounters. Process research studies have isolated these three factors as key to how EFT achieves its effectiveness across a variety of different clinical contexts. (See Greenman & Johnson, 2013; Wiebe & Johnson, 2016, for reviews of these studies.)

T, for Task Aspect of the Therapeutic Alliance

The therapeutic alliance contains three inter-related yet separable components: A warm trusting bond between therapist and client; agreement as to therapeutic goals; and perceived relevance of the tasks presented in therapy (Bordin, 1979). That clients experience the tasks of therapy to be

DOI: 10.4324/9781003242673-3

directly relevant to their concerns is found to be highly important to success in EFT (Johnson & Talitman, 1997). A study examining predictors of success in EFT found that the quality of the therapeutic alliance accounted for 20% of the variance in outcome, and that it is the *task* relevant aspect of the alliance, in particular, that is a powerful predictor of relationship satisfaction and positive outcome of therapy. It matters, for example, that partners find the "tasks of EFT, which promote emotional engagement, as relevant to their problems" (Johnson & Talitman, 1997, p. 146). Knowing that "clients' reactions to and confidence in the interventions that [therapists] use ... are related to outcomes" (Greenman & Johnson, 2013, p. 46), EFT therapists take note of clients' reactions and explicitly invite them to express how they feel about the therapy process.

Emily catches her breath and ponders over this realization:

> I certainly need clarity and confidence to engage my clients in tasks that demand a lot more of them than a simple conversation! I need to build their trust that what we are doing will help them get to where they want to go. I need to be transparent about what I am doing when I try to engage them in identifying the repetitive pattern that is blocking them from their goals. Likewise, I need them to discover the value of the challenges of deepening emotional experience and participating in direct encounters with a partner (EFCT) or an imaginal other (EFIT). The more I practice and come to see that these tasks do indeed make a difference, the more patient and empathically persistent I am becoming.

(For guidance on practicing, see *Workouts for Stepping into EFT: Exercises to Strengthen Your Practice.*)

Task alliance can be defined as clients sensing that the tasks of therapy are directly relevant to their concerns. It is fostered and maintained with an EFT therapeutic stance of empathic understanding, unconditional positive regard, and therapist genuineness (Furrow et al., 2022; Rogers, 1980). These Rogerian core conditions are essentially the secure base, safe haven of which Bowlby wrote, and which Johnson portrays as accessibility, responsiveness, and emotional engagement in the acronym ARE, to denote *Are you there for me?* (Johnson, 2008, 2019, 2020).

Emily seeks to be transparent with her clients about how they can work together. She shares that she is working from the perspective that change begins with building trust and understanding, and identifying goals and hopes for therapy. While showing a path toward change that begins with identifying their current pattern, she also invites exploration of how the larger social context is impacting them and their self-protective response pattern.

During sessions, EFT therapists are open about the therapy process. They listen to and validate clients' discomfort with deepening emotions and shaping in-session encounters, while being flexible, culturally responsive, and patiently focused on these key tasks of EFT. If clients do not come to perceive the relevance of identifying and stabilizing the automatic pattern, deepening emotional experience, and engaging in in-session encounters or they do not trust that the therapist is engaging in these processes in culturally responsive ways, then therapy may not progress.

Task alliance is built with an empathic, validating, genuine presence that includes naming how clients' best attempts at saving a relationship or managing depression are the very things that are triggering and triggered by their distress, heightened at times by factors of contextual oppression. Clients frequently express feeling awkward when they are asked to slow down and stay with emerging emotion or to disclose newly distilled emotional experience directly to another. Validating the discomfort and being transparent about the process build trust. In couple therapy, for example: "I know this can feel awkward. I know you just told *me*, however, turning to share this same message with your partner will be a different experience. Will you please give yourselves a chance to have that experience?" When a partner finds it too difficult to turn and disclose, the

EFT therapist accepts the struggle and remains focused on the task, slicing the request more thinly, "Tell her then, please, 'It is too difficult right now for me to tell you how I shut you out when you look so angry'." The process is similar in individual therapy, where a client may be asked to stay with newly emerging emotion, and then to disclose to an imaginal other or to repeat the disclosure to the therapist. In addition, EFT therapists build task alliance by maintaining control of sessions, validating reactivity, redirecting to create safety, and by reframing aggressive reactions as attempts to regulate underlying attachment fears and emotion with an EFT micro-skill known as *catching a bullet* (Johnson, 2020).

Emily attunes to clients' reactions to and confidence in the interventions she uses, knowing this is related to therapeutic outcomes (Greenman & Johnson, 2013). She reflects on their reactions and invites them to express how they feel about the therapy process. She is prepared to be open about the process anytime throughout therapy. She invites their feedback at the end of sessions, reflecting and validating discomfort if there is any and offering genuine transparency. Reflections of present process, as in EFT Tango Move 1, are central to establishing and maintaining task alliance. EFT Tango Move 5 also contributes significantly to task alliance as the therapist summarizes and integrates clients' work in each session, savoring the shifts and relating the movement of each session to clients' goals and longings. In Chapter 7, I expand on forming an informal therapy agreement and being transparent about the therapy process.

E, for Depth of Emotional Experiencing

Client depth of experiencing has been identified across therapeutic orientations to be the most promising predictor of outcome (Pascual-Leone & Yeryomenko, 2017). Emotion that includes a bodily felt component is a key variable leading to therapeutic change (Gendlin, 1961). To deepen emotional experiencing, EFT therapists engage clients at a manageable working distance from their emotions. Clients flow between distance from and closeness to emotional experience. Tracking and validating this flow can increase awareness and depth. Gradually, within the client's *window of tolerance* (Siegel, 2012), the therapist seeks to increase their client's attunement to their inner felt flow. EFT therapists contain the dysregulated client or evoke and heighten the experience of the client who is detached from their inner experience. Basic empathic reflections and EFT Tango Move 2 affect assembly and deepening are rich tools for doing this.

A helpful process map for clinicians to attune to clients' level of experiencing is the Experiencing Scale (EXP; Klein et al., 1969, 1986). It was developed for research purposes, but therapists familiar with it can use it to assess clients' depth of emotional experiencing and their degree of focusing on internal referents. The scale measures the degree of client involvement in attuning to their inner experience as they explore new meanings, new feelings, and new action impulses. It is the single most widely used measure of intrapersonal process and of effective in-session process (Pascual-Leone & Yeryomenko, 2017).

At low levels of emotional experiencing (Levels 1–3), a client is distant from inner emotional experiencing, talking about events, ideas, or others, without expressing emotions or they may talk *about* emotions and thoughts, without experiencing them. Hyperactivating and deactivating strategies typically block a client from present-moment experience.

A medium level of emotional experiencing (Level 4) is a minimum for experiential therapy. At Level 4, a client is self-reflective, engages with the felt flow of inner experiencing, and experiences emotions in an alive, vivid manner in the present moment, with some attention to the flow of bodily-affective-cognitive-action-impulse experience.

At higher levels of emotional experiencing (Levels 5–7) new depths, emerging edges, and felt shifts of emotional experiencing emerge. Clients gain awareness of previously implicit feelings

---

Box 2.1   Levels of Emotional Experiencing Scale (EXP) Klein et al. (1986)

Abbreviation for Easy Access

Levels 1–3 – Detached from inner experience, impersonal, abstract, general, external descriptions.

Level 4 – **Attending to felt flow of inner experiencing, connecting body, meanings, action impulses**. Considered the minimum level for experiential therapy.

Level 5–7 – Expansive – increasingly concrete, vivid, alive. Felt shifts emerge, increasing trust of inner experience (as a reliable guide). Fresh way of knowing; new action tendencies and new meanings evolve.

EFT therapists are constantly seeking to increase clients' capacity to integrate cognitive reflection with affective experience. By orienting clients toward reflecting consciously on moment-to-moment experiencing, therapists prime them for the most profound newly emerging shifts in experience, new meanings, new action tendencies, new resiliency and the restructuring of attachment security that occurs in Stage 2.

---

and meanings and engage in new depths of experiences and perspectives. Corrective emotional experiences occur at these levels. At Level 5, clients focus on emerging edges of vague, implicit experience, seeking to elaborate it. At Level 6, they explore emergent experience that is increasingly active, vivid, immediate, shifting or resolving. At Level 7, clients experience an expansive, trustworthy source of new meanings and actions, a fresh way of knowing.

A simple example of Ella, an exhausted withdrawer, moving from low levels of experiencing to an emergent, more expansive awareness of inner experiencing, could be characterized as follows:

- Low levels of experiencing: "Criticism flies constantly! There is endless ranting and raving even about the way I drink my tea!"
- Medium level of experiencing, as in Level 4: "It's so hard when I cannot please Sophie. So difficult whenever I see she is not happy."
- Higher levels of experiencing: "For me, it's a series of crushing defeats – I keep hitting the ball, but I never get to first base. My gut is in knots with fear that I'm not her precious one."

As Ella's inner emotional experiencing deepens, she moves from vague frustration to a precise struggle related to her partner Sophie's unhappiness, her crushing sense of defeat at failing to please her, and her core attachment fear of being ultimately rejected. The expanding awareness at Levels 5–7 mobilizes her core attachment fear and grief at the distance between them into motivation to disclose assertively and vulnerably, and to risk stepping into emotional intimacy with her partner.

An EFIT example can be seen with Sahra who has a somewhat fearful avoidant pattern – revving up in panic and clamping down to control the pain. She blocks herself from feeling, particularly when flashbacks and re-experiencing of past trauma occur.

She describes a mirroring within/between pattern of being judged by others (*between* pattern) and of judging herself (*within* pattern). She speaks in a nonchalant manner as she reports (Level 3) that she has had no contact with her father since he left the family when she was eight years old and that she has no interest in a relationship with him. Later, she deepens into new considerations and longings (Level 4) that she might still want to locate him and have a relationship with him. Deepening into Level 5, more emotional reactions emerge – anger at the myriad of unanswered questions about his departure, heartbreak over how he crushed her life and broke the family, and vague fears at the thought of seeing him. At Level 6, she accesses specific fears of unbearable pain, judgment, rejection, and abandonment that she had "boxed up and put away." She engages deeply at Level 7 in an imaginal encounter with her father when she expresses her pain, a complexity of rage and heartbreak, for how deeply he hurt her by disappearing unexpectedly from her life when she was only eight years old! This Level 7 experience shifts her internal working model of self from sensing that she was unlovable, to a new experience of feeling worthy of love and care. She moves through bodily felt heartache and rage to clearly sensing that she deserved and still does deserve to have a responsive, accessible, and loving father.

Emily recognizes that much of her training has focused upon clients' thoughts, behaviors, and feeling words, and that much less focus has been upon learning to tune into clients' levels of internal emotional experiencing. Reviewing the Experiencing Scale (EXP) helps her to consciously bring her focus to the moment-to-moment process. She continuously looks for indications of each client's engagement with, or disengagement from, their inner experience. She is developing confidence in responding to clients' long pauses, noticing that nonverbal indications that a client is engaging internally frequently look different than signs a client dissociating outside of their window of tolerance. Nonetheless, Emily will check in with a client when she is unsure if they are getting overwhelmed or if their silence is because they are processing internal shifts.

Sahra frequently has long pauses of silence, particularly during encounters. Emily monitors closely to check if Sahra is getting overwhelmed. Sahra gives clear signs that she is within her window of tolerance, making eye contact with Emily, and saying, "I just need time to find the courage and the words."

In EFCT Emily engages the partner for support when a client is engaging deeply. When Julie touches on a deep terror and Rick reaches out and takes her hand, Emily comments, "Rick just reached out and took your hand – just notice how that feels to have him so close during this moment of your fear bubbling up!"

Deliberately attuning, staying with, reflecting, and expanding emotional experience is how an EFT therapist helps clients to attend to and reflect on their felt flow of inner experiencing and to then reprocess emotion and shape new ways of responding. Process research on EFT has identified that more intense emotional experiencing in clients is related to the second active ingredient of change – affiliative responding in engaged encounters. Corrective emotional experiences occur during encounters of affiliative reaching and responding at heightened levels of emotional experience.

A, for Affiliative Interactions

The third key process variable is the client's manner of interacting, particularly during therapist directed encounters. Increasingly affiliative statements – open, vulnerable, emotionally engaged disclosures (in EFT Tango Move 3) and understanding, warm, caring responses (in EFT Tango Move 4) – are associated with successful outcomes, particularly in Stage 2 (Greenman & Johnson, 2013). An affiliative posture is defined as warm, caring, tender, sensitive, curious, nurturing, and appreciative. In contrast, a posture lacking affiliation is hostile, domineering, dismissive, cold, ignoring, belittling, or blaming. EFT therapists monitor, foster, and heighten affiliation in Tango Move 3, shaping emotionally engaged, vulnerable, disclosures, and warm and caring responding in Tango Move 4. Given the transformative impact of affiliation in engaged encounters, an EFT therapist relies upon the EFT process for shaping safe encounters throughout all steps and stages of client change (Brubacher, 2022; Furrow et al., 2022; Johnson, 2020; Tilley & Palmer, 2013).

Open, Vulnerable, Affiliative Disclosures – Variations on a Theme. While shaping engaged encounters in Tango Move 3, Emily has been surprised to discover that open disclosures can include assertiveness and congruently expressed anger. Assertiveness can be experienced as emotionally engaged and vulnerable, leading to affiliative responding. For example, when she guides Wayne to tell Jessica that before he walks away in silence, he is annoyed about her complaints, Emily experiences how risky and vulnerable it is for Wayne to *own* this. This rather simple encounter facilitates increasing clarity and coherence. Wayne owns his action tendency to walk away in silence and links it to an underlying core, assertive annoyance. New behaviors and meanings begin to emerge. It is new to turn toward Jessica, instead of silently walking away, and to tell her that her complaints do annoy him and typically send him away, dreading that he will hurt her if he expresses his annoyance. The new meaning that begins to emerge for Wayne with this more coherent message is, "This trigger of Jessica's complaints does not need to send me away. I can have a voice and perhaps we can talk differently during these difficult moments without me fearing I will hurt Jessica." As Emily checks in with Jessica in Tango Move 4, Jessica responds warmly to Wayne, "I want to know what's going on for you! Stay with me – let us talk – I don't want my complaints to send you away!"

In Tango Move 4, EFT therapists hope to elicit this sort of warm, attuned responding. Ella and Sophie have an affiliative interaction when in Stage 2, Ella discloses her fears of being a disappointment in Sophie's eyes. Her risking to ask for acceptance and comfort draws a warm and compassionate response from Sophie.

Validate Authenticity to Contain Non-affiliative Responses. While affiliative sharing is the goal, EFT therapists do not encourage inauthentic responding. Instead, they validate and contain non-affiliative responses in Tango Move 4. Emily is learning to be prepared for situations where the responder is not warm and attuned. It is not uncommon for partners in EFCT or for imaginal others or part of self in EFIT to initially react to a new disclosure with disorientation or disbelief (Johnson, 2020). They may interrupt in a dismissive or accusatory manner. For this very reason, Johnson created the micro-skill known as *catching the bullet* to patiently catch aggressive or dismissive interruptions, validating the reactivity, and reframing the aggression or harshness. (See Chapter 4 for details on *catching a bullet*.) EFT therapists work with what is most alive in the moment, containing and validating to maintain safety and to move gradually toward the goal of affiliation, or resolution for permanent distance, as is the case in some EFIT encounters with abusive and unreliable others.

In the example of Sahra, her congruent, vulnerable disclosure to an image of her father was not met with an imagined affiliative, warm, supportive response. To the contrary, she perceived a response of dismissal and minimizing. The therapist's validation of this authentic, yet disappointing encounter, nevertheless shifted Sahra's sense of self as deserving of love and support and helped her to shift her internal working model of others. She consolidated a growing capacity to distinguish between others who are unreliable and dangerous (father) and those who are reliable and trustworthy (her close friend and the therapist).

In the absence of affiliative interactions, EFT therapists continue to process present moment experiencing. Postures of hostility or dis-affiliation call for a therapist to show increased empathic curiosity and validation to facilitate more vulnerable self-disclosure in Tango Move 3 and more engaged, attuned responding in Tango Move 4. Hence, while affiliation is the goal, clients are helped to share authentic disclosures and responses.

TEA provides a simple reminder of the three active ingredients or tasks central to success in EFT: **T**ask alliance where therapy tasks feel relevant to clients' concerns, depth of **E**motional experiencing, and in-session **A**ffiliative interactions with partners in EFCT and in EFIT, with imaginal others, with the therapist and between parts with self. EFT couple therapy research and

EFT research with individual survivors of complex trauma has consistently shown that depth of emotional experiencing and more affiliative interactions in EFT sessions predict better outcomes in emotion regulation, trauma resolution and relationship satisfaction (Greenman & Johnson, 2013; Johnson & Greenberg, 1988; Pascual-Leone & Yeryomenko, 2017). EFT therapists' transparency and openness with clients about the process help to build and maintain clients' confidence that these therapeutic elements are relevant to meeting their needs. EFT therapists employ the EFT interventions, outlined next, with an ongoing awareness of these three process factors for successful outcome.

The EFT Macro-Intervention: The EFT Tango

All interventions are employed with an attachment perspective. That is, in couple therapy, in the context of the specific couple's relationship, the focus is on how partners are impacting one another. What fosters or blocks emotional accessibility, responsiveness, and engagement between them? In individual therapy, from an attachment perspective, the concern is about what blocks or fosters secure connections and optimal engagement "with their own experience, with others, and with the existential dilemmas of life?" (Johnson, 2019, p. 75). The attachment perspective in EFT focuses on the *relational matrix* (Magnavita & Anchin, 2014; Shore, 2014) which includes the clients' socio-cultural context, significant others, attachment figures past and present, the therapist, and disconnected internal parts.

Employing interventions in an attachment context also features *how the interventions are operationalized.* The nonverbal aspect is considered to be as important or more important than the actual words the therapist says. The prosody, intonation and pacing of the therapist's voice, and the moment-to-moment nonverbal communication between therapist and clients are salient in attachment-based therapy (Shore, 2014, p. xxxiii). This aspect of *the manner* in which the EFT interventions are done is explicitly discussed in each of Chapters 7–11, through the steps and stages of EFT.

Each stage of EFT has different intensities, but throughout each session and each stage of client change, EFT therapists employ – in an artfully constructed flow – the five moves of the EFT macro-intervention, the EFT Tango (Brubacher & Johnson, 2017; Furrow et al., 2022; Johnson, 2019, 2020). EFT therapists work slowly, simply, softly, specifically, somatically, and vividly, reflecting and validating the present realities and engaging in the incremental change process with variations of these five moves:

EFT Tango Move 1: Mirror and reflect present process (within and between).
EFT Tango Move 2: Assemble elements of emotion and deepen core emotion.
EFT Tango Move 3: Shape an engaged encounter to share newly accessed emotional experience.
EFT Tango Move 4: Process the encounter with both the discloser and the receiver of the message.
EFT Tango Move 5: Integrate, validate, and summarize the experience that has just occurred.

Emily is coming to rely upon the five basic moves of the EFT Tango to guide her in her work. Mirror; Assemble and Deepen; Shape; Process; Integrate. "These moves are a very reliable guide," she muses. "They help me to begin with mirroring the present-moment experience of a client – individual or couple – and then to move forward by ordering, deepening, and reshaping experience and strategies for interacting."

Before exploring the micro-interventions or skills in detail, let us drop into a Stage 1 session of Emily with Jessica and Wayne. The EFT Tango Moves are labeled and some micro-skills, which will be expanded on in Chapters 3 and 4, are indicated within the EFT Tango Moves. The moves of the tango need not be followed rigidly and linearly. The more familiar a therapist becomes with the moves, the more flexibly and artfully they can flow between them. During this Stage 1 session, however, Emily steps in a rather orderly fashion through the EFT Tango Moves.

Before each session, Emily reviews her notes and highlights a few salient images or *emotional handles* (images or evocative words and phrases) that capture the process from the previous session. She enters the session with a clear picture and a felt sense of where they have come so far and where she hopes she can guide them in this session. From there she flows with a couple or an individual through the moves of the EFT Tango, exploring, expanding, and reshaping their present-moment experience.

In the previous session, Jessica and Wayne explored how the racist world plays out in their relationship. The same caution that Wayne experiences in society, where his physical form is perceived as a threat, is a part of his daily life in his relationship with Jessica as well. He is constantly keeping a tight control on all his responses, constantly toning down his responses to survive in the world. Wayne acknowledges how this same dynamic plays out with Jessica – continually keeping a tight control on himself, fearing his communication is not landing well with her, always afraid of hurting her or appearing as a threat to her and then *getting hurt in the crossfire*.

Wayne: A Black man knows that when he knocks on a door, he should always take a few steps back before the door is opened – so you're in full view and don't pose a threat and get caught in the crossfire…. I still don't know how to talk to her so she doesn't get hurt – gotta talk so carefully or she gets hurt and then I get caught in the crossfire. Like this morning, I tried to tell you something and your face told me a story.

Jessica: Well, you told me to put my plate in the sink with such a sarcastic tone – I felt a jab – like a thorn in my side. I knew you were jabbing at me –that was the look. I felt jabbed and to avoid an argument I said nothing, but I was mad at you!

EFT Tango Move 1: Reflect Present Process

Emily: It still feels unsafe to show up in the relationship with your whole self, yes? (Empathic reflection; Wayne nods.) The more carefully you tread, Wayne, not to hurt Jessica and try to tone yourself down, the more the little comments you make seem to trigger her looks which tell you a story of disapproval. And the more Jessica, you sense frustration in his tone and dissatisfaction with you for something as small as a plate you left on the counter, the more hurt and annoyed you feel, and after giving a look which speaks volumes to Wayne, you go quiet to avoid an argument. (Tracking sequences of interactions – cues, perceptions of threat, action tendencies, meanings made.) Both of you holding back (action tendency), feeling unsafe in the face of the other's disapproval, hurting, alone, feeling the sting of alienation from the other (Empathic reflection, conjecture with tentativeness, validation, heightening.) Am I getting it? (Checking for confirmation.)

Jessica: Oh my God! – I've never really understood him being as guarded in our relationship as he is in the world!

Emily: (To Jessica.) You sound startled… (empathic reflection) …almost horrified to hear that he carries this threat not only out in the world but back at home with you as well (empathic conjecture, tracking/linking core emotion with partner's message). It is such a shock to hear that he feels he needs to be careful around you!

Wayne: (To therapist.) It is there – always there – my dread of triggering a harm response in her and then causing harm to both of us and to our relationship!

Jessica: (Cycle begins to escalate.) I am not going to hurt you! Sounds like you are blaming me! Do I have to be happy all the time?

Emily: (Catching a bullet from Jessica, before moving forward with a Tango Move 2 with Wayne.) Wayne just said he dreads making the wrong move – saying something wrong that will harm you, and you stepped in to say, "Wait a minute!" It is difficult to hear him speak about his dread of triggering a harm response from you, yes? You want to step in to say, "Don't be afraid of me," yes? (Jessica nods.) You long so much for him to feel safe to speak out in this relationship and not hold back from you, yes? (Jessica interjects: Absolutely!) So, it is difficult to hear about his dread of harming you and triggering you to hurt him, causing harm to the entire relationship, yes? (Jessica nods again.) You've said often that you long to hear more from him, so I'd like to hear more from Wayne just now, ok? (Jessica nods.)

In the midst of this Tango Move 1 of reflecting the present process, Emily followed the simple formula for *catching bullets:*

- Interrupted Jessica.
- Reflected present process: Wayne expressed dread and Jessica stepped in.
- Reframed by conjecturing at the micro-moment that triggered Jessica: Wayne says he dreads triggering a harm response in Jessica and it is difficult for Jessica to hear this.
- Validated reactivity and conjectured with empathy at Jessica's positive attachment intention: Jessica wants Wayne to not hold back, dreading that she will hurt him. She longs to hear more from him.
- Checked for confirmation with Jessica.
- Refocused to continue to hear what Wayne was in the midst of expressing.

EFT Tango Move 2: Assemble Emotion and Deepen Core Emotion

Emily: Jessica just stepped in to say, "Don't dread me harming you. I won't hurt you," and you are saying, "But I do – I do – I continually dread I will somehow threaten her and she will hurt me back" – or as you've said, her reaction is like getting caught in the crossfire. (Tracking, validating. Wayne responds, "Exactly!") And you said one of the times your dread comes up is when you see a look on her face – like this morning, yes? (Evocative question to identify the cue.)

Wayne: The look like just before a sudden collision – like it's all too late – nothing more I can do – she's upset – I wasn't careful enough.

Emily: And when you see that look on her face – a look that looks as dangerous as a collision about to happen what do you feel in your body?

Wayne: Tension – my entire body goes stiff – especially my back stiffens – bracing – like it will all be destroyed.

Emily: (Assembling, linking elements of emotion with tracking and heightening.) You see a look on Jessica's face (cue), that says, "She is upset – and I'm about to get hit in a collision and we will spiral into destruction." That's how it feels (meaning). And your entire body stiffens (body), and says, "It's too late – I've blown it – she's upset – it is going to hurt" (more meaning). Is that right? (Wayne nods.) You think, "Danger, danger – too late – I've done it now – she is upset by what I said and now I'm gonna get hurt. We're both getting hurt." And what you typically do in those moments is_____? (question to evoke his action tendency)

Wayne: I shut down all together. I measure everything – constantly on guard that the relationship will crumble before our eyes.

Emily: You shut down completely to protect the relationship (validation). You live with this constant caution, "Be careful, be careful, keep tight control of myself or I might be seen as dangerous and we might both get hurt, and everything between us will crumble!" (heightening)

Wayne: I shut down completely!

Emily: Wow – when you get the sense from the look on her face (cue.), that you have up-set her (meaning), your entire body tenses (body), you tell yourself, "There I've done it – too late, she is hurt, and everything is going bad. Everything will crash. Everything will crumble" (meaning). "Jessica is turtling away and I've done big time harm to our relationship," and you shut down completely (meaning, action tendency). You go into hyper-cautious get-out-of-the-way mode, yes? (Wayne nods.)

EFT Tango Move 3: SHAPE an Engaged Encounter

SHAPE forms a perfect acronym to identify the key elements of choreographing an encounter: Sharpen, Heighten, Anticipate, Present, Engage.

Sharpen the Message.

Emily: Wayne, I'd like to help you shape a message to share with Jessica about your dread of upsetting her and causing her to turtle away from you – and the entire relationship being harmed, perhaps irreparably. This dread is on the edge all the time for you, yes? That you could upset Jessica and have her pull away entirely from you?

Heighten the Message.

Emily: (With proxy voice.) Dreading that look of – *the collision about to happen* – almost like a panic – My body goes stiff and I shut right down, trying to analyze how to do better by you! Dreading causing you harm – and you turtling away and giving up on me!

Anticipate Sharing the Message.

Emily: Can you imagine turning to tell her now, "Dreading all the time that if I speak up – show you who I really am, that I will harm you and you will turtle away and com-pletely reject me. Convinced that if I get it wrong, there will be no more chances – so I shut down completely when I see any look of disappointment on your face"? (More heightening, with proxy voice, repeating core message, asking him to imagine sharing this message with her.) Jessica, can you let Wayne tell you this dread he lives with? (Checking with partner as part of anticipating. Evocative question to let him know she is receptive.)

Jessica: Sure

Present the Message.

Emily: (Directing Wayne to present the message.) Can you turn and look at Jessica and can you tell her about this enormous dread – so cautious not to cause her harm, that anything which looks like she is upset sends you into tense body-panic. "Oh no I've upset her and now she's giving up on me!" (heightening with repetition, focusing, directing)

Wayne: I thought she knew this – I don't shut down completely just to be cold.

Engage, Following an Exit.

Emily: That's right – your shutting down is all about this dread. Can you go back to that tension in your body – the tight back and gut – can you feel it again? That rigid tension that says, "Oh no! I've done it – my words have harmed Jessica so much this time – she is giving up on me – turtling away in her shell." Can you tell her please?

Wayne: I do – it's true – I live on guard all the time of harming you and then when I see that look on your face, my body freezes and I shut down completely. Always on guard like out in the world – don't be a threat – don't be so big – don't appear – you'll be in danger – you'll get caught in the crossfire (pause). So I shut down – it is safer than facing your rejection.

EFT Tango Move 4: Process Impact of the Encounter with Discloser

Emily: Wayne, how was that to look right at Jessica and tell her about this huge, constant dread that you will threaten her, that you will harm her and then when you see her look of upset, your body freezes, so sure you've harmed her so much and she is rejecting you! How was it to share that with Jessica just now? Jessica who is looking right at you with some curiosity, it seems?

Wayne: A relief – a big relief actually – so good to let her know how bad it is!

Emily: Wow – amazing isn't it? You've told her how big your dread is – how cautious you are of making the wrong move and of her turtling away from you with disgust and rejection! You looked right in her eyes and shared this – and you feel relief!

EFT Tango Move 4: Process Impact of the Encounter with Recipient

Emily: And Jessica, how was it to hear what is going on inside Wayne when he shuts down and stops talking with you? How it is to hear he has this dreadful sense that his words have harmed you, upset you, and that you are turtling away, rejecting him for what he's said or done? How was it to have him share this with your so clearly?

Jessica: Wow – I didn't know – I am so sad for you Wayne. I didn't know. I am heartbroken for you – for us. I want you to feel safe with me. I don't want you knocking at the door and stepping back so you don't get caught in the crossfire. I just want you to feel safe to come right through the door to me!

(Tango Move 4 continues with the initial discloser)

Emily: How is this Wayne? You feel relieved to tell her of your enormous dread of Jessica sensing you as a threat, somehow scary, and her turtling away, rejecting you! And she is touched to hear this fear – and she is inviting you in, wanting to be the safe one you can come straight through the door to! How is that for you?

Wayne: That is a grand romantic gesture… She wants to see all of me – inviting me to bring my whole self forward. Wow! – Wow!

EFT Tango Move 5: Integrate and Summarize

Emily: This is amazing what you just did! Wayne, you shared how your dread is triggered by a look on Jessica's face that tells you the collision is about to happen or she is about to turtle. And you take it to mean you have somehow threatened or hurt her or done some-thing wrong – and you feel her rejection – as though you are unacceptable to her. You worry she will turtle away from you – totally reject you – and your entire body goes tense and you shut down completely. And Jessica when you hear this fear – initially you get defensive, "Don't blame me" – and then when he turned to you and told you himself of his constant dread of hurting you or upsetting you and you turtling away from him – you were filled with sadness and heartbreak for Wayne. You cringe to hear that he so much dreads your rejection– that he frequently shuts down even before you speak. Just your disappointed look can be enough to freak him out and send him into panic that you are rejecting him. Hearing this pulled you closer to him.

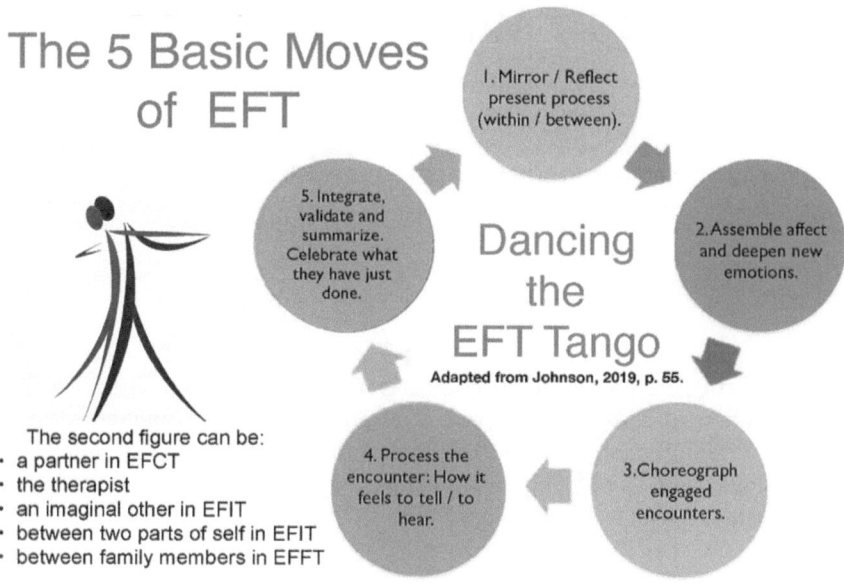

Figure 2.1 The Five Basic Moves of EFT: Dancing the EFT Tango.

Figure 2.1 illustrates the macro-intervention of the EFT Tango. These five moves contain experiential micro-skills for accessing and reprocessing emotion, and systemic micro-skills for tracking current interactions, linking elements of emotional experience, and using newly discovered emotional experience to create new interactions. With the five moves of the EFT Tango as a backdrop, the rich set of EFT micro-skills that are employed across these five moves will be detailed in the following two chapters. There is much integration and overlapping of experiential and systemic micro-skills, but we will explore them separately.

3 Experiential EFT Micro-Skills

Experiential, individually oriented EFT interventions are used in all moves of the EFT Tango. They are used to create an alliance, to assemble and deepen, and to access and reprocess emotional experience. The experiential micro-skills of empathic attuning and reflecting; validation; evocative reflections and questions; heightening; empathic conjectures; and therapist transparency are detailed and demonstrated with examples from Emily's clients.

Empathic Attuning and Responding

Empathic attunement and responsiveness, clearly associated with the Rogerian, experiential tradition, form the essence of EFT (Johnson, 2020). They are needed in each move of the EFT Tango. Forming an empathic reflection/response begins with attunement and full emotional engagement on the part of the therapist. Johnson (2020) calls this *intense concentration* and *empathic absorption*. As Rogers (1980) said, the therapist needs to enter the world of the client and move around in it, to feel and sense with one's entire mind, heart, and body what it is like to be in this client's world and to sense the *intended emotional meaning* of the client's verbal and nonverbal message (Martin, 2016; Shore, 2014). Sensing the intended message means to attune to the nonverbal aspects of the client's expression, to the larger context of the client's experience, and to the key *emotional handles* (phrases, images, and poignantly expressed words that can open into increasingly alive, felt experience). To immerse oneself in another's world, an EFT therapist attunes to the client's nonverbal, implicit messages, as well as to their words, while also using their own inner experience as a reference point to resonate with and get a felt sense of the clients' stories. "We recognize changes in emotional states of others based on perception of subtle shifts in their facial expressions or posture, and recognize changes in our own states based on somatic or kinesthetic experience" (Bucci, 2002, p. 194, quoted in Shore, 2014, p. xxxiii). An attitude of cultural and contextual humility compels therapists to recognize their limitations to accurately, empathically enter another's world. Culturally humble therapists are empathically curious, inviting client's stories, and seeking to grow in awareness of their client's context. They invite clients to express their misgivings if they feel misunderstood or disrespected, and they attune to and inquire about signals from clients that they may not be feeling accurately understood.

Empathic attunement is a process that happens between client and therapist before the therapist finds words to describe what they are resonating with and understanding. K. Arnold (2014) describes empathic listening as a shared activity or a dance between client and therapist. He suggests that Rogers conceptualized

> empathy as an iterative relational process. Empathy is a *way of being* with another person. Empathic listening is inherently interactional, not an isolated state inside the mind of the therapist. It is not only an inner process, but a verbalizing of provisional understandings to the client, who

DOI: 10.4324/9781003242673-4

then has the opportunity to amend or reject them. Insofar as the client's feedback better attunes the therapist to the client's inner process, empathic listening is something that the therapist and client do together. The client helps the therapist to listen better. (p. 365)

Empathic responding is an active process in which EFT therapists constantly engage. First, they tune in to get a felt sense of the client's experience; then they find words to capture the core, most poignant part of the message; and finally, they invite feedback from the client as to whether their words accurately match their experience. That is, does the client experience that they have received empathic understanding?

Emily pauses to reflect on the power of empathic listening as a shared activity:

As a new therapist, I used to think that my job was simply to listen to clients share their stories with me. Now, I am learning that it is *in the telling and being responded to* that their stories and the accompanying emotional experience come alive and begin to make sense in new ways, not only to me, but to them as well. And then, of course with couples, there is the added benefit of helping one partner share a newly assembled experience with their partner, and to begin to see empathic understanding emerge between partners!

In couple therapy, Emily frequently experiences partners presenting very different experiences, yet both needing to be attended to, attuned with, and validated for their unique experience. At the same time, she also attunes to her own bodily emotional reactions to each partner. Present-moment resonance with nonverbal and verbal experience occurs before the therapist finds words to empathically reflect the impact the couple's negative cycle is having on them as a couple, and on each of their individual experiences of the relationship.

Empathy is an active, moment-to-moment, continuous process that serves several functions. For this reason, I will provide more detail on the combined attitude and skill of empathic responding than on the other EFT micro-skills. Although they are interrelated, I will discuss five separate functions of the simple, yet powerful, intervention of empathic responding, that is foundational to EFT. **Empathic responding, it must be noted, is an indispensable aspect of each of the other EFT micro-skills. Active empathic attunement and responding is a precursor to the experiential micro-skills of validation, evocative questions and responses, heightening, empathic conjecture, therapist self-disclosure, re-focusing, and redirecting. The systemic or relational micro-skills of tracking and reflecting, reframing, shaping encounters, *slicing thinner, catching bullets, and seeding attachment* are also fully dependent upon empathic attunement and responsiveness.**

[S]ensitively communicated empathy enhances a client's sense of safety, promotes a focus on the construction of experience and its meaning, and so enables new responses. The therapist is a processing partner who, through various forms of empathic responsiveness, *assembles, orders* and *deepens* each client's experience... Empathic attunement and responsiveness can be a demanding task. The EFT therapist has then to be willing to engage with and attune to each client's experience, and to *resonate* with this experience. (Johnson, 2020, p. 54, italics in original)

Empathy as a Shared Activity Centers the Clients' Context

Emily has been immersing herself in the Rogerian adage of *using one's empathic imagination to see the world through a client's eyes* (Rogers, 1961). "But stop!" she says to herself:

As a white woman, can I see through the eyes of another who does not have the advantages I have? Can I *see through the eyes of one who lives with* discrimination and oppression because of the color of their skin or their sexual orientation? My capacities for grasping another's life experiences may be limited. I cannot assume I fully understand but must attend to each person with cultural humility and a beginner's openness.

When there are intersectionality differences, whether they be cultural, sexual orientation, gender, racial, neurodiversity or others, therapists need to be especially mindful of their own limitations. Their best empathic resonance may not be enough to grasp the racial, cultural, and power differences between them and their client(s) or between partners. Therapists need to be open to attune to a client's story, not assume their attunement or tentative reflections are accurate, and be mindful to always check for confirmation. They also need to be aware that a client may well have a larger story that they are not yet ready to share. Comfort with being transparent about one's social location as a therapist (Jones, 2016) and with the broaching of intersectionality differences (Day-Vines et al., 2020) helps a therapist to own their limitations and convey humility and hospitality that center clients' stories.

Consider Wayne's words discussed earlier:

As a black man, I am perceived as a weapon in the world. My experience in the world is to constantly minimize my behaviors, constantly toning myself down – like knocking on the door and then stepping back so I am in full view – to alert the person opening the door that I am here without alarming them, so I don't get caught in the crossfire.

Emily wonders if there is a response she could make from her social location that would resonate with empathy and cultural humility and also validate that she cannot possibly fully grasp his experience. In an attempt to do this she says to Wayne:

As a white woman who can move more safely through this world and not need to tone myself down all the time, I can never fully understand your sense of threat – the frustration and the danger! But I am listening, always open to being corrected, hoping to understand, and to help Jessica understand your experience better as we work together. If I am hearing you correctly, you are saying that your experience in the world and in this relationship too, is that you are constantly on guard – fearing you'll be perceived as a threat and get caught in the crossfire if you show up. Am I getting it? And then with Jessica, you are saying that you are constantly holding back to not get caught in the crossfires of her complaints, never quite knowing if it is safe for you to show up. Yes?

Empathic Reflections Make the Leading Edge of Experience Explicit

A therapist is always listening on the leading edge (Johnson, 2015; Rice, 1974) of what the client seems to be saying but may not always put into words (Martin, 2016). Empathic reflections are attempts to mirror the client's core message, especially the most emotionally poignant and attachment-significant aspect of the message (Johnson, 2020; Martin, 2016). There are several parts to this simple definition of empathy: First, to hear and understand the person's intended message; second, to communicate that understanding; and third, to check if the client perceives that they are understood. This is a collaborate process where the client, in a context of emotional safety, is frequently finding words for experience that has not previously been formulated. *Evocative empathy* (Rice, 1974) opens up clients' experience, bringing to life the implicit or leading edge, first articulated by Rogers (1975):

[Empathy] involves being sensitive moment to moment to the changing felt meanings which flow in this other person, to the fear or rage, or tenderness or confusion or whatever, that he/she is experiencing. It means temporarily living in his/her life, moving about in it delicately without making judgements, sensing meanings of which he/she is scarcely aware, but not trying to uncover feelings of which the person is totally unaware, since this would be too threatening. (1975, p. 4)

Martin (2016) provides more of Rogers' perspective:

When the therapist has communicated an effectively empathic response, the client's reaction is likely to be "That's exactly right!"…When the therapist is exceptionally effective and has caught the subtle meanings on the edge of the client's awareness, the client's reaction is likely to be first a pause, then a gradual appreciation: "Yes, I think you're right! I had never thought of it in just that way before, but that is what I've been feeling and experiencing. And now I see some more". (Rogers, 1980, p. 2155, as cited in Martin, 2016, pp. 9–10)

It is always important to be somewhat tentative in a reflection, to give the client time to absorb the impact of hearing the therapist's understanding of what was just said and then to confirm whether or not this reflection matches their experience. Slow pacing and repetition are key in communicating empathic reflections and confirming the accuracy of the therapist's understanding. An experience of being accurately understood communicates, "You are with me. You get me. Perhaps I can come to trust you."

EFCT Example of Empathic Reflection. Partners sometimes communicate appreciation that the therapist understands the other partner, "I don't get my partner—I'm just frustrated with them. Their tantrums make no sense to me—but you seem to understand them and also seem to get me, and that already gives me a glimmer of hope." The simple example below illustrates how empathic reflections, on *the leading edge of attachment-related experience* are also validations.

Wayne: She seems upset with me much of the time!
Jessica: Well, I don't start out upset! I am just so lonely, and I am trying to get your attention!

This is not a time to explain, coach, or negotiate. The intervention of empathic reflecting comes first in EFT. First, each partner needs to experience that his/her reality is safely understood and validated, at least by the therapist. Empathic reflections to each partner begin the ordering and distilling process that fosters a safe haven and secure base for exploring and repairing a distressed relationship.

Emily to Wayne: You sigh as you say she seems upset with you much of the time—as though it is very difficult sensing that *this woman you love* is unhappy *with you*! (Attachment frame is in italics.)

Emily to Jessica: You are *very lonely, missing Wayne so much*, that sometimes you turn up the volume just *to get his attention?* (Even though that statement is not a question, the question mark is used to indicate a raised tone, to convey tentativeness and an invitation for Jessica to confirm or disconfirm if the reflection matches her experience. The tentative tone implies the question, "Is that right?")

EFIT Example of Empathic Reflection. Emily hears anger in Sahra's tone of voice, but upon reflecting the anger, Sahra says she is not angry.

Emily: Your voice sounds angry when you talk of the expectations your mother had of you.
Sahra: No, I'm not angry, I just wish she'd have taken better care of herself.

Race and cultural expectations may be a factor here. Emily suddenly realizes that *anger* may have been the wrong word to use, since it could portray a disrespectful racial stereotype of a woman of color. Empathically attuning to what seems like a misunderstanding, Emily rewords her reflection. Staying as close to the client's experience as possible, she continues to seek words to match what she hears, until the words accurately match Sahra's experience.

Emily: It sounds so very *disappointing* for you that your mother gave and gave to others, and yet seemed to ignore her own needs, yes?
Sahra: Exactly! I am disappointed and… (pause) …well, I am angry too! She modeled being this caring person for everyone but herself – and then it all came back to me – because I was the one who supported her and tried to help her keep her head above water… and she still died from what I think could have been prevented! But I hate feeling angry with her (head in her hands).

The anger that Emily detected on the leading edges, does fit for Sahra, when she has time to absorb feeling understood and respected. Now that the leading edge of her experience – emotion she did not want to face – has been articulated and accessed, she can move into further, increasingly coherent exploration.

Empathic Reflections Order and Distill Experience

Empathic reflection is especially important in Tango Move 1 and in the assembly part of Tango Move 2. By reflecting, repeating, and savoring clients' core emotional experience, emotional processing becomes increasingly orderly and meaningful. There is something intriguing about Rogers' comment that a reflection is more than repetition; it is a revelation. In fact, many empathic reflections are indeed simple repetitions of some of a client's words, but the words repeated are chosen carefully for their attachment and emotional significance. Repetition slows everything down. The therapist's prosodic tone validates and keeps alive what was just expressed.

Working with Ted, a critical pursuer, and Jed, a withdrawer guarding himself from Ted's angry outbursts, the therapist says, "Ted, you just turned to your partner, Jed, and said, 'I would do anything for you, but…' and tears are filling your eyes. 'I would do anything for you but'."

After the therapist's second repetition of the client's words, while also mirroring the tears filling Ted's eyes, Ted takes a huge risk to articulate a fear he had not yet expressed. He says, "But, but… and this is so hard to say (pause; more tears) I don't know if he'd do the same for me. I don't know if he is really committed."

As happened for Ted, repetition of a client's key image or words often becomes a huge revelation for a client who might not have previously attended to this personal experience so closely. Likewise, the client might never have experienced someone so intimately engaged with this particular aspect of their experience. An empathically engaged therapist's prosodic reflection of the client's core experience brings it to life in a new way, thus opening to the possibility of change.

In an experiential therapy, slow, emotionally resonant repetition is tremendously evocative. Repetition retains a present-moment focus and deepens present-moment experience. When a client responds with, "Exactly!" it confirms that they feel deeply understood and that the experience is coming more fully alive. The impact of the repetitive nature of empathic reflections is something that therapists new to EFT might not have experienced before and could be inclined to minimize for its seeming simplicity. It can also seem threatening to do therapy at this slow pace, engaging intimately with clients' moment-to-moment experience.

Empathic Reflections Access Core Emotion within the Content

Content can be distracting and overwhelming, but empathic reflections go to the core emotional experience underlying the content details. Repetition and reflection of the most poignant part of the message slows processing and encourages deepening engagement in core emotional experience. The most poignant part of the message is frequently found by tuning into the attachment channel and hearing, for example, how much one partner is affected by the response or lack of response from their partner.

Tuning into the most poignant part of Wayne's message, Emily hears how he is triggered by any sign that Jessica is unhappy or upset with him, and she offers this empathic tracking reflection, "You see that look on her face when you are trying so hard to get it right with her and you feel like you are sinking in quicksand!" Wayne responds, "Exactly!"

Jessica, sensing she cannot find Wayne or get his attention, says, "Feels like my teammate is caught somewhere up in the rafters." Emily reflects in a proxy voice, "It seems like my teammate is lost in the rafters and *I cannot find him*!" (adding the attachment significance of not being able to find him).

EFT therapists find that, with increased practice, their hearts and ears become naturally tuned to the attachment channel. Clients are the best teachers because, as Chapter 5 will describe, everyone has an attachment story to unfold. We are designed for co-regulation and thus, everyone's story of distress involves some sense of threat or loss, some unmet needs for connection, a loss of humanness or *dehumanization* (Karantzas et al., 2022). Lacking human companionship is the most dehumanizing experience, suggested Nelson Mandela (1995) in *Long Walk to Freedom*.

Empathic reflections keep therapists and clients focused on core experience when they could easily become derailed by content. For example, when Jessica says, "I get so annoyed that my husband spends so much time gaming on his computer," non-empathic responses or questions would detract from the experiential process. Asking, "What would happen if you'd tell him to stop?" or, "Why don't you develop your own hobbies?" would move entirely out of present-moment process. Another non-empathic example that will divert the process could be a question that might imply judgment, such as, "Is it hard for you to let him have his own life?" Yet another could be a question about what kind of gaming he does, or how much time he spends gaming. All these non-reflective, non-empathic responses would distract from the person's present-moment experience and ignore her core attachment message.

An empathically reflective response could be very simple and yet retain focus on attachment significance of the present moment, while communicating understanding, care, and safety for Jessica to stay engaged with her own core experience. For example, using some of Jessica's poignant, attachment-significant phrases, also called *emotional handles*, Emily reflects:

> It's very difficult for you that Wayne spends so much time on his computer. You feel *empty inside* that this most important person in the entire world is *turning away from you*! How very painful *to feel invisible to him*!

Another simple reflection which tracks her experience internally and interpersonally (within and between), and stays very close to her words is, "You start out feeling lonely, missing Wayne, and then you become fiercely determined to get his attention."

Mona, an immigrant from Iran, who is struggling with self-confidence, muses, "I did graduate from college when I was in Doha, but I still have bad dreams of not being able to graduate. This is the darker side of my life. I had a twin brother and he was very smart. And I was always compared to him …always bothers me that my parents never believed in me… I was never enough… it hurts so much."

Emily pauses to tune into Mona's core message and resists congratulating her for graduating, sensing her core message is her present-moment pain and not the fact that she did succeed at college. "As you say, 'I have never felt I was enough', your voice chokes. You hurt so much!" (Personalizing from the more general, "it hurts," to, "you hurt.") "As you relive this message you received from your parents, 'You're not enough; you won't make it,' pain shows on your face. Your tears begin to flow, and your voice sounds like a mix of anger and sadness, like you are saying, 'I needed their belief in me and they did not give it!'"

Mona responds, "Exactly! Lots of sadness and a little anger at them too for the doubts I carry to this day!"

Empathic Reflections Slow Processing

Empathic attunement, repetition, and reflection slow processing and encourage present-moment engagement. To do this, empathic reflections need to be concrete, vivid, and specific. There is a drugstore in the USA with that very acronym: CVS. Being concrete, vivid, and specific with an empathic reflection moves clients out of the vague, cerebral realm of content into a deeper awareness of emotional experiencing. Reflections also need to be offered in a slow, genuine manner, from a therapist who is engaged in attempting to obtain a felt sense in their own body and an imagination of the client's attachment experience. For example, "I get that this is infuriating. I see a lot of pain in your eyes as you say it and I feel a rock in my own stomach as I listen." A therapist resonating in their own body with the client's experience can increase empathic attunement and deepen client's emotional experience (Kailanko et al., 2021b).

Jessica: I just get so mad at him, and then feel awful that I am this prickly porcupine.
Emily: When he is absorbed at his computer – in something other than you – it sounds like you walk off in anger and then feel so badly that you've just blasted the man you love and long to have close and to feel safe with you!

Emily's vivid and specific reflection concretely reflects the attachment-significant trigger for Jessica's angry reaction – that Wayne is absorbed in something other than her and, by implication, unavailable to her. It also captures the attachment context of Jessica's present-moment emotion of feeling badly for blasting the man she loves and longs to have close. The attachment context helps to normalize her attachment need for a response, and to de-pathologize what might be perceived as "neediness." It also helps her to access the softer, more vulnerable emotion underlying her reactive anger.

Jessica: I am missing him, yes! It is so lonely when he's busy with something else. And I can't blame him—who'd want to come close to a porcupine!"
Emily: You blame yourself for getting angry, and underneath is all this pain and loneliness. (An empathic reflection that captures her core message of loneliness and also tracks her behavior of self-blame for getting angry with Wayne.)
Jessica: I do feel really bad, yes. But it really helps to know I'm not all bad.

Emily: It helps you to know that this fury you feel, this pain that you've been stewing in for an hour or so, is code for, "I'm afraid there isn't room for me in your heart right now." You're saying it's kind of helping to grasp that underneath your outrage is this fear that perhaps he doesn't have room in his heart for you anymore, yes?

A basic concrete, vivid, and specific reflection in the attachment frame helps to order and distill her experience. It also brings it alive in the present moment, deepening Jessica's emotional experiencing. Reflecting her core fear that he has no room in his heart for her helps to reframe her porcupine self-image into one that is soft and well-intentioned. At the end of the reflection, Emily checks to see if her reflection matches Jessica's present-moment experience.

EFT therapists understand that empathic reflections of a client's core message have the power to hold a client in present-moment awareness, to move them inside to reflect more specifically on their emotional experience, and to get an emerging, expansive felt sense of the words that have just been spoken. Empathically attuned responding *"directs the client's attention to the unfolding of inner experience, [and] sharpens the client's grasp of the experience… Reflection can be seen as a way of turning and turning an experience to the light so that new facets appear"* (Johnson, 2020, p. 86, italics in the original).

Validation

The prerequisite to formulating a validation is empathic attunement (Johnson, 2020). Validating statements typically begin with the words or implication, "It makes sense that you would feel a certain way or act a certain way," given the specific context the client is experiencing. Validations function to affirm the elements of the client's emotional experience as legitimate and understandable, given the clients' relational and social contexts. Validating comments situate clients' emotional experience and reactivity in their cyclic interactions, frequently linking action tendencies and reactive emotions to other elements of emotional experience. An example of validating a client's withdrawal or avoidant strategy by linking to fears, perceptions, and meanings is, "It makes sense that you hesitate to share your pain when you fear it will trigger her to back away even more." Or, "It makes sense you block your memories of the accident, when you fear the images will overwhelm you."

The EFT therapist is continually watching for markers (signs) of underlying emotions that are on the leading edge of awareness. For example, Sophie expresses reactive emotion about her partner, Ella, "I am so exasperated with her! I have tried ten ways to get her attention and she doesn't hear me!" The therapist's first task is to validate the reactive emotion (frustration), and the attachment meanings Sophie makes, "Of course you are frustrated with her when it seems to you that she is not taking time to hear you." This helps the client to feel seen and immediately brings down the level of anxiety/reactivity in the room, which then opens the door to furthering exploration and linking the elements of emotion to each other.

The attachment context is essentially the rigidly, repetitive, cycle of mis-attempts at secure connection, the habitual strategies for connection of criticize–demand, withdraw–defend, the negative attachment meanings each one makes of the other's actions, and the unmet longings and fears. Validations match the emotional intensity of expressed emotion and make sense of reactivity. For example, "You end up feeling rejected and not at all important to him, and this hurts, and so it's no wonder that you fly off the handle!"

Two partners are likely to present very different experiences, and both need to be attuned with and validated for their unique experience. An EFT therapist seeks to validate each partner's emotional experiencing in the context of the cycle of interactions. Validations combine with empathic reflecting and also link specific elements of emotion together, creating greater emotional coherence and normalizing in an attachment context.

The attachment context is relevant for formulating validations in EFIT as well. Lyndon enters therapy with various compulsions and obsessions related to saving stray animals. After hearing several of his stories of loss and grief that he claims not to have thought about for years, Emily is able to validate what Lyndon describes as a disturbing, all-consuming obsession. She validates his frenzy to save every stray animal as making sense in the context of his having survived grief that felt too difficult to bear and having become caught in a pattern of disregarding his own pain and loss by focusing outward on saving others in need. Validations are much more than general statements claiming, "Of course that makes sense." They are specific, concrete, empathically attuned responses that normalize and make *emotional sense* of client's experience. Chapter 3 Support Material (routledge.com/9781032151335) has many examples of forming validations by linking specific elements of emotion, thereby conveying coherence, agency, and implying hope and new possibilities.

Evocative Reflections and Questions

Empathically attuned reflections with repetition of images and key words are evocative, inviting leading edge elements of emotion into awareness. They "open up the experience and provide the client with a process whereby he can form successively more accurate constructions of his own experience" (Rice, 1974, p. 290). Reflections and evocative process questions are deliberately directed to each element of the *trigger-perception-feeling-meaning-action process of emotion* (M. Arnold, 1960). A series of simple questions (also presented in Box 6.2) evokes each element that M. Arnold identified: What is the cue? (trigger); How does it touch you? (limbic perception); What does your body do? (bodily arousal); What does it say to you? (meaning-making); What do you do? (action tendency) (B. Goettle, personal communication, circa 2012).

Evocative Reflections and Questions to Assemble Emotion

In addition to empathic reflective responses that are innately evocative, an EFT therapist uses evocative questions specifically targeted to the different elements of emotional experience. Emotional experience (expanded on in Chapter 6) contains a cue (or trigger); an immediate preconscious, limbic perception of that cue as safe or dangerous; bodily arousal; meaning-making; an impulse to action; and, in addition, core affective experience that may or may not be clearly noticed. There are both reactive, surface, self-protective emotions and underlying core emotions. Many of these elements remain outside clients' awareness, until the therapist helps them to access them, one element at a time. One could say these elements are on the leading edge of a client's experience but require a therapist's deliberate assembly for a client to experience them explicitly and coherently. EFT therapists replay key moments, followed by questions targeted at specific elements, and together clients and therapist assemble, order, and normalize otherwise chaotic or numb experience.

For example, when Sophie realizes Ella is not coming home for dinner yet again (*cue/ immediate perception of danger*), it tells Ella, once again, that she is at the bottom of Sophie's priority list (*meaning*). She becomes enraged and shouts angrily into her cellphone (*reactive emotion and action tendency*). She does not recognize in the moment that her underlying fearful perception of not mattering to Ella is driving her rage.

"What happens inside when you hear that Ella will not be home for dinner?" is an evocative question to evoke her bodily response or the perception triggered by her partner's action.

To assemble emotional experience, the therapist sandwiches evocative reflections and validations with evocative questions such as the following, to access the different elements of emotion:

- "What do you see that tells you they are not listening?" or "When do you get the message that they are ignoring you?" (To evoke the danger cue that triggers an emotional reaction.)
- "What sensations do you feel in your body when this happens?" (To evoke awareness of physiological arousal.)
- "What do you feel like doing when …?" (To evoke the behavioral reaction or the impulse to action, even if it is not mobilized.)
- "What does it tell you when she turns away from you?" (To evoke the attachment meaning the client makes of another's action. This could be a perceived view of self, such as, "*I am unlovable*," or of other, such as, "*They cannot be trusted.*")

Sophie's core fear of abandonment from Ella comes to life as Emily helps her to link and assemble these elements. Emily helps her to uncover this fear at the core of her outrages toward Ella.

Sophie: (To Ella.) I feel like a monster when I am yelling at you – but all this fuss is code for my fear of not mattering to you enough that you will stick with me through our conflicts. I want to discuss my fears more instead of just flying into a rage.

Underlying core fears are like nuggets of gold to be discovered. When core fears (of rejection, abandonment, or annihilation) can be acknowledged and shared, emotional shifts begin to happen. New meanings and action tendencies arise.

Evocative Questions to Evoke Attachment Significance

Emily is discovering an evocative question can evoke the attachment meaning underlying content which otherwise threatens to bog therapy down in a *content trap*. For example, when partners insist the real problem is a disagreement over domestic chores, she can ask, "What would it say to you if he were to do the vacuuming?" Or, "What would it tell you if she would help more with the garden?" Partners are then likely to touch on attachment-related themes such as longings to feel important, appreciated, supported, and to know the other is there for them.

Evocative Questions to Evoke Content that Needs to Be Named

While content traps can block exploration of the emotional process, there is content that needs to be made explicit in order to more fully explore the process. Content that needs to be specifically evoked is the content of one or more attachment injuries and content about socio-cultural context.

Attachment Injury Content. When a client such as Aida in Chapter 16 says, describing the impact of an attachment injury, "My world changed that day. I have never been the same since. I have never looked at Eric the same way again," Emily hears there was a pivotal moment that changed everything, shattering her view of self and other. A curious evocative reflection, "Everything changed in that moment!" leaves the door open for the client to name it specifically. Or a specific evocative question, "Can you tell me what took place that changed your world in an instant?" elicits naming of the pivotal life-altering event. The specific content matters.

Contextual Content. Evocative reflections and questions can also open the door to important contextual nuances, that could be overlooked. Emily says to Wayne, "You just said, 'Christmas was very difficult in her white family's suburban community'." Before asking an evocative question for a specific example, this empathic reflection of something he had shared previously conveys attunement and brings emotional experience alive:

> You've talked before about how unsafe you feel as the only black man in this white community and how you automatically tone yourself down. You've mentioned that when you hear "something that rubs you the wrong way," you feel you have to leave it alone.

These evocative empathic reflections are followed by an evocative question. "Were you able to notice a moment of your automatic toning it down (racially required self-protective action tendency) that you were then able to tell Jessica about?" This evocative question invites explicit naming of a specific interactive pattern and of a possible step outside of the typical pattern to share it with his partner.

Evocative Questions for Clients without Access to Feeling Words or Bodily Sensations

Clients who are highly intellectualized or who reflexively default to rigid down-regulating strategies can be challenging for EFT therapists. Conjectures about affect are not likely to appeal to or effectively elicit these clients' experience. They are not focused on affective experience, however, action impulses and meaning-making are elements of emotion that are typically quite accessible to intellectual and more avoidant clients. By reflecting and engaging with what is within a client's awareness and linking these elements to the interpersonal trigger (*cue*), an EFT therapist can assemble a more complete gestalt of a client's emotional experience.

A client may insist, "I don't feel anything." To engage such a client, repeating the distressing cue and then asking an evocative question about an aspect of emotional experience other than bodily felt affect or a feeling word is likely to be more effective. Action impulses and meaning-making are commonly within reach. "What do you feel like doing when _____?" Naming the cue can evoke the action tendency part of emotion that is an entrance into assembling the experience of a more shut-down partner or individual client. "What does that (the trigger) say to you…?" will evoke the attachment meaning a client is making. If the trigger (cue) for the *cascade of emotion* has not been identified, the following evocative questions can help to access the trigger:

- "*What happens just before* you stomp out of the room?"
- "*When* do you get that sinking feeling?"
- "*When* do you feel like getting out of the way?"
- "*What do you see/hear* that tells you to be careful?"

Emily cannot get Julian to use any feeling words or to locate any emotion in his body regarding his wife, Geri. "I'm not upset," he insists, "but she has a problem. Nothing but complaints! It is irrational to rage and bluster about how I wipe the counters or how I close the door!" To be respectful and to get closer to his emotional experience, Emily repeats the cue and evokes the meaning he makes: "When you hear she isn't happy with how you wipe the counter or close the door, what does that say to you?" This evokes the meaning Julian makes, which is, "Nothing I do will ever be enough." With that awareness, Emily hears fear of rejection on the leading edge and Julian can gradually access this underlying fear that he has had no words for previously.

Alternately, Emily *evokes his action tendency, repeating the cue,* "What do you feel like doing when you hear she doesn't like how you do things?" Julian responds with acknowledging his action tendencies of throwing up his hands, giving up, and walking out. An EFT therapist does not seek to correct clients' perceived emotional experience or to suggest alternate responses, but rather, to assemble their experience to help them more fully attune to their experience and formulate the core emotion driving their self-protective, repetitive pattern.

Emily assembles the emotional elements of Julian's experience in a kind voice, "What a difficult experience – when Geri expresses dissatisfaction with how you do something (*cue*)! You hear you can never make her happy (*meaning*), and you throw up your hands (*bodily arousal*) and feel like giving up and walking away (*action tendency*). It matters so much for you to make her happy!" (*Hint of attachment fear of her rejection for letting her down.*) Julian recognizes this assembly as his own experience and his present-moment awareness deepens, as he exclaims, "Yes – it is difficult, I guess. I do want her to be happy with me! And when I can't make her happy, I do get discouraged – start to think she may not want me anymore!"

Evocative Questions to Order Confusion and Ambivalence

To order confusion and ambivalence, and explore blocks in clients' experience, EFT therapists are relentlessly curious and compassionately courageous to walk right into confusion and chaos. The more specific and granular the experience, the more calming and empowering it is.

For example, when a client speaks vaguely or disjointedly, "I was unhappy for years but I never said anything, and now I'm just numb – not at all interested sexually," a therapist can move closer by evoking specifics. "You never said anything about what – your unhappiness?" and, "What is it like to be so numb right now? How do you talk about your lack of sexual interest? Was there a time when your interest in sex changed? What are the parts of your sexual relationship that you once enjoyed? Can you talk about your sexual relationship with your partner?" These evocative questions would not be asked in a series but would be followed by reflection, validation, and more exploration.

When a client says, "Maybe I'm not even attracted to my partner anymore but I would like to repair our marriage," a therapist can evoke, "*When* do you feel an interest in repairing this relationship?" (To evoke the cue for this longing.) "What are the parts of your relationship that you value and want to preserve?" Evoking more specificity makes it ok to be hesitant and to have conflicting feelings. It gives permission to address confusion and to name the uncertainties and ambivalence.

Evocative questions help to move clients out of generalities and confusion into specificity and emotional granularity that calms and engenders more of a sense of agency. Evocative questions are useful to envision and shape specific goals and longings for change. For example, "What would repairing this relationship look like for you?"

In summary, evocative reflections and questions help to assemble emotional experience and to bring it alive in the present moment in a focused manner that is specific and grounded in what matters most, the attachment, social contexts of clients' lives. Emotion is contextual (Knudson-Martin et al., 2015) and EFT therapists assemble emotion to order it into "a coherent and relational whole" (Furrow & Bradley, 2011, p. 21; Johnson, 2020). This ability to formulate experience in an understandable way adds to the security and safety needed to explore and reshape attachment bonds, instigate *broaden-and-build emotion regulation strategies,* and restructure working models of self and other.

Heightening

Heightening functions to engage and intensify emotional experience. While it can be used through all the moves of the EFT Tango, it is especially useful in the second part of Tango Move 2 (deepening) and in the heightening part of Tango Move 3 (SHAPE an encounter). The vocal tone, pacing, and timing of interventions are significant parts of what makes EFT interventions effective (Greenman & Johnson, 2013).

RISSSSSC Manner

The acronym RISSSSSC, implying *risking* deeper emotional experiencing (Johnson, 2020), best represents *how* the intervention of heightening is done: with **R**epetition, **I**magery, **S**imple, **S**oft, **S**low, **S**pecific, **S**omatic signals, and use of **C**lient's words.

R: *Repeat* "emotional handles" – key, poignant words and phrases such as "shattered" or "feel like a ghost."
I: *Images* or word pictures evoke emotions more than abstract labels. "Like walking a gangplank; one slip and the sharks will devour me!"
S: Frame responses in *simple, succinct* phrases.
S: Speak at a *slow* pace.
S: A *soft*, low, soothing tone of voice creates safety for deepening; at times, a firmer tone will be used to deepen a client's emerging edges of assertion, for example.
S: Continually seek *specific*, more granular nuances of client's precise emotional experience.
S: Repeat *somatic* cues – clients' bodily movements, reported sensations, voice tone and pace. This deepens awareness of meanings, bodily felt arousal, action impulses, and core emotion.
C: Use *clients'* words and phrases in a supportive and validating way.

The micro-skill of heightening requires empathic attunement and responding in order to be effective. A soft, slow, low tone with simple words and images speaks to the limbic system and deepens clients' emotional engagement. Paradoxically, even more than the spoken words, a prosodic, soft, melodic tone and accompanying facial expression both heighten emotional risk and vulnerability, and convey soothing to calm a dysregulated brain, making it possible for a person to process clearly. Repetition potentiates the gradual process by which clients can move closer and closer to their own frightening and unfamiliar emotions. Examples of using the RISSSSSC manner with the withdraw/withdraw trauma survivor couple, Phil and Julie, are given in the online Chapter 9 Support Material (routledge.com/9781032151335).

Images Heighten Emotional Experience

Images, perhaps the most vivid type of *emotional handle,* frequently drop clients into an experiencing mode. Attachment images are italicized in Emily's reflection to Sophie, "Sophie, when the phone rings and you hear Ella say, 'Sorry, I am not going to make it home for dinner. My mother needs some help,' you *picture her chatting and laughing with her mother and sister, while you sit at home, alone.* Her message stabs your heart with *loneliness and doubt about her love for you!*" In this EFT Tango Move 1, Emily mirrors the moment, repeating Sophie's attachment image of Ella enjoying the comfort of her family, while Sophie sits at home alone. She validates how Ella's message feels like a stab in her heart of loneliness and fear that Ella may not love her.

An intellectualizing defended withdrawer speaks rapidly and distantly from his experience. The therapist, barely able to make contact or to get a word in, says, "It's as if you're a *fast-moving train*—nothing can stop you." Immediately, the image engages both partners in their present-moment emotional experience. "I don't dare stick my hand out the window," he adds, "it will be cut off" (a probable reference to his wife's critical pursuit). "And he just sees a crazy lady running after the train," adds his partner. "He doesn't see I am terrified he's leaving me behind." Given that images "capture and hold emotion" (Johnson, 2020, p. 110) better than abstract words, circling around this imagery heightens underlying attachment emotions and fears. The shared laughter at this image also increases safety and heightens awareness, as the withdrawer adds, "And then, when she catches me, she slugs me with her handbag for leaving her." Underlying attachment emotions emerge from these images: She fears he is leaving her; he fears she is catching him to hurt him.

In response to Jessica's outpouring of grief about her husband's computer gaming, Emily repeats softly, simply, and slowly, Jessica's vivid attachment images of Wayne slipping away, building a new world of peace without her, "This is very frightening! You just said, 'I'm afraid you're going to *slip away from me.* That you're *building a different world – a peaceful world that doesn't come from me.*' What a clear picture of your fear of losing him and of your longing to be *his safe place!*" (Attachment images are in italics.) Validation and heightening come together when the therapist heightens the core emotion and longing and validates them in the attachment context. Validation and heightening also come together when a therapist heightens a Stage 2 bonding moment. When partners spontaneously discuss a bonding moment that happened between sessions, an EFT therapist will slow down to validate and heighten, savoring the moment to ensure the new attachment seedling takes root. Newly accessed and heightened emotional experience is shaped into a direct message to another, in Tango Move 3.

Reflecting Somatic Signals Heightens Emotional Experience

Recent research validates (Kailanko et al., 2021a, 2021b, 2022) the importance of reflecting clients' somatic signals as an explicit part of the RISSSSSC acronym for heightening emotional risk and experience. When an EFT therapist explicitly reflects the slightest bodily movement, such as a flick of a wrist, the tightening of the jaw, or slight laughter, a client is helped to connect to the bodily element of their present-moment experience, and to discover more clearly what is happening. Internal somatic experiences, expressed in images, can also be very useful handles to repeat and deepen emotion. For example: *A cube of hate in my heart, a stab in my back, dizzying chaos, eats away insid*e.

Balance Heightening with Emotional Containment

While heightening is a key EFT intervention, an EFT therapist is continually monitoring the intensity of clients' experience to help them remain within the optimum emotional *window of tolerance* (Siegel, 2012). If the emotion is too great, some clients will shut it down and others will become overwhelmed. Empathic responsiveness modulates emotional intensity and creates a working distance from emotion (Johnson, 2020). Whenever emotion is suppressed or dysregulated, the safe context for exploration is not there and the useful information embedded in emotion is out of clients' reach. An EFT therapist continually seeks to balance heightening with containing, so as to help each client be in touch with, but not overwhelmed by emotional experience. The more a therapist empathically attunes to the attachment channel and recognizes attachment-salient emotional experience and key triggers for each person's reactions, the more adept they become at recognizing when emotional experience needs to be heightened and when it needs to be contained to prevent a client from becoming overwhelmed and unable to process.

Amygdala Whisperers. Finding the optimum balance between heightening and containing emotion is important for EFT across all modalities and is particularly important when working with trauma survivors (Greenman & Johnson, 2012). Similar to the gentle role of a *horse whisperer* developing trust with abused, traumatized horses, EFT therapists are *amygdala whisperers,* helping clients to engage with frightening emotional experience, little by little (Johnson, 2019). Trauma survivors need finely tuned support to be engaged at a working distance from emotion, since they have probably survived by fluctuating between suppression and hyper-activation of emotion. When an emotion is too intense, an EFT therapist will "slice it thinner" slowing down the process and engaging with one manageable piece of experience at a time. To reduce intensity, a therapist can also replace heavy words like "terror" or "fear," with "worried" or "dread" or "a little concerned" and gradually increase intensity to a level with which the client can remain engaged (Liu & Wittenborn, 2011).

Attachment Figures as a Resource. Attachment figures, real or imagined, can help a client encounter difficult, unacceptable emotions within their window of tolerance. Ella tells Sophie in a structured encounter that she pulls away when they argue, to calm down and come back to Sophie in a better way. While Emily is processing this encounter with Sophie (Tango Move 4), Sophie protests, "Too hard to believe… don't trust she wants to come back to me!" Emily validates, "As Ella tells you her withdrawal is code for wanting to calm down so she can come back to you in a better way, your warning bells say, 'No – don't trust that… too afraid she doesn't really want to come back to me,' yes?" Sophie nods, drops her head and is quiet, then adds, "I need a break." Emily sees Sophie is overwhelmed – apparently exceeding her window of tolerance. Ella reaches out and takes Sophie's hand and says to Emily, "It's too much for her." Emily's heart sinks, "Did I heighten her fear too much? Did I make a mistake?" She looks at the couple in front of her: Ella, who in moments of distress tends to withdraw and turn away, is reaching in closer to Sophie, just as they both acknowledge Sophie is *feeling too much*. Emily moves out of her own self-doubts into being fully present with the couple on the screen in this online session. Realizing Sophie needs emotional balance, she decides to heighten Ella's response to Sophie's dysregulated anxiety, "Ella, you are so tuned into Sophie right now – reaching out to her when you see she is too frightened to speak. Sophie, just notice if you can feel Ella holding your hand. Can you feel her hand?" Moments later, after she had calmed down somewhat, Sophie says, "That was new! This was the first time that I was overwhelmed and couldn't speak, that I could actually feel Ella holding my hand. The first time I was having trauma flashbacks and didn't totally go numb! I could actually feel Ella's presence while I was shaking on the inside. That was new for me. I wasn't totally overwhelmed!"

Emily sighs a breath of relief and reminds herself to continue to draw on the regulating power of an attachment figure. She recalls a similar incident of soothing from an attachment figure with a trauma survivor in an EFIT session: During a trauma flashback, Sahra was able to find some soothing to ground her in the present moment by recalling the wordless, loving presence and sensation of her grandmother's loving arms around her.

Heightening Core Emotion Points to Relevant Encounters

Assembling and heightening core emotion with Tango Move 2 organically lead to the choice of a relevant encounter to shape. Emily watches a video of an EFIT session with Adam (pseudonym), a survivor of a traumatic, racially motivated attack; the therapist repeats the kinesthetic image of his anger – a "cube of hatred" in his chest. The repetition of this image serves to heighten and bring forth an emotional experience for which the client had previously had no words because he "didn't want to be an angry man." Adam describes what he endured and the therapist heightens by repeating emotional handles of "on the ground; kicked and beaten; all alone; nothing to hold on to." While heightening the client's attachment emotion with these images, the enormity of horror that he endured and had suppressed for decades comes alive. Together they assemble his rage into a coherent story of loss and trauma. The therapist validates and heightens that the attack which he suffered was indeed a pivotal incident that "changed everything." His emotion becomes more coherent and acceptable as she validates that of course he is filled with rage at this random, brutal attack. Having successfully suppressed his rage, the client discovers, in the context of the emerging safety and coherence provided by the therapist's use of Tango Move 2, that his rage is still there as raw, unprocessed experience, ready to be discovered, assembled, and brought to life.

With the therapist's heightening interventions, Adam deepens into his core emotions of suppressed rage, grief, and sadness at the losses from the event of the brutal attack. The emerging edges of deeply experienced core sadness and loss bring alive a memory with a similar bodily felt, emotion. In an instant, Adam vividly recalls another pivotal event filled with loss, after which "nothing was ever the same." This event is the death of his beloved father. Heightened emotion, fully experienced, is open to revision.

Emily is filled with tears and poignant hope as she realizes she is indeed witnessing the power of deepened core emotion in action! Heightened core emotion frequently brings alive similar developmental or earlier experiences of that emotion. "It is true!" sighs Emily, "*Staying with and deepening* core emotion spontaneously brings alive previously hidden feelings and meanings. New depths of experience, new action impulses, new perspectives, and clarity about which encounter to shape, emerge in this process. Truly, I can trust the process of emotion to guide me to choose the relevant encounter!"

From here, the therapist shapes an encounter for the client to invite his father into the scene of his traumatic attack and share with him the horror he had to endure. In an encounter with an imaginal other (his father), shame, that he had not before recognized, is lifted. He experiences an emerging shift of connection with his father in this traumatic scene where he was absolutely alone and helpless. The therapist continues to validate and heighten the horror Adam has tended to ignore and his justifiable core anger toward his attackers, validating as well, that he can trust his emotions more and feel safe to explore their emerging edges, no longer fearing he will be consumed by his own hatred. Heightening his core emotions within a manageable level of tolerance and safety is the process by which the therapist helps him, in Stage 2, to reprocess his experience: Becoming freer and safer to fully acknowledge and grieve his experience and reshape a positive sense of self and discriminate who are safe others. A session with *Adam* can be accessed at www. steppingintoeft.com.

Empathic Conjectures

Empathic conjectures are tentatively offered reflections which go slightly beyond the leading edge of what a client has been able to put into words. Conjectures could be called *hunches detected through bodily felt attunement to* attachment and context. Made at the leading edge of experience and within an attachment/contextual frame, conjectures function to expand clients' awareness and articulation of experience.

When offering conjectures, it is important to convey tentativeness and to take time to check if the communicated understanding accurately matches the client's expanding experience. Perceived understanding on the part of the client is paramount (Barrett-Lennard, 2013). If a therapist is too far on the leading edge with a conjecture, a client is likely to deny the accuracy or else agree intellectually but not be engaged. Conjectures are evocative, empathic reflections of what we hear hinted at in the entire context of what the client has shared, verbally and nonverbally. They are not hunches about "why" someone acts or feels the way they do. Conjectures evolve out of the therapist's attuned listening, to their own bodily felt sensing of the client's story and to what attachment theory tells us about human needs for connection and safety. Emily is learning to tune into her own bodily felt sensing – what Glanzer (2014) calls *edge-sensing* – as she attunes to her clients. In EFT, we are not searching for reasons or explanations; we are seeking to expand each client's emotional experience and their capacity to put words to their newly emerging experience.

Emily feels a pang of tension in her own heart before validating and offering an attachment-based conjecture to an irate client. With a tentative tone to convey an invitation for the client to check if this understanding fits and to freely disconfirm if it does not, she offers, "Of course you are angry that he has betrayed you, and I also notice you fighting back tears as you say how furious you are that he lied to you over and over. I wonder if there is unspoken pain and sadness beneath your fury?"

A conjecture is an attempt to capture the leading edge of experience. Many iterations of collaborative and respectful clarifying can be made between client and therapist before an accurate description of the client's present-moment experience is captured. The therapist attunes and offers their best attempt to convey understanding, always open to having the words tweaked or adjusted for a perfect fit to the client's experience. If a client agrees with an empathic conjecture intellectually, it is important to check *how,* specifically, this matches their felt experience.

The most engaging and emotionally alive conjectures are those where the therapist speaks in a proxy voice, as though they were in that client's skin. For example, "Under all of this anger, Sophie, I'm wondering if I am also hearing a lot of fear." Then, switching to a proxy voice, "'I'm terrified that Ella is going to just slip away from me and find she prefers her family over being with me. I'm terrified she doesn't want the fussing, fuming person I'm becoming!' Am I close?"

Three specific conjectures – *slicing risks thinner, catching bullets* and *seeding attachment* – are described as systemic EFT micro-skills in Chapter 4.

Therapist Transparency

Therapist self-disclosure is used judiciously in EFT. It has several functions, all of which strengthen the therapeutic alliance. First, self-disclosure is a particularly important way that therapists can share their social location to open doors to discuss intersectionality. Chapter 7 describes examples of therapist transparency to convey openness to discuss lived experiences of privilege and subjugation. Second, self-disclosure is a way of operationalizing therapist genuineness when a therapist says, for example, "I felt the pain pierce through my heart as you talked about the anguish you feel for having betrayed your partner as you did." Third, brief self-disclosures can help to deepen client emotional experiencing while also demonstrating the therapist's genuine engagement. For example, a therapist says, "Did I just imagine it or did I hear a catch in your voice as you said, 'I'm on a path…'?" The client responds, "Yes – you did. I almost cried." With transparency, the therapist replies, "I almost cried too, with you." Fourth, ease and comfort with brief self-disclosures from the therapist help to normalize the dilemmas of being human, and to foster the therapist's non-expert role as a process consultant collaborating with a couple, individual, or family. "Disciplined self-disclosure to normalize and prevent shame is part of EFT" (Johnson, 2019, p. 172). Finally, to fosters task alliance, therapist transparency about the therapy process functions to build and maintain client's trust that the therapy is relevant to their concerns.

Conclusion

All experiential interventions described above require that EFT therapists check regularly with clients whether they are accurately understanding their experience. EFT therapists continually seek to attune to clients' experience and to use words that match their experience. In their very thoughtful guidelines for working with cultural diversity and emotional experience, Liu and Wittenborn (2011) aptly remind us that the goal of accessing core emotion is not as much to find language to *label* an emotion, as it is for clients to have safe access to their "more vulnerable states without becoming defensive or avoidant" (p. 305). Slow pacing is needed to give clients time to hear the therapist's experiential interventions and to check inside if the therapist's words and emotional tone accurately match their experience. Empathy is an interactive process and a client needs time to receive or adjust the empathic understanding that is offered to them (K. Arnold, 2014; Martin, 2016).

Experiential micro-skills focus on and work specifically with the emotion that has control precedence (Tronick, 1989, 2007). That is, the focus is on the emotions that drive the pursue–demand and defend–withdraw actions of a couple's repetitive cycle or that drive an individual's repetitive patterns of anxious hyper-activating or avoidant deactivating. The focus is on engaging the core fears and needs driving the imprisoning patterns. Lingering longer to reprocess these fears in Stage 2 is what leads to lasting change, restructuring connections into ones of security and views of self and other into positive working models. Experiential micro-interventions are the therapist's tools for actively engaging clients with their core emotional experience at a *working distance* from that experience (Gendlin, 1981; Lietaer et al., 1990). Before examining the systemic or interactionally oriented interventions in the following chapter, notice how all of the above experiential interventions contribute to the fundamental focus across all modalities of EFT: To track, assemble, and deepen emotion "within the scaffold of a safe therapeutic relationship in which the therapist is an active moment-by-moment co-regulator and processor of emotion, and then to order and distill it, placing it in an attachment and interactional context" (Johnson & Faller, 2011, p. 174). The ongoing flow between experiential and systemic micro-interventions is how corrective emotional experiences are shaped in EFT. An EFT therapist "constantly helps partners to expand inner emotional awareness, especially of the deeper, softer emotions, and to send new signals ... that evoke new and more positive responses" (Johnson et al., 2015, p. 394). Expanding inner emotional experience in order to send clearer messages is also at the heart of the change process in EFIT. Chapter 3 Support Material (routledge.com/9781032151335) provides summaries and tips about the EFT experiential micro-skills.

4 Systemic EFT Micro-Skills

Systemic, interactionally oriented EFT micro-skills are used in all moves of the EFT Tango and across all steps of client change. EFT therapists use systemic micro-skills to identify patterns in Stage 1 of client change, to restructure patterns for interaction and regulating emotion in clients' Stage 2, and to consolidate and strengthen the broaden-and-build patterns in Stage 3. We will explore the following systemic micro-skills: Tracking reflections, reframing, refocusing/redirecting, followed by shaping encounters, processing encounters, and summarizing/integrating. The latter three micro-skills, frequently listed in EFT literature as micro-skills, are also essentially Tango Moves 3, 4, and 5. We also examine the special conjectures used in shaping and processing encounters: *Slicing it thinner, seeding attachment, and catching a bullet.*

Tracking Reflections

Tracking reflections, sometimes referred to as *tracking and reflecting*, can be said to focus primarily on systemic patterns of interacting as distinguished from *empathic reflections*, which focus on inner emotional experience. Emotion, by its very nature, is systemic – a constant interplay between self and system. Patterns of interaction are a weaving of interpersonal and intrapersonal experience. Thus, tracking reflections capture this interplay in the *patterns of interacting*, while empathic reflections mirror and expand *inner experience*.

When EFT therapists offer tracking reflections, clients are helped to identify current problematic patterns and to integrate new patterns of interacting and newly emerging meanings and experience. Tracking reflections usually include action tendencies and triggers, as well as emerging underlying emotions and meanings. Replaying a typical interaction between partners as it occurs in session, linking action tendencies, triggers, and other explicit elements in the cascade of emotional elements, conveys an accepting picture of the pattern as the problem. As time goes on, the replay of this process becomes more elaborate and more coherent. Clients are able to take ownership for how they get triggered into the pattern. As the underlying emotions that are driving the pattern become clearly differentiated and expressed, readiness for Stage 2 emerges.

In Stage 2, EFT therapists offer tracking reflections, sometimes replaying the old pattern when it takes over again but this time with an increased capacity to see what is happening; more often replaying how shifting core emotions are pulling for new dance moves. Tracking reflections of new patterns of *between and within* interaction helps to integrate and consolidate Stage 2 restructuring.

A tracking reflection is a key micro-intervention used in several EFT Tango moves. It is used in Move 1, reflecting present process, in the assembly part of Move 2, and in the integrating and summarizing of Move 5. An EFIT example in Move 1 and an EFCT example in Move 2 are given below. Reflections that track the behaviors or steps in a couple's typical dance make explicit the partners'

DOI: 10.4324/9781003242673-5

positions of pursue or withdraw and their typical repetitive pattern. Empathic attunement and responsiveness are, again, prerequisites for this micro-skill of tracking repetitive moves in a client's self-protective pattern. Empathy "allows the therapist to track and to taste the client's moment-to-moment experience" (Johnson, 2020, p. 55), while attuning to a couple's pattern of interaction or to an individual client's patterns of interpersonal interactions and internal emotion regulation patterns.

An EFIT example of tracking reflections of interactional patterns in Move 1 reflecting present process:

Max: My partner leaving me is throwing me into turmoil that I have tried to avoid for the past 20 years! I can't seem to block my emotions any longer! This fear of having a conscious memory of my friend's body – he died when I crashed the car – is always there at the back of my head. I know from the amount of trauma my body suffered that he must have looked awful! (Client's eyes fill with tears. After looking down a few seconds, he raises his face to the ceiling for five seconds.)

Emily: Your partner's unexpected departure (trigger) is evoking emotional turmoil. For decades you've blocked your biggest fear of remembering how Léo's body looked (action tendency: blocking fear) but with your partner's sudden departure (repeating trigger), you can't seem to hold the fear back anymore (repeating action tendency of trying to block the fear). Am I getting it?

An EFCT example of tracking reflections to assemble the unfolding process of emotion in Tango Move 2:

Jessica: When I walk into the room and Wayne is absorbed in his gaming, he barely notices I am there, so I say nothing, walk out of the room, and stew for an hour before returning like this prickly porcupine!

Emily: (Attachment-related images and behaviors are in italics.) You stew at your sense that Wayne is all absorbed in something (cue) *and there's no room for you* (attachment threatening meaning). You tell yourself that he doesn't even know *how lonely and upset you are* for that entire hour of your stewing (bodily arousal). After you can't stand the stewing *in your own loneliness without Wayne*, you go back to him and erupt in anger, *demanding his attention* (action tendency).

Reframing

Reframing is an important EFT intervention. It could be considered the backbone of this depathologizing model of therapy which sees the problem not in the person, but in the rigid, repetitive patterns of interactions that couples, individuals, and families become caught in, in their best attempts to preserve relationships and regulate emotions. Reframing experience in terms of attachment meanings and motivations changes the view of a seemingly negative response or pattern. Reframing can be used in Moves 1 and 2. It can also be used in Move 4 to *catch bullets* – an EFT micro-skill designed to protect a client from a partner's verbal aggression (in EFCT) or from self-criticism (in EFIT). Reactivity to a partner's disclosed message or a judgment against oneself is reframed with a positive attachment intention, shifting the view of other and self to a positive portrayal.

The classic reframe in Move 1 for a partner's critical pursuit is *trying to get a response or to pull your partner close*:

Sophie, your turn up the volume and get louder and harsher in your desperation to find Ella and to get a response from her, don't you? It's not that you are out to hurt her, but you are actually doing everything in her power to pull her close, yes?

The classic reframe for a defensive withdrawer such as Ella is *pulling away, not out of indifference or nonchalance, but because they are overwhelmed and care so much about being accepted as they are*:

Ella, when you shrug your shoulders and say to Sophie, 'Don't let it bother you so much,' it's not that you don't care, it's that you care so much about keeping her happy that you start to get rattled inside when she is upset, and you try to come up with a quick way to settle her down, yes?

Attachment reframes contain an element of conjecture about the attachment significance or attachment intention, such as preserving a significant relationship. For example,

Emily says to Ella, the more withdrawn partner:

You had no idea that she turns up the volume because she very much wants to be with you! You sensed you had blown it again, had somehow become that person she is fed up with, and that any day she might hurt you irreparably. And now you are hearing that, in fact, it is *you* she wants – just as you are, not to *change* you, just to connect with you the way you are.

Emily says to Sophie, the more pursuing partner:

You turn up the volume to call Ella towards you. You sense that she withdraws to her study or her family because you aren't important to her. That frightens you so much that you do everything you can to get close to her. The despair and fury that you feel is really code for 'I'm afraid there isn't room for me in your heart right now'.

An attachment reframe can be used to soften the blow of Jessica's cry, "I don't want him starting up another hobby! He just wants things that make him happy!" *Catching the bullet* with an attachment reframe in a proxy voice, Emily conjectures softly:

Are you saying, 'I get so afraid of him finding a new activity that makes him feel good, and I'll not be a part of it?' When you don't know how to share this fear, I wonder if it all comes out in blaming him for being selfish?

In summary, common reframes in EFCT are that critical pursuit is a desperate attempt to find the partner and make them respond and that withdrawal is being overwhelmed with a sense of lacking approval or acceptance from the partner.

Likewise, there are common reframes in EFIT for attachment strategies: Anxious hyperactivating is framed as a search for safety and connection; avoidant deactivation as a protective attempt to move on without getting hurt or hurting another; and erratic fearful avoidance is framed as seeking support, yet being understandably cautious and mistrusting of others.

Sahra, in EFIT, blurts out in exasperation:

For years my mother said I just need to be single and now my friends are saying that too. Just because my last partner was abusive, why do they want me to suffer alone? Just feels like everyone is judging me and I need to push them away!

Without invalidating her experience, Emily seeks to reframe Sahra's sense of helplessness and isolation to one of agency and being part of a caring matrix by saying, "Other's comments and advice have you stuck in a pattern of pushing them away to protect yourself, yes? You long for their support, yet it is difficult to let them be close to you, when their advice hurts, yes?"

Max judges himself for being disingenuous and living in denial, saying, "I see now that was not the right way to do it." Emily gently reframes to retain a strength-focus:

> You see now that there is another way to cope with difficult experience. You feel safe now to walk into the scene of the accident with your eyes wide open, rather than avoiding it or suggesting you were not the driver.

Reframing shifts "a client's perspective from a problem-reinforcing mindset to one that expands awareness and acknowledges underlying attachment vulnerabilities" (Johnson, 2019, p. 70) and intentions. Two EFT micro-skills that combine reframing with conjecture – *catching the bullet* and *seeding attachment* – are explored in the descriptions of shaping and processing engaged encounters below.

Refocusing/Redirecting

This intervention is characterized by the phrase, "Stop – can we go back?" It is used when a client exits or distracts from exploration of present-moment experiencing, or in EFCT when a partner interrupts their partner just as they are beginning to explore core emotional experience in a new and alive manner. For example:

> Phil, I noticed just as Julie's voice dropped and she said, almost in a whisper, that she is still frightened about your pulling away, you interrupted to say she has nothing to worry about. Can we go back to the moment she took this huge risk to share this with you? What happened inside for you, as you heard Julie say she does have this fear?

An effective way to refocus on the alive moment of core emotion is to replay the cue or some emotional handle which re-evokes the earlier moment of engagement. Sahra chuckles after she says, "I feel like an empty pitcher, nothing left inside to share so I'm breaking off pieces of the pitcher itself!" To redirect her back to this poignant emotional handle of her fatigue, Emily says:

> Let's go back – feeling like an empty pitcher, breaking off parts of yourself to give to others! Wow – just notice how that feels in your body to be giving, giving, giving, when you feel you have nothing left to give!

Refocusing or redirecting has been described by Johnson as *changing channels* (2019). In addition to the above example of refocusing on the channel of emotional engagement, when a client exits or gets interrupted, there are various other ways an EFT therapist will refocus and redirect clients:

1. To move from past to present-moment experience:
   You are describing how the fight played out last week, and I wonder, in this moment as you describe it, whether you are feeling some of that same fear of being judged?
2. To move from the individual to the relational:
   As you speak of how exhausted you are, I am still struck with your comment that your partner noticed your fatigue and stopped to ask if you were ok. Can we stay with that experience of how it is for you when your partner notices your distress?

3. To move from content to the process in the content:

   Max, you speak in a rather distant, factual manner about the time you spent in jail, yet I notice a slight quiver in your voice as you mention being under someone's else's control 24/7. I sense there is something very difficult about recalling that time, yes?

4. To move from a label (for example of others being self-centered or fake) or a diagnosis (of depression or weakness) to a specific, acceptable, behavioral description:

   a. EFCT example: "Ella, you've never felt accepted by Sophie's family and it's very difficult to talk with Sophie about this. It's easier to hold in the pain and just tell Sophie to go to her family dinner without you!"

   b. EFIT example: "Sahra, you mentioned it is lonely living by yourself and at the same time it is so difficult to trust that your friends' invitations are genuine. When you find yourself turning down opportunities to get together with friends, your mother's accusations that you are crazy and difficult start booming in your ears, yes?"

5. Johnson (2020, p. 112) provides a useful and succinct guide for refocusing and redirecting. Specific focus on these elements enhances the capacity of all EFT interventions to foster depth of emotional experiencing. Move from:

   - Vague to vivid
   - Obscure to tangible
   - General to specific
   - Then to now – immediate present
   - Global to personal
   - Passive to active
   - Abstract to concrete

Refocusing and redirecting are also important micro-interventions for shaping and processing engaged encounters, as shown below. In particular, the intervention of *slicing a risk thinner* is a refocusing/redirecting micro-intervention to titrate the request to share personal experience into a more manageable task.

The next three systemic micro-skills that I will present – *shaping encounters, processing encounters, and summarizing and integrating* – as mentioned earlier are essentially Moves 3, 4, and 5 of the EFT Tango.

Shaping Engaged Encounters (Move 3): The Core Restructuring Intervention

Traditionally called *enactments* in couple therapy, the core restructuring move across all modalities of EFT with couples, individuals, and families is an *engaged encounter*. An engaged *encounter* is a specific dialogue shaped in a predictable manner by the therapist using what is known as EFT Tango Move 3. This move contains several micro-interventions, notably, *empathic reflections, tracking reflections, evocative responding, heightening, seeding attachment, refocusing/redirecting, reframing, and slicing the request thinner.* Engaged encounters are essential to shaping corrective emotional experiences that create lasting change. A therapist requests direct sharing of a clearly distilled message from one partner to the other in couple therapy and between a client and an imaginal other in EFIT. Encounters are structured for various purposes at different points in therapy, depending on the stage of change in which clients are engaged.

Functions of Engaged Encounters

Engaged encounters serve several functions. First, in early therapy, encounters are choreographed for clients to share their awareness of their typical protective positions of distancing or pursuing in their repetitive dance such as, "I do shut you out," or, "I do blast you when I get so lonely." Disclosing these action tendencies "brings them into the light" (Johnson, 2019, p. 70) and helps a client to fully own, "This is what I do. This is the strategy I default to when I am not feeling safe." Individuals, similarly, are helped to disclose in an engaged encounter to an imaginal other, "I push aside my thoughts of you. I don't let myself feel how much I miss you," or to a part of self, "I ignore your pain. I am afraid it will be too much to face."

Second, engaged encounters function to deepen emotional experience and clients' sense of agency. Ownership of action tendencies and all expressed, distilled emotion is intensified during the carefully structured process of sharing directly with another, real or imagined.

Third, later in therapy, encounters are shaped to turn newly accessed emotional experience into new signals. For example in EFCT, "I get scared when you shut me out—afraid you aren't wanting to be with me." Sharing core emotion, fears, and distress, in a clear manner is risky, and is the gateway into the specific change events of Stage 2. A withdrawn partner in Stage 2 deepening may say, "I am so petrified of your judgement, that my mind spins and my body freezes."

Fourth, by dipping into this raw, clearly distilled core emotion, clients are helped to access their unmet attachment need, embedded in that emotion and to make a specific request to have this need met. Encounters with a specific request create the specific change events in Stage 2 of EFT. Partners reach in new ways to have their deepest attachment needs met. For example, from an engaging withdrawer, "Can you accept me as I am, with all my failings?" and from a softening pursuer, "Can you assure me I'm not too much for you? That I am precious to you?"

In EFIT, individuals reach to an imaginal other, to the therapist or to a part of self to ask for a core need to be met, asking, for example, "Can you assure me you see my goodness, my worthiness?" A need expressed toward an abusive or dismissive other may be for total distance. As noted in Chapter 1, sharing the core fears and distress is the client's Step 5 and the vulnerable reach of asking for needs to be met is the client's Step 7. Between those encounters is the real or imaginal response from the other, known as Step 6.

How to Shape Encounters

The predictable nature of how to choreograph encounters can be described with the acronym **SHAPE** (Brubacher, 2022). This acronym provides a reliable guide for a task that many therapists and clients can initially find quite daunting.

S: Sharpen the Message. Newly accessed emotion is distilled/sharpened into a simple direct message in EFCT to the other partner and in EFIT to an imaginal other or between two parts of self. EFCT example: Emily helps Jessica to crystallize the core of her emotional experience underlying her outbursts at Wayne. The more Wayne disappears to his computer games, the more lonely and then angry Jessica becomes. Emily sharpens the link between Jessica's outbursts and her underlying fear of Wayne slipping away into another world.

H: Heighten. The emotionality in the sharpened message is heightened with repetition. In EFCT, Emily repeats the image of Jessica's fear of Wayne slipping away into another world. In EFIT, heightening may include feeling the fear or the anger toward an imaginal other, while also picturing how this person looks in that moment. Alternatively, it may include heightening the compassion or feisty protectiveness one feels, looking into the sad eyes of a younger self.

A: Anticipate. Inviting a client to anticipate or picture themselves sharing this clear, emotionally alive message invariably heightens the emotion and intensifies the risk of anticipating how the other will respond to their disclosure. The therapist seeks to keep the emotional risk alive within a window of safety. In EFCT, Emily asks Jessica to anticipate sharing her newly accessed fear of losing Wayne, directly with him. Repeating the key words which Jessica has used to keep her focused on her own experience, and not get derailed in talking about what Wayne does, Emily says, "Imagine turning to Wayne just now and telling him about how afraid you are of him slipping away, and how, when you get that fear, it comes out in what you call your *torrents of words*." She does not ask a question for Jessica to answer that would likely disrupt her experiencing, such as "What would it be like to share this with him?" She simply asks Jessica to notice what comes up in her body as she prepares to share her fear with Wayne.

One way to heighten through anticipation in EFCT and to ensure safety is to check if the partner is willing to receive this disclosure. If they are unwilling or reluctant, then the therapist will attend to this barrier and re-establish safety before proceeding.

In EFIT, the anticipation can include, "Picture how the imaginal other or part of self looks, just now, as you imagine sharing." Before directing the encounter, the therapist first confirms that the client is engaged in their experience and checks if the imaginal other appears open and safe to receive their message. If the client doesn't want to hear back from a hurtful imaginal other, the therapist supports them to make that assertive claim and to establish that boundary of safety, before confirming they are ready to proceed with the encounter.

P: Present the message. Therapist directs a client to *present* the message, when the other, in EFCT, is ready to receive the disclosure, or, in EFIT, the client perceives there is sufficient safety to disclose.

In EFCT, after Jessica is engaged with her underlying emotional experience, has anticipated sharing it with Wayne and has had confirmation that Wayne is ready to listen to her, Emily directs her to disclose. "Can you turn to him right now? Can you look at him and tell him about this fear?" Jessica accepts the invitation and shares with Wayne:

I am afraid you're going to slip away from me. That you're going to build a world where your peace and calmness doesn't come from me. I get so afraid you won't want me anymore and I explode in an outpouring of rage to manage this fear.

In EFIT as Sahra prepares and anticipates an encounter to an imaginal abusive other (Chapter 16), she makes it clear that she wants to hear nothing back from him. Emily *slices the risk thin* to increase safety and helps Sahra to present her first message of securing this boundary. Emily directs Sahra:

Can you picture him there now, at a safe distance from you, and can you tell him, 'I am going to say my piece and I do not want to hear back from you. I will tell you how badly you have hurt me – and then I'll tell you to leave!'?

E: Engage. When there is hesitancy or distractions, such as exiting the process, an EFT therapist will engage the client by *slicing the request thinner* or by refocusing and redirecting.

In EFCT, if Jessica had been hesitant, Emily would have gently persisted, "I'd like you to try." If the hesitancy is overwhelming and Jessica refuses, Emily will slice the request thinner, "Can you tell him, 'It's too difficult to tell you about this fear I have'?" Emily remembers not to back away or to lose focus. She remembers to *slice the risk thinner* into a manageable amount of disclosure that a client can tolerate, such as, "It is too scary or too hard to tell you right now." Either way, the objective of the enactment is achieved and partners have *made contact* in a new, substantial, and congruent way.

If Jessica had *exited* from the present moment during the disclosure, Emily would have engaged her by refocusing and redirecting, by offering:

> You were just about to turn to Wayne and tell him how afraid you are that he will slip away and that when this fear gets so big you explode at him to manage your fear. And then you turned and said, "What's the point. He'll never change." Can we go back to the moment where the fear felt so alive?

Client reluctance is respected. Emily reminds herself to respect reluctance but not to shy away from the process. She often relies upon the intervention of *slicing the request thinner* to reduce the risk without diverting from this powerful moment of interpersonal encounter.

In EFIT, with Sahra, Emily can also *slice the risk even more thinly*, by saying, "Can you tell him, for now, how hard it is to speak to him?" For an encounter with her mother to slice the risk thinner, Emily says:

> Can you tell this image of your mother, "I am just too angry with you right now to tell you how loudly your criticisms ring in my ears!" Can you risk telling her you are too angry at the moment to tell her?

It is not uncommon in EFCT for the recipient of a disclosure to interrupt during the encounter. When this happens, an EFT therapist slows the process, interrupts, offers a tracking reflection of what just happened and then refocuses. The refocusing can be done by repeating the triggering moment or by validating the client's felt need to interrupt the process, while re-engaging the disclosing partner in their present-moment process.

Engaged encounters are carefully choreographed by the therapist, who then validates the risk taken by the client and immediately invites clients to process this vulnerable experience. The exploration of the experience of sharing and receiving the disclosure is known as Move 4.

Processing Encounters (Move 4)

EFT therapists carefully evoke each client's experience of the moment of interpersonal contact in an encounter. Most often, the encounter is processed first with the one who has disclosed the message and secondly, with the recipient or the imaginal recipient of the message. There is an art to Move 4, in that, most often, the processing begins with the discloser, to keep alive their experience and provide time and space for them to reflect out loud about it. There will be times, however, when addressing the receiver of the message first may seem the best way to keep the emotional experiencing alive. Either way, it will be processed with one and then the other, in turn.

Many micro-skills can be used in processing encounters, notably *evocative questions, tracking reflections, heightening, refocusing/redirecting,* and *catching bullets.* The level of emotional experiencing is deepened most effectively when the therapist repeats the core message just shared. The discloser is invited to linger and notice internally how it is to have put this message out loud to the other and then is asked to express how it is to share it. Following the slow, intentional process of exploring how it was to share this message, the one who has received the disclosure is invited to describe how it was to receive it. Receivers are guided to tune into their internal experience and then to put words to the impact of receiving the disclosure. An additional encounter can now be choreographed for the recipient of the message to share their experience.

EFCT Example of Processing with the Discloser

First, Emily asks Jessica, "What was it like to tell him about your big fear of him slipping away from you that bursts out in your troubled lists of complaints?" Repeating the key words of Jessica's disclosure helps to retain and heighten the focus on the core message just disclosed.

EFCT Example of Processing with the Recipient

Next, Emily invites Wayne, the receiving partner, to tune into his internal experience of Jessica's disclosure, "What was it like for you, Wayne, to hear Jessica share with you that under her out-pourings of anger is this deep fear you could slip away from her, and she would be without you?" Again, Emily repeats key words used, to keep the focus and heighten the attachment frame.

If Wayne diverts with, "She doesn't need to be afraid of that," Emily validates and refocuses him:

> In your mind, she doesn't need to be afraid and yet she is. Can you go back—what happened inside for you, Wayne, when Jessica shared with you about all this terror she has underneath, terror that she could lose you? How is it for you to look in her eyes and see how frightened she is?

Wayne, acknowledges, with tears, "I'm shocked—I had no idea, she is afraid of losing *me*! I thought she was just fed up with me."

If Wayne, the receiving partner, responded harshly in this moment of disorientation with, "That's rubbish! I'm supposed to believe all these complaints are about fear of losing me?" Emily would use the reframe known as *catch the bullet*. She would interrupt the escalation and reflect present process, including the key message that triggered him. Reflecting in a non-judgmental, soothing manner regulates reactivity. This soothing could calm him enough that he could take in this new information from Jessica, while also protecting Jessica from getting stung by his reaction. Emily would catch the bullet by saying:

> Jessica just said that under all her outbursts is this hot terror of losing you, and you stepped in to say, wait a moment, it's very hard to believe you are afraid! It is so difficult, so surprising to hear that she has this terror of losing you – so hard to believe that when she complains to you, she is terrified of losing you. Am I getting it?

EFIT Example of Processing an Encounter

Similarly, in EFIT, if the recipient is an imaginal other, the experience of what it was like to share is processed, as well as the client's imagined response from the other. Following an encounter with Sahra's imaginal mother, Emily first invites her to express how it was to tell an image of her mother that her harsh criticism continues to tear at her soul. After Sahra responds, Emily says:

> And how do you experience your imaginal mother is responding as she has just heard her weary, self-doubting daughter share that her harsh criticism tears at her daughter's soul? How do you experience your imaginal mother as she hears your bravely shared words?

Sahra is invited to express her perception of how her imaginal mother responds, and how this impacts her.

Conjectures for Shaping and Processing Encounters

Special conjectures used for shaping and processing encounters, include *seeding attachment* to heighten and contain the risk of disclosing, *slicing risks thinner* to engage clients who are hesitant to share, and *catching bullets*, to contain aggression from the recipient of the disclosure. *Slicing risks thinner* is described earlier as a way to engage clients in encounters. *Seeding attachment* and *catching the bullet* are described below.

Seeding Attachment

The particular conjecture named *seeding attachment* was first promoted as an intervention to be used in Stage 2 softening change events. Seeding attachment simultaneously heightens and validates a client's core fear, while at the same time, seeds a picture of the soothing antidote to that fear. With this micro-intervention, a therapist seeds a picture of risking reaching that has, up until now, been blocked by fears of rejection or abandonment. This helps to facilitate the key Stage 2 change events. For example, "Sophie, you could never, ever reach to Ella when you are fearing you are not her precious one and ask her to come and be with you?" An image of risking reaching toward one's partner is seeded to simultaneously heighten the fear of reaching, so the client can access the need embedded in the fear that holds her back, while at the same time, paint a vivid picture of the antidote to that fear – reaching toward the partner and being safely held. Heightened fear is mixed with hope that risking reaching may satisfy one's deepest longings. For example, to help a partner take the risk of asking for their attachment needs to be met, a therapist can *seed attachment* by saying in a soft, slow voice:

> You just couldn't imagine sharing how very small and weak you feel, and asking for reassurance that she still loves you? You can't imagine she would want to come close to you when she sees you like this and to take you in her arms and hold you?

The image can heighten the vulnerability and clarity of what one needs, as well as plant a vivid image of risking to reach and being securely reassured. Seeding attachment can also be used to shape an engagement change event, such as by offering, "You couldn't imagine showing up with your assertive voice and having your partner welcome you and show the acceptance and interest you are longing to experience?"

The conjecture of seeding attachment, created for Stage 2 change events, can also be used in Stage 1. Evoking a picture of secure attachment can give clients hope and it can help with formulating goals at the outset of therapy with a couple or an individual. It can be used to evoke compatible agendas in early assessment by painting a picture of where a couple might want to end up, in the colors and hues that match their readiness. One or both partners might not be ready, in early therapy, to picture intimate, close connection, but they may both resonate with longing to feel important and accepted by the other. For example, "It sounds as if you both long to feel comfortable in one another's presence, without fearing judgement – trusting the other has your back and cares to hear from you." (See Chapter 7 on assessing for compatible agendas.)

Similarly, in EFIT, seeding attachment can be used in Stages 1 and 2. During goal setting with Max, Emily assembles his emotion:

> You are so fearful of reviewing all the damage you have done to others that you have managed to block many events from your memory. Now you are saying, "I want to face the things I've lived through – I want to talk about these traumatic events, even the tragic street-racing crash where I was badly injured and one of my passengers was killed. I can't imagine it yet – but I

want to face the pain and the grief of my whole life without disappearing in shame or nothing-ness. I want to face what I've done and lived through and find my dignity again."

His strategy of denying his responsibility has kept him from facing his experience in the tragic event and has triggered a lot of shame. He wants to "come to terms with" his traumas of sexual abuse, scenes of death, time in jail, and the car accident which changed his life. Emily seeds attachment in this goal setting phase:

You want to clearly face these events – especially to feel safe enough to look in your imagina-tion at your friend at the scene of the accident. You want to feel a safe bond again with this deceased friend – where you can look at him and feel both responsible for his death and also forgiven by him, yes?

In a Stage 2 encounter that Emily shapes with Sahra, she seeds attachment as she conjectures:

You can't imagine that you can speak to an image of your father who abandoned you at a cru-cial moment of need, and that he will actually listen to you and let himself be touched by your pain and his responsibility in hurting you. Never, ever can you imagine him actually listening to your pain and showing remorse!

This seed of attachment heightens her present-moment fear of speaking to an image of her father, while at the same time, seeds a possibility of safety in being clear and direct with an imaginal father for an attachment injury she was never able to address with him in real life.

Seeding attachment deepens emotional experiencing, heightening the very fear which blocks secure connection, while also imagining the antidote of secure responsivity and connection. Fi-nally, in Stage 3, the seedlings of attachment that are already growing are watered and fertilized, and the partners discuss how to grow their future love story with their newly secure attachment bond (Chapter 11). EFIT clients also consider how the seeds of new interaction patterns are open-ing them to new, more vibrant, and secure experiences.

Catching the Bullet

This intervention is needed when the recipient of a disclosure is aggressive or dismissing (John-son, 2020). Combined with an attachment reframe, this conjecture functions to contain aggression and regain safety when one partner's aggression or discounting would otherwise make it unsafe for the more vulnerable partner. It also functions to validate two partners in a heightened moment of different perspectives. In EFIT, it can be used to soften the blow of an individual's harsh criti-cism toward themselves so that they can calm down and become open and curious again about their experience.

To catch aggression toward a partner in couple therapy or toward oneself in individual or couple therapy, a therapist will: Interrupt to contain the aggression; then reflect, without judgment, the process that just unfolded; then reframe the reactivity by conjecturing at confusion, attachment threat, disorientation or disbelief; validate this reaction; if possible, the therapist will also conjec-ture at a positive attachment intention; and finally, will check for confirmation of the conjecture(s) to find out if their words fit for the client's experience.

Imagine a more pursuing partner beginning to disclose that buried beneath her shrill complaints are her desperate attempts to pull the partner close. Suddenly, the more withdrawn partner inter-rupts with, "I don't believe it. This is hogwash!"

The therapist interrupts, "Excuse me – but I'm going to interrupt you for a minute. Right now, as she began to share that her loud complaints are code for trying to call you closer to her, you moved in to stop her" (reflecting present process). Catching the bullet, the therapist continues. "It is so new for you, unbelievable actually, to hear that under her complaints, she is trying to call you close?" (conjecture at disorientation as a reframe for his abrupt, aggressive interruption). "You have felt unwanted for so long and it is too hard to trust that it is you she wants?" (attachment reframe). Repeating this key phrase of *how much she actually wants him* and of how hard it is for him to trust when he has felt so rejected for so long, validates both partners at the same time.

There are bullets to catch when one partner minimizes another's experience of racial discrimination, such as when Jessica minimizes Wayne's experiences of minority stress. The case example in the Chapter 16 Support Material (routledge.com/9781032151335) on attachment injury repair and racial trauma, also illustrates catching several bullets.

Sahra, in an early EFIT session, flushes with embarrassment as her words pour out:

> I stay in relationships far longer than I know is good for me. Whatever is wrong with me? I am just too obsessed with relationships! UGH! I will clearly, clearly see a red flag with somebody I am with and actively choose to ignore it. I think to myself – we can work it out! UGH!! This is ridiculous – to actively choose to continue to pursue a relationship with someone who is hurting me!

To catch this aggression toward self, the therapist interrupts, "Let me slow you down, ok? You've just talked about how important it is to be in a relationship – and suddenly you are almost scolding yourself, for staying in hurtful relationships" (reflecting present process). "It's almost an automatic self-protective move to turn against yourself when you are so let down by yet one more partner, yes? So difficult to notice your own hurt and your legitimate longing for a safe relationship, yes?" (validating this pattern with an attachment reframe/positive intention and checking for confirmation).

Outside of encounters, there are many occasions that call for an EFT therapist to move in to interrupt and catch aggression. Containing aggression and being in charge of the therapy process are paramount to keeping therapy safe.

Summarizing and Integrating (as in Move 5)

Following the processing of an encounter, in EFCT, the therapist summarizes, validates and integrates to give an overview of this interaction between partners to further capitalize on the moment of clear reaching and responding between them. In EFIT, a new interaction with an imaginal other, between parts of self or in dialogue with the therapist is summarized. Micro-interventions in Move 5 include empathic reflections, tracking, heightening, evocative questions to elicit clients' reflection on their work, and seeding attachment to envision the impact of going forward with the change they have just created.

Summarizing and integrating engaged encounters, weaves these moments of interpersonal dialogue into the change process and consolidates the corrective emotional experiences however incremental or life-changing they may be. Move 5 summarizing and integrating is done not only at the end of sessions, and not only after an encounter, but throughout sessions as well to validate and clarify incremental shifts and the interpersonal change processes in which clients are engaging. Chapter 4 Support Material (routledge.com/9781032151335) provides summaries and tips about the EFT systemic micro-skills.

Conclusion

With this integration of the micro-skills in Move 5 of the EFT Tango, we have come full circle, combining EFT experiential micro-skills described in Chapter 3 and the EFT systemic micro-skills detailed in this chapter. Studying and practicing all the EFT micro-skills used in the EFT macro-intervention, richly laid out in Chapter 2, is an ongoing growth process for every EFT therapist. Mastery and confidence in all moves of the EFT Tango and in the specific micro-skills can be enhanced tremendously by exploring the companion volume to this book: *Workouts for Stepping into Emotionally Focused Therapy: Exercises to Strengthen Your Practice.*

5 The Revolutionary Science of Love as an Attachment Bond

> [R]elational–cultural theory (RCT) is built on the premise that, throughout the lifespan, human beings grow through and toward connection. It holds that we need connections to flourish, even to stay alive, and isolation is a major source of suffering for people, at both a personal and cultural level. (Jordan, 2018, p. 3)

An experiential felt sense of the adult need for emotional connection is illuminated in this chapter which defines love as a secure bond, similar to the bond that exists between infant and parent. Bowlby claimed that a need for a personal secure base extends throughout life.

> This concept of the secure personal base, from which a child, an adolescent, or an adult goes out to explore and to which he returns from time to time, is ... crucial for an understanding of how an emotionally stable person develops and functions all through his life. (Bowlby, 1988, p. 46)

In EFCT, threats to an attachment bond are viewed as the element that casts romantic love into peril. The attachment foundation of EFT portrayed in this chapter answers the questions, "How is romantic love an attachment process?" and "How does attachment theory provide a clearly articulated theory and science of adult love and emotion regulation?" "How does a therapy model that validates fostering secure connections provide the path out of individual and cultural disconnection, isolation, and emotional pain?"

Two new elements included throughout this second edition – The impacts of race, ethnicity, and culture (REC), and emotionally focused individual therapy (EFIT) – highlight the broader perspective of adult attachment theory, not only as a theory of romantic love, but also as a theory of emotion regulation (Mikulincer & Shaver, 2019; Simpson & Rholes, 2015) and a theory of trauma (Bowlby, 1973, 1980; Cassidy & Shaver, 2016; Johnson, 2002, 2019). Attachment as a theory of emotion regulation and of trauma has been a part of the EFT couple modality since its inception; however, these dimensions take on new meaning when we focus on EFIT and on the need to embrace the contextual, systemic impacts of culture and the trauma of oppression more explicitly. While much of the adult attachment literature focuses on romantic relationships, it is of particular interest to note how various individual therapies and movements for social change, such as Relational-Cultural Therapy (RCT; Jordan, 2018), also validate that human beings grow *toward* connection and *in* connection, and that we need those connections with others to survive and to thrive, and to move from *protective disconnection* back into *growth-fostering connection*.

As a theory of emotion regulation, attachment theory provides a model for conceptualizing health and dysfunction. Attachment theory is the foundation for a model of restoring healthy functioning with individual clients, beginning with assessing strategies for emotion regulation and patterns of interacting *with others and internally* (aka *between and within*). Emotional and relational distress are related to a lack of *effective dependency* and negative working models of self and

DOI: 10.4324/9781003242673-6

other. Emotional resilience and fitness are rooted in effective co-regulation and attachment security, whereas lack of secure attachment "is a vulnerability often predictive of poorer life outcomes, …manifested in slightly different ways in different cultures, which may result in culturally-specific forms of adaptation and social development" (Simpson & Karantzas, 2019, p. 179). "Individual mental health problems such as depression, anxiety, trauma survival reactions, relational conflict, substance use and other addictive processes can all be framed as ineffective attempts to cope with separation distress" (Brubacher & Johnson, 2017, p. 8), in the absence of available and responsive sources of social engagement for comfort and support. For example, from an attachment perspective, borderline personality disorder is "seen as fearful-avoidant attachment" (Johnson, 2009a, p. 420) and overt narcissism can be seen to have links to avoidant attachment (Mikulincer & Shaver, 2016). Depression and anxiety can be explored for patterns of anxious and avoidant strategies for connection. Addictive processes can be framed as an attachment disorder (Flores, 2004; Maté, 2010) where, in the absence of safe human sources of comfort and support, an individual reaches automatically to *faux* attachments which replace human connection. By providing an alternative to diagnostic labeling, the culturally attuned attachment base of EFT frames the problem and the context for healing as systemic feedback loops of strategies for connection. Individuals' best attempts at regulating emotions can perpetuate rigid, repetitive patterns of survival strategies that may no longer be helpful in the present context.

Attachment theory, as a theory of trauma, holds that isolation and loss at individual, relational, and cultural levels are traumatizing (Johnson, 2002; Jordan, 2018). Survival depends on human connection as an antidote to threats of rejection, abandonment, and injury. The two worst things for a mammal are isolation and restraint (Porges, 2016). Individual and couple clients marginalized due to racial, ethnic, and cultural identities, and/or heteronormative oppression or neurotypical expectations, live in an ongoing traumatic context, with chronic triggers of discrimination and constant vigilance for threat. Systemic discrimination compromises health, healthcare, education, wealth, employment, justice, physical safety, and so much more, creating enormous additional threats to safety and security in the world, and thus, within self and within relationships. EFT therapists openly invite exploration of the emotional and relational impacts of living with constant vigilance for threats of minority stress, death, and discrimination (Day-Vines et al., 2020; DeGruy, 2017; Guillory, 2022; Hardy, 2022, 2023). Culturally sensitive EFT therapists in positions of dominance or privilege attune and explore how historical and present-day discrimination stressors are playing out in clients' strategies for engaging with life. They also need to acknowledge that leading a conversation is a white privilege that needs to be balanced with culturally humble listening. We need to listen more and listen more deeply (Guillory, 2022; Stern, 2004).

My intent in this chapter is to immerse you in an attachment view of adult love so that a culturally sensitive attachment orientation can become your guiding companion from the first session through the entire change process. For this purpose, we explore:

1. An attachment perspective on therapy, acknowledging contextual impacts of REC.
2. Lived experiences of attachment theory.
3. Principles of attachment theory: Laws of human love and bonding.
4. Common roadblocks for therapists seeking to internalize culturally humble attachment theory as a guiding paradigm.

A Culturally Humble Attachment Perspective

Attachment theory has created a paradigm shift in how therapy is conceptualized and in how it is practiced (Johnson, 2007, 2019). The attachment perspective of adult romantic love as a bond similar to that which exists between infant and parent marked a revolutionary departure in couple therapy from the traditional view of intimate relationships as *quid pro quo* bargains, where costs and benefits need to be negotiated. Viewing romantic love as a bond, the goal of couple therapy becomes one of creating a secure bond and the therapist functions in the role of a process consultant. A process consultant helps partners to discover the repetitive pattern weakening their bond and facilitates change events that can transform distressed relationships into secure and lasting bonds. This therapeutic role differs significantly from coaching partners to learn to compromise, or teaching communication and conflict resolution skills, as well as from approaches that explore insight as the solution to relationship distress.

The paradigm shift that EFT offers to therapists begins with the attachment theoretical view that the attachment system is activated

> when individuals experience distress, fear, loss, pain or separation, all of which are cues that trigger proximity-seeking. During development, different attachment patterns (in children) and orientations (in adults) form largely in response to the quality of care and support individuals receive from their attachment figures, with higher-quality care/support typically resulting in attachment security. (Simpson & Karantzas, 2019, p. 178)

When individuals feel a threat to the bond with their primary attachment figure(s), they react in predictable ways to secure that bond. Bowlby (1973) called these predictable behaviors *separation distress* responses. When these reactions fail to evoke the needed response, they become repetitive, destructive, cyclic patterns. The patterns can be validated as understandable attempts to regulate distress and protect an attachment bond that is under threat. When their reactions do not succeed in bringing forth needed support and calming, individuals get stuck in ineffective strategies of emotion regulation. The attachment lens normalizes the fact that emotional and relationship distress do not result from a lack of skills or understanding, or from laziness, stupidity, random stubbornness, or meanness. Rather, from an attachment perspective, emotional and relational distress trigger and are triggered by negative patterns of best attempts at protecting a primary bond or coping with a lack of secure connection. As Bowlby noted (1980), these negative interactive patterns become habitual and automatic and thus become orientations that are very difficult, but not impossible, to change.

Fortunately, even though attachment orientations tend to be stable over time, they can change in response to life events or therapeutic intervention (Simpson & Karantzas, 2019). EFT outcome studies validate that attachment orientations can change and remain stable post-therapy (Wiebe, Johnson, Burgess Moser et al., 2017; Wiebe, Johnson, Lafontaine et al., 2017).

Emily has heard that the attachment perspective keeps an EFT therapist "on track"; yet, she remains unsure how understanding attachment can continuously guide her work. She wonders:

> How can attachment theory provide a no-fault definition of relational distress and repair? How can it help me formulate an individual client's emotional distress and path toward desired goals? How can attachment theory compel me to become more culturally humble and open to discuss impacts of culture and race? How can it guide me moment-to-moment through the moves of the EFT Tango?

She sees herself at the bottom of a very tall hill, daunted by the enormity of the task of finding a culturally humble attachment lens! The hill imagery, however, makes her smile. She relaxes, recalling that she is one of thousands of therapists worldwide facing this hill and learning together. Tension in her body eases as she remembers she is not alone in this endeavor. She feels like a participant in the well-known study by Beckes and Coan (2011) that illustrates the impact of interpersonal closeness on regulating distress and threat perception. In the study, participants standing at the bottom of a hill, wearing a heavy backpack, were asked to judge the slant of the hill they were about to climb. They estimated it to be less steep when they stood next to a friend than when they stood alone. Their perception of the steepness was mediated not by consciously thinking, "It won't be so difficult because I have you with me." Their perception was influenced *preconsciously* by the proximity of their friend. Interpersonal connection "decreases the cost of climbing both the literal and figurative hills we face, because the brain construes *social* resources as *bioenergetic* resources, much like oxygen or glucose" (Coan & Sbarra, 2015).

Words from "The Hill We Climb" by Amanda Gorman (2021) a young African American and the youngest American poet laureate, come to Emily's mind, and encourage her in what sometimes feels like a daunting task of learning to practice the EFT model. The poem reminds Emily of the power of interpersonal connection to ease the load on the hills we climb, and to ensure we will succeed as EFT therapists, not because we won't have times of feeling defeated or discouraged, but because we are not alone. Emily relaxes, as she muses:

> I am not alone as I seek to follow the map of attachment. Since I know from research and experience that co-regulation is more efficient and more effective than conscious self-soothing (Beckes & Coan, 2011; Coan, 2016; Coan & Maresh, 2014), I will invite and offer support to make this a successful climb. I will continue to record my work, review my sessions, and consult with colleagues.

Focused on the sense of being part of a community of professional learners, Emily switches in her reflections to the "we" pronoun as Gorman does through much of her poetry and reflects specifically on the poem, "Call Us What We Carry." This poem replaces her questions of, "Can I learn this model well?" with the assuring thought that, "We carry the task of shaping secure connections, not as isolated individual therapists, but as an interconnected community, perfecting our craft together."

"Step by step," Emily thinks to herself:

> We climb this hill towards creating corrective emotional experiences for couples and individuals in distress. We validate and mobilize the power of emotional connection as we follow the emotional interplay of attachment insecurity and *cultural trauma*. Together we can challenge that independence, competition, and strength-in-isolation do not need to be the hallmarks of maturity (Jordan, 2018). We can help each other grasp that a partner's angry outburst or abrupt turn away from their partner is an understandable reaction to some perceived threat to the relational bond. Together, we can go beyond my safe world of white advantage to hold the weight of cultural discrimination and pervasive survival threats endured by the majority of our human family. We can help each other to listen to the strengths of cultural patterns and values, to grow in cultural humility. We can learn together to formulate individuals' *emotional disorders* (Barlow et al., 2018) within an attachment frame, and to identify and normalize ineffective strategies and patterns of emotion regulation in the absence of *interpersonal dependence.*

The Radical Notion of Our Innate Need for Connection

Emily feels encouraged to learn in community with her colleagues about what it means to *follow attachment* but continues to puzzle over the bold claim of EFT that attachment theory can keep a therapist *on track*. When Bowlby proposed to his psychoanalytic colleagues in the 1950s that human beings have innate needs for emotional connection, it was a radical notion. Normalizing human needs for connection was a direct challenge to the popular view that a child bonded with their mother simply because she fed them. By proposing that humans have a survival need, across the life span, to have a protective loved one to count on for support and care, Bowlby challenged the individualistic view of human nature that venerates independence and self-sufficiency by emphasizing the human need for affectional bonds. Survival, Bowlby proposed, depends upon seeking comfort and protection when in distress. He claimed that it is wired into our genes as social animals to seek proximity when in danger or distress, and to heed danger cues and alarm bells that signal a threat to our most important relationships. His study of the nature of the child's bond with its mother (1958) offered a way to normalize and de-pathologize the predictable sequence of separation distress responses that occur when an attachment figure is not accessible and responsive: Frantic clinging and seeking is followed by angry protests, despair, depression, and finally, detachment. Bowlby's (1973) contributions highlight that our survival as individuals and as a species depends on avoiding that which threatens our primary relationships, and on seeking the comfort and protection of our trusted attachment figures when we are in need.

Interpersonal loss is dehumanizing (Karantzas et al., 2022). During centuries of colonization, genocide, slavery, and apartheid, far too many parents were blocked from caring for their children; children were stolen from parents; partners were torn apart; women were raped (Guillory, 2022; Hannah-Jones, 2019; Wagamese, 2012). Far too many cultures in their entirety have been robbed of comfort and safety from their attachment figures, a basic survival need, according to attachment theory. Morrison (1992) challenges us to listen to the deafening "silence of 400 years … the void of historical discourse on slave parent-child relationships and pain" (p. 22). Culturally competent, humble EFT therapists have the tools to help clients create secure bonds of connection that create resiliency and help to buffer against experiences of minority stress and dehumanizing losses (Guillory, 2022; Mikulincer & Shaver, 2021).

Recognizing the need for secure connection as the essence of who we are as human beings, Johnson radically invited attachment theory onto the center stage of psychotherapy, revolutionizing and refreshing the field with new possibilities (2019, 2020). Never before has such an optimistic and clear view of relational and emotional distress and repair been the foundation of a model of therapy. Johnson instigated a couple therapy model based on a clearly researched theory of adult love and close relationships (Johnson, 2007; Mikulincer & Shaver, 2016, 2019). By extending this model across modalities of couple, individual, and family therapy, Johnson has reshaped the field of psychotherapy to be focused on the healing power of emotional connection (2019). This new era of psychotherapy began with her focus on the attachment theoretical claim that it is primarily when attachment security is threatened – when individuals feel uncertain or afraid – that interactions begin to go badly. When romantically attached partners are not accessible, responsive, and emotionally engaged with one another (Johnson, 2008), one partner experiences loss or threat and the attachment behavioral system – seeking closeness to a significant other – is activated. When partners are able to connect or to repair a moment of disconnection, the relationship can thrive. However, if the attachment system is activated and a partner's reach for connection is blocked, ignored, or rejected, the predictable dynamic of separation distress ensues. Bowlby (1973) wrote the entire second volume of his trilogy on attachment on this dynamic of separation distress during moments of threat of loss. Separation distress responses, in romantic relationships and in individuals' coping strategies for regulating distressing emotions, are at the core of the EFT model (Johnson, 2013, 2019, 2020).

These emotionally driven patterns of separation distress are similar to what Johnson and Greenberg (1988) named couples' *negative interaction cycles* – a dynamic where one partner demands and pursues connection, and the other defends and withdraws. This typical negative pattern has also been identified by Gottman (1991). Johnson and Greenberg's original EFT model of change was based on reprocessing the emotions fuelling these negative patterns. With her integration of attachment theory into the EFT model, Johnson added clarity to the target for therapeutic change: Reshaping bonds of attachment security. She sharpened the focus on the problem in couple therapy as the slippery slope of separation distress responses that emerge when attempts to find safety with one's partner are thwarted. Similarly, in EFIT, she proposed an attachment frame for individual distress: Without adequate social supports to regulate emotional distress, individuals get caught in coping patterns of anxious hyperactivating or avoidant deactivating. These patterns then "impair the sense of security and the regulation of emotions" (Mikulincer & Shaver, 2019, p. 8) and block interpersonal caring and support. Vivid metaphors of the attachment strategies in these patterns are in the Chapter 5 Support Material (routledge.com/9781032151335). It must be noted that down-regulating emotions is a valid survival strategy in some contexts. Down-regulation, like all second-ary strategies, can become problematic when it becomes an entrenched pattern, used automatically and rigidly across contexts. For example, down-regulation, necessary for survival in a racist context, may interfere with developing intimacy in a relationship where vulnerable self-disclosure is valued.

Attachment Embraces Race, Ethnicity, and Culture (REC)

Attachment theory holds that all human beings need and deserve the dignity and respect of safe human connection. A therapy grounded in this attachment orientation is, thus, compelled to attune to and explore the trauma of systemic racism and institutionalized oppression within clients' level of comfort and window of tolerance.

It is important to be mindful that, "People of color are not a monolith, and reducing clients to their race or making assumptions based on a stereotypical understanding of their race can be in-credibly harmful" (Galán et al., 2022, p. 588). LGBTQIA+ individuals' experiences are not alike; neurodiverse individuals and those with differing abilities have endless differences; refugees and immigrants each have their own unique story. The key issue is for therapists to be skilled and open to discuss impacts of marginalization on client's strategies for engaging with others and with self. To be a culturally sensitive EFT therapist it is helpful to explore one's own unconscious biases and propensity toward *subtle acts of exclusion* (Jana & Baran, 2020; Williams, 2020). Given the "societal tendency to deny or rationalize the presence of racism" (Williams et al., 2014, p. 105), therapists can overlook contextual impacts and mistakenly pathologize clients. When therapists dis-regard contexts of trauma and REC identities, they are apt to mislabel trauma survival strategies as personality flaws, negative family traits, or undesirable cultural characteristics (Menakem, 2017).

Intersectionality literature (Crenshaw et al., 1995; Hill Collins & Bilge, 2020) highlights that different social identities and social positions, such as race, gender, sexual orientation, religion, age, and neurodiversity lead to different experiences of the external and internal worlds. When the intersectionality perspective becomes integrated into EFT, it can make explicit what has been only implicit in EFT: Taking interest in the impacts of contextual and racial differences. EFT interven-tions place clients' stories and experience above all else as the expert voice. When we explore our own social identities and positions of privilege, EFT interventions provide the tools to explore emotional impacts of racial trauma and socio-cultural marginalization and to be culturally sensi-tive process consultants that help clients order and shape their experience in the direction of their needs. Cultural humility and empathic curiosity are integral to the egalitarian, collaborative, un-conditionally accepting stance of the EFT therapist.

Guillory (2022) leads the way in challenging EFT therapists to become culturally humble by learning about the bonds of African American love in hostile environments and integrating a cultural lens into the empirically validated EFT model. The stories of black love illustrate the human propensity to form bonds of love during the most inhumane conditions of slavery and imprisonment, where societal discrimination and inequities prevail. Guillory challenges EFT therapists to balance attending to both attachment threats and racial danger cues. Throughout this chapter are attempts to integrate attachment with contextual awareness. The chapter ends with Emily's description of her journey towards a culturally humble attachment orientation as she continues to expand her grasp of EFT.

EFT is expanding to make room for discussing REC and to weave the dehumanizing impacts of these contextual variables on clients' relationships and sense of self into the healing process. Emily follows leaders in the field such as Guillory (2022), Nightingale et al. (2019), and Hardy (2022, 2023), to find a way to explicitly integrate racial, ethnic, and cultural strengths and trauma treatment in EFT. She also follows gender-affirming colleagues to educate and sensitize herself to create culturally competent, safe therapy for LGBTQIA+ clients (Trimane, 2022; Yoshino, 2007). She seeks to broaden Guillory's (2022) call across all marginalized populations, including the neurodiverse community, to pay attention to the "deep unconscious love, resistance to unfairness connected to spirit, intelligence, and knowing of White American culture that also survived generations of the worst human cruelty. The therapist's curiosity about these deep rivers, racial wounds, and adaptive beauty, will significantly enhance… therapy" (p. 185).

Stepping into Lived Attachment Experiences

Emily recognizes that she is easily distracted from the EFT tasks by the content of clients' stories. She feels compelled to offer simple suggestions to solve couples' presenting problems. She senses that if she could only immerse herself in the legitimacy of the basic human need for emotional connection, she could listen with more empathy and more acceptance, and could engage more naturally and effectively with her clients as an EFT process consultant. She has heard Dr. Johnson say that what is happening in a distressed couple is that they are literally "Scaring the hell out of each other!" But it is a giant stretch for her to see that her client, Sophie, is afraid, as she yells angrily at her timid wife, Ella. It is equally difficult to recognize that stoic Wayne or logical Phil could ever be afraid of anything at all. In fact, Phil actually told Emily that he has a well-developed protection against ever becoming afraid again. Wayne says he can identify with James Baldwin saying that being Black and conscious in America is to be in a constant state of rage (Simons, 2020). Emily does not see fear in these individuals, yet she yearns to tune in, more fully, to the *attachment channel* and the larger socio-emotional contexts of marginalization (Knudson-Martin et al., 2015). She is looking for her own felt sense of how the negative behaviors between partners are, at the core, about emotionally desperate reactions to attachment fears and unmet needs, while also seeking to attune to the threats of racial and minority stress (Allan et al., 2022). She is also seeking to grasp how depression and anxiety are rooted in isolating, ineffective, and self-reinforcing patterns of emotion regulation.

You may share some of these challenges of staying tuned to the attachment channel. The following section provides opportunities to step into attachment experiences from several perspectives. First, explore lived experience of attachment dynamics, beginning with young children. Second, reflect on your own experiences of adult love against the backdrops of the attachment foundation in EFT and the explosion of studies of adult love and attachment theory in the field of social psychology. Third, notice your internal response to evidence from the field of affective neuroscience that shows that by increasing attachment security the brain's response to threat actually changes (Johnson et al., 2013). Discover if you can resonate with the perspective that anxiety, depression, and post-trauma reactions are repetitive patterns of insecure strategies for regulating emotion and engaging with the existential challenges of life (Barlow et al., 2018; Bowlby, 1980).

Attachment between Children and Parents

Attachment theory emanates from Bowlby's study of juvenile delinquents (1944) and from his col-leagues' observations of children and their parents (Ainsworth, 1967; Ainsworth & Bowlby, 1991; Ainsworth et al., 1978; Bowlby, 1973; Robertson, 1952). Your personal experiences may be rich with examples similar to those that Bowlby and his colleagues observed.

Step for a moment into memories of interacting with your own child or of observing a parent–toddler interaction in a grocery store or local park. Recently, in a busy airport, I saw a toddler in a stroller clapping her hands happily while her dad checked his iPhone. After a few minutes she began to call, "Daddy, daddy!" Her father's attention was consumed with just a few more emails and he did not look up. She continued to protest, volume increasing incrementally and tears beginning. Her back arched as her cries dissolved into sobs, and still her dad did not look up. He reached out with one hand and pushed the stroller back and forth, with no eye contact, and no response to her increasingly loud and now heartbroken cries of distress. Suddenly, he put his phone away. "Oh baby I am so sorry—you were calling daddy, and I didn't answer you!" His face reflected her anguish as he unlatched her harness and folded her in his arms. "Ah—you are so sad—you were calling and calling, weren't you?" Wiping her tears, he planted kisses on her cheeks, and she gasped heavily as her final sobs were released. Her body melted into his and she wrapped her arms around him. "Look! Slides," she squealed, pointing at the climbing structure down the way. "Yes! Would you like to go and play there?" Her dad's tone mirrored her look of enthusiasm. She happily took his hand and ran toward the play structures. Momentary distress was soothed and signs of secure attachment evidenced. I hope this temporary rupture, followed by a repair of attunement and engagement, reminds you of your own experiences as a child or as an attachment figure for a child dear to you. As Karen (1994) in *Becoming Attached* says about love, "You do not need to be rich or smart or talented or funny; you just have to be there" (p. 416). Emotionally engaged presence makes all the difference between disconnection and security.

The child who does not reliably have this repair after disconnection does not recover so quickly. You have seen the anxious child – the one who protests relentlessly, receiving no response, and eventually sobbing themselves to distraction – shutting down all emotion and, without expression, turning away from the adult whose attention they had been seeking. You might also have seen the avoidant child, the young child who appears remarkably independent and untouched by their parent's disappearance or reappearance, when lost in a store, for example. Mikulincer and Shaver (2016), social psychology leaders in adult attachment studies, capture the distinction between these predictable patterns of attachment behaviors as shown in secure vs. insecure scripts. These implicit scripts, recognizable in children, are also seen in adults. The secure script is:

> If I encounter an obstacle and/or become distressed, I can approach a significant other for help; he or she is likely to be available and supportive; I will experience relief and comfort as a result of proximity to this person; I can then return to other activities. (Mikulincer & Shaver, 2016, p. 189)

However, when an attachment system remains in a perpetually activated state, preoccupied with threats, there are two different insecure coping responses. The avoidant (dismissive) approach "includes rapid self-protective responses to danger without examining one's emotions, consult-ing other people or seeking to receive help from them" (Mikulincer & Shaver, 2016, p. 190). The implicit script is, "If I am in distress, I will carry on with other activities" (oblivious to anyone else and with a pseudo-positive sense of self). In contrast, the anxious approach is described as sentinel, constantly on guard for threat, and having difficulty receiving comfort. The implicit script is, "If I am in distress, I will reach for you and reach for you and reach for you, endlessly and to no avail."

The film, *A Two-year-old Goes to Hospital*, made by social worker John Robertson (1952), a colleague of Bowlby, is a gripping visual of how a child responds to parental separation. To protect herself from her growing grief and despair, the child gradually alters her behaviors and reactions to her parents when they visit during prescribed visiting hours. Harvard developmental psychologist Tronick's research protocol, known as the "still face experiment" (Tronick, 2007), shows a child experiencing, in just a few moments, precisely what Robertson's two-year-old experienced, and what Bowlby (1973) described as normal separation distress responses: A progression from frantic clinging and seeking, followed by angry protests, despair, depression, and finally, detachment. A training video of a couple with pseudonyms Robert and Marsha (at www.steppingintoeft.com) shows a withdrawn partner who experienced this distress as a child. Married for over 30 years, this couple was caught in a rather rigid withdraw-pursue pattern. His wife would walk off in anger because Robert didn't engage as she needed him to. Robert would be flooded with the same panic of, "Don't leave me – stay with me!" that he felt as a child left alone in the hospital without his mother. In an engagement change event shown in this training video, after expressing his fears of rejection and isolation, Robert is able to express this core need to his wife. "When I let you down, please don't leave me – stay with me."

Similar to the African collectivist value of *Ubuntu* (Asiimwe et al., 2021), sometimes described as, "It takes a village to raise a child," it takes a team to develop and promulgate a theory. It has been said that were it not for Canadian psychologist Mary Ainsworth, who worked closely with Bowlby beginning in the late 1950s, his work might have merely gathered dust in a library in England. Ainsworth (1967) did her first studies of attachment in Uganda, a collectivist society where children had an attachment network of caregivers. She can be credited with bringing attachment theory to life (Bretherton, 1992). Bowlby formulated the basic tenets of attachment theory and Ainsworth piloted the means by which to test the theory empirically.

More recent cross-cultural attachment studies followed Ainsworth's example (Mesman et al., 2016), including studies done in Africa, East Asia, Latin America and Israel. The studies validate the attachment-theory hypotheses of universality (when given an opportunity, infants will become attached to one or more specific caregivers), normativity (most infants are securely attached *in contexts not threatening to health and survival*), sensitivity (attachment security is dependent on sensitive and prompt responsiveness), and competence (secure attachment leads to developmental competencies). In essence, whether a child has one, two or a network of specific caregivers, the universal need for sensitive caregiving and responsiveness is fundamentally important! Despite the findings of these studies, Mesman (2021) cautions against claiming the cross-cultural validity of attachment theory.

Ainsworth's research protocol, the *strange situation* highlights the attachment concept of the attachment figure as a secure base (Bowlby, 1988) and the view that when a child has a secure base connection, the exploratory system is activated. Observing infants and mothers in their homes and in the laboratory, Ainsworth saw three basic patterns of interaction: secure, anxious–ambivalent, and avoidant (Ainsworth et al., 1978). She noticed that the majority group of children with secure patterns of interaction had very harmonious relationships with their mothers at home and in the laboratory, and sought comfort and soothing from their mother upon her return after having left the room. They were readily reassured and calmed, obviously trusting her, and very quickly left her lap to resume exploration of the toy room. Securely attached children were clearly the most resilient.

Children with anxious/ambivalent patterns of interaction were obviously extremely anxious about their mother's presence. These children were highly distressed when their mother left the room, but then, upon her return, were quite ambivalent, reluctant to receive and trust her comfort. Children with avoidant patterns showed very low or no separation anxiety at all. This is what Bowlby referred to as an erroneous impression of maturity – a pseudo-independence as a defense against feeling the sadness, anguish, and pain of rejection (Bowlby, 1988; Bretherton, 1992). These basic patterns of interaction are also seen in adult romantic relationships.

The striking parallels between infant–parent attachment and adult attachment processes are clearly shown in a YouTube video entitled *Love Sense: From Infant to Adult*, created by Johnson and Tronick (2016). More clearly demonstrated than ever before, one can see, in 11 minutes, the striking similarities between the core moves in the emotional dance that plays out between parent and infant, and those that play out between adult lovers, in this instance, a bi-racial couple. The steps in the dance are illustrated as:

1. Partners naturally reach to invite connection.
2. When there is no response, the more pursuing partner protests and pushes.
3. In the face of continued lack of response, the pursuing partner's next move is to turn away and shut down to protect from the pain of rejection.
4. Next, an emotional meltdown of frantic demanding, anguish, and despair occurs.
5. Finally, in a secure relationship, partners reconnect.

Your childhood memories and the stories of your ancestors may contain recollections of comfort and security or narratives of resilience and enduring love, during race-based stress and the most hostile circumstances in the human story. The unspeakable tragedy of a mother whose daughter was abducted during a raid on their village in Sierra Leonne tore through my heart as this immigrant family, mother, father, and son, joined my family at our dinner table. The mother looked kindly, lovingly at my 12-year-old daughter and with unfathomable poignancy whispered, "You are the same age as our daughter." Their daughter, abducted in Sierra Leonne by rebels, lost to them forever, may or may not be alive or safe. She is forever torn from her parents, yet in their broken hearts is forever loved and cherished.

While writing his book on EFT with African American couples, Guillory (2022) gripped my heart with the moving *slave narrative* of a young boy who never saw his mother in daylight. Each night, after working all day in the cotton fields, she would walk the miles from her plantation to his, and sleep with him. By morning she was gone again. Quoting Andrews & Gates, 2000, Guillory (p. 9) gives us this child's story of secure connection during cruel times:

> I do not recollect of ever seeing my mother by the light of day. She was with me in the night. She would lie down with me, and get me to sleep, but long before I waked she was gone. One night I was too hungry to sleep. The friendless hungry boy, in his extreme need and when he did not dare to look for succor … found himself in the strong, protecting arms of a mother: A mother who was, at the moment more than a match for all his enemies. I will never forget … that night I learned the fact, that I was not only a child, but somebody's child. The "sweet cake" my mother gave me was in the shape of a heart, with a rich, dark ring glazed upon the edge of it, I was victorious, proud; and in the morning she was gone.

As you seek to tune into the attachment channel more naturally, consider the power of the bonds between children and their attachment figures. The need for this bond is alive in every client you meet, for the duration of their lives. When you find yourself reacting with confusion or judgment to a response that a client makes, imagine a young child in separation distress and see if it helps you to attune to the adult's present-moment reaction.

Adult Attachment Experiences

At the same time as Johnson was busily integrating attachment theory with the clinical realm of EFT couple therapy, there was a surge of adult attachment research in the field of social psychology. Drawing on Bowlby and Ainsworth's theory of the formation of affectional bonds, Hazan and Shaver (1987) applied Ainsworth's classification of patterns of attachment interactions to adult romantic relationships. Their first study began with a "love quiz" placed in the *Rocky Mountain News*, their local Denver newspaper. The original questionnaire was based on the three attachment styles identified by Ainsworth in her studies of mothers and infants. Later, this questionnaire was expanded by Bartholomew (1990) to include a fourth attachment strategy, that of fearful avoidance (the sequential shifting between anxious pursuit and avoidant withdrawal). Hazan and Shaver's (1987) questions on the attachment-style prototypes – secure, avoidant, and anxious – can be found in Mikulincer and Shaver (2023b) and they also appear in the relationship style questionnaire (RSQ) with Bartholomew's addition of "fearful avoidance" in Mikulincer and Shaver (2016). There are various other questionnaires for measuring attachment in close relationships with partners, in client-therapist relationships, with pets, organizations, and God (Mikulincer & Shaver, 2023b).

Since Bowlby and Ainsworth's original writing, adult attachment research has burgeoned to become "one of the broadest, most profound, and most creative lines of research in 20th- and 21st-century psychology" (Cassidy & Shaver, 2016, p. x). Simpson and Karantzas (2019) describe adult attachment as a "dynamic field with a rich past and a bright future" (p. 177) and Magnavita and Anchin (2014) build on the *relational matrix of* attachment theory as the basis for a unifying paradigm for psychotherapy. The empirically validated theory of adult love continues to normalize dependency (Simpson & Rholes, 2015), elucidating the emotions and dynamics that are key to relationship distress and renewal. Attachment as an "inborn regulatory system" (Mikulincer & Shaver, 2016, p. 26) has ongoing clinical relevance for therapists. It broadens the understanding of the insecure strategies for coping with normative fears and relational needs, helping therapists to empathize more accurately with individuals' attachment fears and needs, and to effectively restructure patterns of distress into growth-fostering connections and secure bonds. Attachment theory is expanding to include multiple sources of security, such as attachment with pets, organizations, groups, schools, medical settings, therapist-client relationships, spiritual figures, and attachment networks in nonconsensual monogamous relationships (Mikulincer & Shaver, 2023a, 2023b).

Johnson creatively strengthened the original empirically validated EFT model (Johnson & Greenberg, 1985, 1988) by expanding it, theoretically and pragmatically, with attachment science. With this expansion, every aspect of EFT became centered in attachment theory as a theory of adult love. Imagine Johnson and Greenberg in the process of developing EFT for couples, observing a video of Jessica and Wayne. They hear Jessica complaining that the problem lies mostly with Wayne's failure to care about her as much as he cares about shiny clean counter tops and a meticulously organized household. They also see Wayne sighing with muted frustration as he looks again and again at his watch to see if the session is nearly finished. As Johnson and Greenberg observe, they see how the therapist's empathic understanding of each partner's experience begins to create a secure base for the couple to safely explore opposing perspectives. They notice that as the therapist validates Jessica's distress when her husband stays silent, she calms down enough to hear the therapist validate Wayne's alarm at hearing she is losing faith in their relationship.

They track the couple's cyclical dynamic, where the more Jessica complains and intensifies her criticism and despair, the more Wayne sighs, throws up his hands, and pleads with her, "Be more reasonable, Jessica. We don't need warfare in our home." In turn, the more Wayne attempts to block Jessica from complaining, the more insistent she becomes. They are also likely to discern that it is when the therapist remains emotionally engaged with each partner in the present process that change begins to happen. Johnson and Greenberg's discoveries from observing video recordings of their own couple sessions led them to document, *from the bottom up*, how couples transform distressed relationships.

Johnson's perspective of the relationship as an attachment bond highlights recurrent attachment themes and she is likely to hear attributions and fears of rejection, separation, and loss, rather than seeing a contractual relationship needing conflict resolution strategies. She hears that Jessica is taking Wayne's silence to mean he does not care about her. Wayne's frustration and impatience for the session to end make sense in terms of how difficult it must be to hear that he is disappointing Jessica, and worse, that she is losing faith in him. Through her attachment lens, Johnson would see Jessica's panic that Wayne might be abandoning her when he does not respond, and she would see Wayne's silence and efforts to shut Jessica down as his best attempts to avoid hearing one of the most dreadful of attachment messages, "She is rejecting me because I am disappointing her."

We have learned, since the 1980s, when EFT was developed, that a therapist needs to also attend to the racial stressors on the couple's relationship. Wayne's silence and attempts to block Jessica's complaints are part of a larger story of his experience as a black man in an unsafe world, where emotional down-regulation is an adaptive survival strategy. A culturally competent EFT therapist is empathically curious and comfortable to invite clients to share their personal experiences of racial and ethnic minority pride and stress (Davis et al., 2018; Guillory, 2022).

The individual client, rigidly caught in a pattern of isolating while also pining for meaningful relationships, is not unlike couples caught in repetitive patterns of best attempts to get the safety and acceptance they are seeking. Imagine Johnson watching a session of Emily with Max. In EFIT, as in couple therapy, Johnson would see Emily following the moves of the EFT Tango. As Emily works with the power of present-moment experience, she shapes corrective emotional experiences, beginning with Move 1, reflecting Max's present patterns of attempting to suppress his daily, decades-old fear of recalling the scene of his friend's death. Emily assembles, with Move 2, the elements of emotion in Max's avoidant patterns and deepens his core emotional experience to shape relevant interpersonal encounters with Move 3. Emily shapes imaginal encounters for Max to send clear, emotional messages to his deceased friend, sharing his remorse for the accident, his love for his friend and owning his guilt, responsibility and fear of being overwhelmed at consciously remembering how his body appeared. In an attachment frame, Emily processes these encounters, with Move 4, by asking Max how it feels to share and how it feels to receive his friend's imaginal responses. Finally, Johnson would see Emily, using Move 5, to integrate and summarize Max's shift in view of self and other, and to consolidate the corrective emotional experience. (A similar EFIT training video of multiple sessions, *EFIT: Transforming Trauma and Grieving Lost Love*, is available at steppingintoeft.com.)

Attachment Security Changes the Brain

Findings in the field of affective neuroscience validate that secure bonds effectively regulate emotion and promote health. The natural capacity of relationships to co-regulate emotional distress and threat is demonstrated in fMRI handholding studies (Coan et al., 2006). These studies demonstrate that the neocortical activation of subjects in an fMRI machine, anticipating and receiving intermittent electric shocks to their ankles, is dramatically reduced when holding the hand of a loved one. Subjects reported that the sensation from the electric shocks was *uncomfortable* when holding the hand of a secure attachment figure, whereas they reported the sensation as *painful* when left alone in the fMRI machine.

The fMRI results comparing female partners' neural response to threat of pain before and after receiving 8–10 sessions of EFT indicated that female partners' neural response to threat of pain was significantly reduced after receiving therapy. By facilitating the creation of secure attachment bonds, which co-regulate emotion more quickly than an individual can consciously self-regulate, EFT can change the brain's neural response to threat. fMRI research shows that EFT goes beyond creating relationship satisfaction to strengthening the attachment bond and changing the brain (Burgess Moser et al., 2015; Johnson et al., 2013; Wiebe, Johnson, Burgess Moser et al., 2017).

Research shows the positive impact of secure bonds on mental, emotional, and physical health and healing (Greenman & Johnson, 2022; Hawkley et al., 2006), and the power of attachment security to lessen response to threats, both from within and beyond relationships (Coan, 2016; Coan et al., 2006; Johnson, 2013). These results are particularly encouraging to EFT practitioners across modalities of individuals, couples and families. The EFT therapist always attunes to clients in their attachment, relational contexts, viewing them as essentially co-regulating beings – functioning best when they have one or two others on whom they can depend. *Effective dependency* (Bowlby, 1988), an ingredient essential to health and well-being, fosters and maintains positive views of some others as trustworthy and dependable and a view of self as lovable and competent.

Principles of Attachment Theory: Laws of Human Love and Bonding

The basic tenets of attachment theory, the laws of human love and bonding (Figure 5.1), illustrate how an attachment bond is a particular kind of relationship where attachment figures significantly impact each other's inner experience and relational patterns. Inner emotional experience and interpersonal interactions shape and reinforce the other. EFT therapists "know how to tune into emotions and not just heal relationships but to shape relationships that heal" (Howard, 2021, Psychiatry UBC interview, introduction of S. Johnson).

When we understand the attachment significance of a person's relational context, all behaviors – even the seemingly bizarre – make sense. Jessica's subtle, yet intractable complaints about her husband's unavailability, in sharp contrast to Wayne's strategies of sighing, suggesting how Jessica could approach things differently and throwing up his hands in resignation, represent a common scene in early couple therapy sessions. The more persistent that one partner's attempts to get a response become, the more silent and resigned or frustrated the other partner becomes. The degree to which one triggers these responses in the other indicates an attachment relationship, however insecure it might be. If there was no attachment between the individuals, then they would have

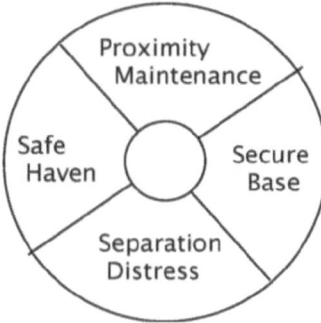

Figure 5.1 Basic Laws of Human Love and Bonding.

minimal impact and little power to trigger these reactions in one another. People who are not important to one another do not expend energy complaining and pushing another to be different, neither would they experience despair and frustration over hearing how the other is feeling let down by them.

Sahra's tendencies to isolate and complain that no one is a source of support or comfort make sense in her attachment, relational context. She withdraws to protect herself from judgment and emotional pain. With no reliable other to rely on, she sinks into loneliness, anxiety, and depression. The more she flips between anxious dysregulation, unable to concentrate on soothing activities, and numbing despair, unable to reach out to anyone, the more she confirms there is no safe other and that she is unlovable.

Attachment theory can be encapsulated by the following eight basic tenets. References to *attachment partners* frequently refers to romantic partners, but can also refer to individuals' attachment figures in EFIT.

Humans Are Innately Wired for Connection and Dependency

According to attachment theory, dependence is an essential part of the human condition (Feeney et al., 2015). Bowlby claimed that the primary need of human beings throughout life is to have a felt sense of relational safety and security that comes from having one or two others upon whom they can depend. This compelling, innate mammalian drive for maintaining connection with a trusted other is seen in the touching story of a baby hippopotamus orphaned off the Kenyan coast after a tsunami. He chose a 100-year-old male tortoise to be his *mother*. This unlikely pair formed a strong bond, eating together, swimming together, sleeping together, and snuggling up close to one another (Hatkoff et al., 2007). Love, defined as secure connection, is an ancient survival code, a need for an "emotional bond that may not be fully recognized until a relationship is threatened, severed, or lost" (Shaver & Mikulincer, 2014, p. 285).

Secure Attachment Provides a Safe Haven/Secure Base

Adults, like children, need both a secure base that serves as a springboard for independent exploration of the world and a safe haven of comfort to return to in the face of life's bruises. The experience of secure base support and safe haven comfort from another fosters confidence, resilience, and creativity. As one woman remarked, "I feel we are tethered together, my lifeline is always there, and I feel empowered! I feel the safety of his arms even when we are thousands of kilometres apart."

Secure dependence complements autonomy. The more connected you are, the more separate and autonomous you can be. "Bowlby suggests there is no such thing as overdependency or true independence; there is only effective or ineffective dependence" (Johnson, 2003, p. 105). The essence of attachment theory is that connection with a secure attachment figure mitigates the impact of fear and uncertainty and fosters growth. An EFIT client "Adam" finds that when, in his imagination, he can invite his beloved father into the scene of his trauma from 20 years earlier, his shame is lifted and the injustice he suffered is manageable for him to face. (See "Adam" training video at www.steppingintoeft.com.) He now has a secure base from which to face and restructure the enduring impacts of his racially motivated trauma.

Emotion Is Central to Attachment

Emotion, defined *as a dynamic cascade of perception-feeling-meaning-action, in response to an interpersonal trigger*, is central to both secure and insecure connections. When individuals feel safe and secure, emotion is regulated, and they experience, joy, safety, curiosity, and passion

(Johnson, 2016b). When romantic partners or individuals live with a sense of distance and uncertainty, however, emotion is not regulated, and a chaotic mixture of anger, sadness, longing, shame, and fear wreak havoc on relationship bonds and a sense of felt security. Consistent with systems theory, emotion is recognized as the link between self and system, the leading element that organizes patterns of interpersonal and internal interaction, and the element that can be reprocessed so as to organize *broaden-and-build* cycles.

Emotional Isolation Is Traumatizing

Loss of an attachment figure is inherently traumatic. Fear and insecurity become absorbing in that all actions and perceptions fuel the fear. Nothing offers reprieve or leads out of this state of panic. Fight, flight, or freeze trauma responses ensue, manifesting in the predictable pattern of separation distress: reaching–seeking–clinging; angry protest; depression–despair; detachment (Bowlby, 1973; Johnson, 2003).

A distressed partner, clearly longing for a safe haven and a secure base connection, captures the trauma of isolation, "It's not the fights that really matter. I could handle disagreements – if I could find you when I need you, but I am all alone in this relationship." Emotion is the central element in both secure connection and relationship distress. A felt sense of closeness and connection is coded as a safety cue in the brain. Individuals speak of feeling their entire body relaxing at the thought of hearing a partner's voice or seeing a loving attachment figure's face. However, signs of emotional distancing and separation from attachment figures are danger cues. A look of disapproval or nonchalance on a partner's or loved one's face, can trigger numbness, panic, or rage. Critical pursuit and defensive withdrawal are typical reactions when such danger cues are perceived.

As a theory of emotion regulation and trauma, attachment theory offers an EFT therapist a frame for understanding emotion regulation difficulties that make up trauma responses, as well as the depression and anxiety that naturally accompany relationship distress (Johnson, 2002, 2003). The lack of emotional response from an attachment figure results in isolation that is, indeed, traumatizing and dehumanizing. Notably, there is enduring trauma on the bodies and emotional lives of generations of shattered attachment bonds for people surviving slavery, colonization, refugee experiences, and modern-day oppression due to racial, ethnic, and cultural marginalization.

Emotional Engagement Defines Attachment Security

Johnson (2008) proposes a simple acronym, which encapsulates the key elements of a secure attachment bond: ARE. The attachment need for an emotional response when one reaches to a significant other for support and comfort is embedded in the question, "ARE you there for me?" meaning, "Will you be there for me when I need you?" or "Can I depend on you?"

"A" represents, "Are you accessible, available, within reach?" A young man openly acknowledges that he is obsessed with online gambling and spends endless hours on the computer. His wife complains of loneliness and of "never being able to find him." "I don't know what you mean," he says, "I'm sitting right beside you all evening, while you prepare your lessons for the next day." Although he was in the room, he was not accessible to his partner. *He could not be found.*

"R" represents, "Will you respond to me when I call?" A successful criminal lawyer routinely has escalating shouting matches with his partner, also a successful lawyer. Recognizing how he makes himself unavailable and unresponsive when they are in a "heated match," he describes it as, "I'm not refusing to talk. I most certainly get upset and things will escalate, but if I'm getting upset, I'll sort of *stop listening*, even if I keep talking. I'm not really engaging. I'm just shut off and upset." This is an example of being non-responsive. Even though he is shouting back at his partner, he is acknowledging that he is not at all responsive to her.

"E" represents emotional engagement. "Will you engage *emotionally* with me when you answer my call?" Already, it is becoming clear how intertwined these three elements are, since accessibility and responsiveness clearly are part of being emotionally engaged. One partner said:

> When I tell you about my worries about my dying mother, I see the compassion in your eyes and the softness in your face. You move just a little closer to me and I feel you are totally with me, feeling my anguish, and then I know I can get through this ordeal.

This is emotional engagement. It is the kind of emotional accessibility, responsiveness, and engagement that builds bonds, and provides a safe haven of comfort and a secure base of support from which to resiliently face the most difficult challenges of life.

Accessibility, responsiveness, and emotional engagement build resilient and lasting bonds between attachment figures. A person who has confidence from repeated experiences of a significant other's availability is much less likely to feel intense anxiety and fear, or to turn away from the relationship to regulate emotions.

Humans Function According to Internal Working Models

Bowlby (1973) described the impact of internal working models. He proposed that safe and secure connection promotes positive internal working models where others are seen as reliable and trustworthy, and the self is experienced as lovable and worthy of love. Insecure connection, however, promotes a negative working model of the other as unreliable or hurtful, and of self as unlovable and unworthy. Negative models limit growth and individuals get stuck in habitual ways of dealing with emotion, and of engaging with, and responding to, significant others.

Internal working models of self and other need not be viewed as permanent. They can be modified throughout life (Bowlby, 1973, 1988). There is growing literature on changes in attachment orientations and internal working models that can occur through psychotherapy and new experiences in specific relationships (Gillath et al., 2008; Johnson et al., 2015). Present interactions can revise working models (Feeney et al., 2015). The process of change in EFT facilitates stronger attachment bonds and changes in relationship specific attachment (Wiebe, Johnson, Burgess Moser et al., 2017; Wiebe, Johnson, Lafontaine et al., 2017).

While internal working models of self and other are amenable to change and security can be earned, a culturally humble therapist needs to be attuned to potential limitations of changes in attachment security and view of self and other. The impacts of racism and other forms of discrimination are likely to block change in a client's perception of the world as a safe place, even as their primary relationships become more secure (Williams et al., 2014). For example, Nightingale (2021) found that during EFT therapy, as their attachment bonds with their partners became more secure, African American men did not experience a reduction in race-based stress in the world.

Strategies for Engagement and Bonding

There are a finite number of strategies for engaging with attachment figures when in need of support and comfort. The primary attachment strategy or mode of engagement that is prominent in secure relationships is to reach for support when experiencing threat or distress, confident that a response will be forthcoming. However, when a person senses that a positive response to a call for support is unlikely, they opt for *secondary* modes of engaging. These secondary strategies, organized around the dimensions of anxiety and avoidance, are as follows.

The ***anxious strategy*** involves hyperactivating and upping the ante with desperate, demanding, and persistent attempts to get a response, "Where are you, where are you?" In this strategy, anxiety is high. This individual, sensing the threat of loss or facing the inaccessibility of the attachment figure (who could be physically present, but emotionally absent), becomes preoccupied with seeking, clinging, and angrily demanding a response, and then resisting comfort when it is eventually offered. If no response is forthcoming, the protest escalates to a mix of tears, anger, and resignation, and is eventually followed by turning away and giving up. Hypervigilance and ruminating prevail.

The ***avoidant strategy*** involves deactivating all attachment needs and emotions by distancing, numbing out, shutting down, and conveying pseudo-independence or strength. In this strategy, avoidance or down-regulation of emotions and suppression are high. Individuals deactivate any longings for response or connection and carry on with no attempt to engage the other. This self-protective mode of acting strong, independent, and rational is a necessary survival strategy for many living with marginalization. For example, "I'm just fine thank you. I don't need anyone." This strategy carries with it a pseudo-positive sense of self and/or disdain for leaning on another. In reality, the individual who defaults to this strategy in times of stress feels safer by avoiding closeness and vulnerable self-disclosures, since closeness has come to be associated with emotional pain. Closeness and connection are legitimately threatening to these individuals. They threaten to destroy one's sense of self. Demands from a partner for more openness, more closeness, more emotional expressiveness can seem like a demand for a personality change. The avoidant strategy frequently breaks down in response to uncontrollable, chronic, severe stress, and avoidant individuals sometimes lose control and show strong negative emotions (Mikulincer & Shaver, 2019).

A third common insecure attachment strategy is the ***fearful avoidant strategy,*** a chaotic combination of both insecure attachment strategies in sequence. For example, "Come here, come here; go away!" or, "I am afraid without you and want your support, and yet I am afraid *of you*!" In this conflicted strategy, both anxiety and avoidance are high. This is commonly seen with trauma survivors who experienced their attachment figures as unreliably present, unpredictably neglectful, or hurtful (Johnson, 2002, 2003; Mikulincer & Shaver, 2016). This attachment survival strategy evolves to manage the harm caused by ruptured attachment bonds and cultural trauma. It is called *fearful avoidance* in the adult attachment literature and *disorganized attachment* in the childhood literature. Considering the pervasive socio-cultural trauma faced by people from marginalized groups, an EFT therapist must be attuned to and elicit exploration of the impacts of socio-cultural trauma on clients' relationships, their patterns of communication, and their emotional connections. Hardy (2016, 2022, 2023) and Williams (2020) challenge therapists to attune to the invisible wounds of racial trauma, including the subtle microaggressions and harmful impacts therapists can have from their own unconscious biases.

The attachment scripts described earlier (Mikulincer & Shaver, 2016) and the metaphors for each insecure strategy given in the supplemental material link (routledge.com/9781032151335) highlight the differences in the strategies. They offer EFT therapists a felt sense of each strategy that clients use when in distress. In Stage 1, EFT therapists use the five moves of the EFT Tango to assemble the emotional process in the self-protective strategies and to promote emotional balance. In Stage 2, they shape corrective emotional experiences of secure strategies of reaching and responding so that *broaden-and-build* cycles of attachment security (Mikulincer & Shaver, 2016) can replace the ineffective strategies and patterns.

Attachment Integrates Caregiving and Sexuality

Adult attachment theory integrates caring, attachment needs, and sexuality (Shaver & Mikulincer, 2006). In an adult romantic attachment bond, caring and sexuality move to the fore at different times in the relationship; however, both expressions of caring and engagement in sexuality are significantly influenced by individuals' typical attachment strategies. Avoidance and anxiety put the brakes on sexuality, leading either to *solace sex* – an anxious pursuit for reassurance – or to *sealed-off sex* – an emotionally avoidant focus upon performance (Johnson, 2008, 2016a). This contrasts with the popular view that novelty and thrill are required to maintain heightened passion and sexual satisfaction. To the contrary, Johnson claims that attachment security is the greatest aphrodisiac, leading to what she calls *synchrony sex*. Sexual response and relationship quality have a reciprocal impact on one another. Relationship security positively affects sexual functioning and increases passion (Birnbaum, 2023), and optimal sexual satisfaction heightens relationship quality. EFT has a model for placing sexual functioning in the context of the attachment view of love, integrating sex therapy as an inseparable part of couple therapy by facilitating the same steps and stages of client change, while explicitly discussing sexual responses between partners (Johnson, 2017; Johnson et al., 2018; Johnson & Zuccarini, 2010, 2011; Wiebe et al., 2019).

In summary, the eight laws of human love and bonding provide an EFT therapist with a compassionate, scientific framework to guide therapy. Compassion and unconditional acceptance are rooted in recognizing that all attachment strategies can be healthy and adaptive in particular contexts but become problematic when applied rigidly in all contexts, regardless of available support (Bowlby, 1980). Contextual impacts and REC wounds need to be integrated into the exploration of attachment strategies. Attachment behaviors, whether they are congruent, secure reaches for comfort and connection, insecure behaviors of anxious pursuit, avoidant distancing, or the chaotic combination of pursuing and turning away, are all clients' best attempts at finding a way to safely engage with a significant other to regulate emotion while in distress. It can be difficult for beginning therapists to recognize angry demands as a strategy for engagement. It may be even more difficult to conceptualize isolating or shutting down and firing back in defense as a strategy for engagement. Only by listening closely within a culturally humble attachment frame and engaging with couples and individuals to unfold their unique contextual attachment dramas, can a therapist deeply understand how staying aloof or criticizing harshly are, indeed, both strategies for engagement – best attempts to regulate emotional experience and create secure bonds of acceptance and support. The key implications of attachment science for creating psychotherapeutic change are that emotion is the agent of change and that change is inherently interpersonal, shaped through dialogues of congruent emotional messages (Johnson, 2019).

Roadblocks to Internalizing Attachment Theory as a Guide

There are numerous factors which can present roadblocks for therapists seeking to internalize attachment theory as a guiding paradigm for therapy. A therapist new to EFT is likely to find it challenging to consistently hold an attachment perspective of a couple's unfolding drama of escalating and shutting down. Similarly, it can be difficult to de-pathologize an individual client's depression and anxiety with an attachment perspective that frames the problem as a self-protective, self-defining repetitive *pattern of disconnection.*

The challenge is compounded when the therapist's own emotions are aroused, and they lose their emotional balance. They may find themselves taking sides with one partner or may get overwhelmed with feeling pressure to solve an individual client's presenting issue (Mikulincer & Shaver, 2023a). Challenges can come from tacit, unexamined theoretical views that stand in the way of adopting an attachment orientation or from personal experiences and unconscious biases that interfere with internalizing a culturally humble attachment perspective. The Chapter 5 Support Material (routledge.com/9781032151335) gives more detail about each of the following potential roadblocks, with guidelines for change.

Tacit, Unexamined Theoretical Views

By identifying your tacit beliefs, unconscious biases, and emotional vulnerabilities, you then have more clarity and agency to challenge and possibly shift some previously implicit views and patterns, should you desire to do so.

An Individualistic View of Human Nature and Therapeutic Change. For many therapists, trained in an ethic self-sufficiency, individual growth, and independence, a worldview of interdependency is, indeed, a huge leap. For therapists who adhere, either tacitly or consciously, to the view that adults can be self-sufficient and must develop a capacity to soothe and love themselves before receiving comfort or love from another, it could require considerable vulnerability and courage to explore the therapeutic power of effective dependency.

An Insight Orientation. Many therapists new to EFT become distracted by trying to help clients figure out why they feel or behave in a certain way, implying that therapeutic change comes from insight. EFT is not an insight therapy. Explanations do not deepen clients' engagement in present-moment experience and interpersonal processes. If you assume that explanations and insight lead to change, you might find yourself becoming distracted from the attachment significance of the present moment. When emotions are running high, you could become easily distracted and unwittingly digress into a client's stories of childhood, beginning to see childhood causes as "the real problem" to explore. An EFT therapist first identifies the problematic pattern and then accesses the underlying attachment fears driving that pattern.

Limited by Diagnostic Labels. It can be challenging for therapists to integrate the attachment alternative to diagnostic labeling. For many therapists it can be an immense paradigm shift to see emotional disorders and interpersonal distress as associated with legitimate, unmet needs for interpersonal connection and not as a personal deficit in a client. It can be difficult to move from implicitly seeing an individual's diagnosis as the problem, to perceiving the patterns of attachment strategies as both exacerbating emotional distress and providing a hopeful target for change. It can be quite radical to relinquish a focus on individual shortcomings and to embrace the interpersonal, attachment view that hope and change begin with becoming fully acquainted with the current interactive distress-cycle.

The "empirical evidence linking attachment insecurities to emotion regulation" (Mikulincer & Shaver, 2019, p. 7) provides a growth-oriented, empowering perspective of various emotional disorders such as borderline personality disorder, overt narcissism, depression, anxiety disorders, addictive processes, avoidant personality disorders and unrealistically positive self-appraisals.

Fear of Imposing Personal Values or Unconscious Bias. Some therapists may be reluctant to follow an attachment paradigm for fear they will be imposing values of intimacy and emotionally vulnerable expressiveness on cultures where this is not the norm. Attachment research is expanding across cultures and continuing to ask more critical questions (Mikulincer & Shaver, 2023b; Thompson et al., 2021). Despite the established universality of attachment needs and responses and the centrality of emotion to attachment bonds across cultural contexts, EFT therapists are increasingly open to yet-unspoken elements and nuances of clients' experiences. Attachment may include networks of attachments, whether they be adult multiple-partner relationships (Edwards et al., 2023; Fern, 2020; Moors et al., 2019) or multiple-caregivers, known as *alloparenting* (Mesman et al., 2016).

Guillory (2022) encourages EFT therapists to consider both attachment threats which trigger cascades of emotion in self-protective patterns, as well as racial danger cues which directly impact one's experience in the world and in intimate relationships. Honoring racial experiences and cultural differences also includes sensitivity to sexual-identity stress (Josephson, 2003; Trimane, 2022; Zuccarini & Karos, 2011) and awareness and respect for different display rules for emotional expression and emotion regulation (Ekman, 2007). Attachment theory supports the cultural sensitivity needed with each client and with each couple, as well the necessary sensitivity toward each client's comfort with emotional expression (Dockett, 2022; Liu & Wittenborn, 2011). Attachment-based EFT therapists seek to attune to the intersecting power relations and challenges of racism, sexism, poverty, and all experiences of socio-cultural minorities (Hill Collins & Bilge, 2020; PettyJohn et al., 2020), while eliciting and attending to emotional experience in conversations with differing experiences of power and privilege.

Personal Factors

Personal attachment experiences and strategies for emotion regulation can also interfere with a therapist internalizing an attachment perspective as a guide for therapy. An EFT therapist needs to become comfortable with strong emotion, able to trust their own emotional experiencing, and courageous to seek consultation. Personal factors, expanded on in the online supplementary material, cover the following areas:

Cultural Humility or Implicit Bias. Attachment theory shapes a particular kind of therapeutic stance. To embody this safe attachment stance (described more in Chapter 7) a therapist needs cultural humility. Barriers to cultural humility are unconscious or implicit biases, such as those explored in *The Enduring, and Invisible, and Ubiquitous Centrality of Whiteness* (Hardy, 2022). Like unacknowledged core emotion, implicit bias resides in our brains (Oluo, 2019) and in our bodies (Menakem, 2017), and informs actions, and leads to rapid judgments, and assessments that we are unaware of making.

Cultural humility and discovery of one's own implicit biases requires a therapist to explore their own positions of privilege and subjugation and to educate themselves through reading, consultation, training videos, and recording and viewing their own work. Openness to learn about their own biases and their clients' culturally specific experiences of attachment is key.

Unfamiliarity with Secure Attachment. Therapists might come to EFT without personally having experienced a secure connection or attachment bond in an intimate relationship. Thus, the target for change – secure attachment – might be little more than theoretical. It is important for therapists to explore and seek support for their own attachment insecurities because they can interfere with successful therapeutic outcomes (Mikulincer & Shaver, 2023a).

An Unfamiliar Attachment Strategy. Therapists find it challenging to integrate the attachment paradigm when they cannot appreciate, or are unfamiliar with, one of the insecure attachment strategies of anxious hyperactivating (pursuing) or avoidant deactivating (withdrawing). They might not be conscious of their own automatic style of coping when under stress, or they might not yet have fully stepped inside the experience of the other strategy. This common, legitimate growing-edge experience in learning EFT can get in the way of validating each client and tracking their repetitive pattern.

Personal Emotion Regulation. Therapists differ in personal styles of regulating their own emotions and engaging with others. They also differ in their personal comfort with intense emotion. Therapists' level of comfort with intense emotion will have a big impact on how closely attuned they can stay with each client and with the present-moment interactive dynamic between partners or between an individual client and their imaginal other.

Some or all of these roadblocks are likely to arise for you in your journey to grow in competence and confidence as an EFT therapist. Self-reflection, consultation, and risking engaging with others who show empathy and curiosity are key supportive activities to expand your facility with integrating an attachment perspective as your EFT guide.

Courage to Embrace Attachment Theory as a Guide

Therapists seeking to work with a culturally humble attachment paradigm embark on an exciting journey that can also require a lot of courage. It could mean identifying and relinquishing some tacit presumptions of human nature, such as, "People need to make self-love and self-care a priority." It might mean stepping back from familiar ways of doing couple therapy. It might mean risking a shift in your sense of the therapeutic role, as you move away from teaching conflict management skills or providing family of origin explanations to becoming a *process consultant*. Therapists seeking to internalize an attachment definition of adult needs and adult love could be compelled to expand or radically change their working theory of therapeutic change. In this quest, they are in good company of courageous and open minds and hearts. They are boldly venturing into new territories, as did Bowlby, Ainsworth, Shaver, Johnson, Crenshaw, DuGruy, hooks, Guillory, and you, dear reader, as you accept the challenge of becoming an increasingly culturally humble, attachment-oriented EFT therapist! "Knowing love or the hope of knowing love is the anchor that keeps us from falling into that sea of despair…Rarely, if ever, are any of us healed in isolation. Healing is an act of communion" (hooks, 2001, pp. 78, 215).

Conclusion

Attachment theory is the thread that binds theory, research, and practice in EFT. As an empirically validated theory of adult love, attachment theory, by its very nature, is experiential (focused on present moment reaching, attuning, and responding, where emotional signals have precedence) and systemic (focused on the interactive feedback loops of interpersonal and contextual dynamics).

In this chapter, I reviewed the innate human need for secure emotional connection and the gravity of the ways human love and bonding have been tampered with in some of this world's most grievous practices, particularly slavery, colonialism, and genocide. Cross-cultural attachment research is asking questions about how attachment processes manifest in different cultures, how culture manifests in attachment processes (Thompson et al., 2021), and whether secure attachment can buffer the impact of racism and discrimination (Mikulincer & Shaver, 2021). Mesman, who initially reported cross-cultural studies that validated the claims of the universality of attachment, is now saying, "We need to ask more critical questions before we can firmly claim cross-cultural validity of attachment theory" (2021, p. 250).

Attachment theory provides a clear target for the end point of therapy for both couples and individuals. Couples strive for secure lasting bonds nurtured by responsive emotional presence. The end point of attachment as a theory of romantic love equips the clinician with a kind of emotional logic or "love sense" (Johnson, 2013) that elucidates what draws partners to treat one another tenderly, protectively, caringly, and joyfully, and to thrill with passion and excitement in each other's presence. It normalizes moments at the other end of the spectrum as well, when unmet needs or mixed signals take over so powerfully that partners flare up in rage or construct concrete walls of silence. The emotional logic of attachment theory makes sense out of the traps of negative interactions in which clients are repeatedly caught (Bowlby, 1973).

Individuals in EFIT move from rigid patterns of anxiety, depression, loneliness, or self-doubts, to being more open to experience and more able to engage with strong emotion. They move into open, responsive engagement with others and a coherent, competent, sense of self, fully alive, and more able to deal with existential life issues and to receive and contribute to secure attachment with others.

Rumi suggests, "Without a guide it will take you two hundred years for a journey of two years" (Amodeo, 2015). An attachment orientation is a reliable guide; love as secure connection is sensible and logical. The EFT interventions and model for change are effective to reshape depression, anxiety, and distressed relationships into open, responsive nurturing bonds with others that foster and are fostered by a sense of competence and flexibility to face the vicissitudes of life. The EFT Tango moves are an accessible guide for therapists to follow to help clients shape lasting change; however, cultural humility beckons us to remember there is more to learn! Attachment research is continuing in many cultures and EFT is continuing to expand.

The attachment orientation of the empirically validated model of EFT compels practitioners to be continually open to deeper understandings of human needs for connection across intersectional differences. Morrison (1992) writes:

> My work requires me to think of how free I can be as an African-American woman writer in my genderized, sexualized, wholly racialized world … imagining is not merely looking or looking at; nor is it taking oneself intact into the other. It is, for the purposes of the work, *becoming.* (p. 4)

There is a hopefulness in her words *imagining* and *becoming.* We need to keep challenging ourselves to expand our empathic imaginations. Both attachment research and the EFT model are expanding and *becoming* increasingly relevant across cultures. EFT therapists need to awaken our blind spots and expand our capacities to tune in deeply to clients' stories – to help them expand their own experience in the telling; to embrace their goals for change; and then to engage the power of emotion to shape corrective emotional experiences that unblock innate tendencies for growth, connection, resilience, and safety with at least some others. Creating dependable, nurturing bonds in *broaden-and-build cycles* that reinforce effective co-regulation and *effective dependency* is the end point of attachment-based EFT.

Addendum to Chapter 5: Expanding Cultural Awareness, Humility, and Competence

Emily recognizes that to answer the overarching question in EFT, "Can I cultivate safety in session?" in the affirmative, she must expand her REC awareness, humility, and competence. She is increasingly aware of her whiteness and shakes her head in realization of how many of her advantages she has taken for granted. She has lived with annoying experiences of male dominance, dismissive comments from others in positions of power, and offensive experience of exclusion due to family member's disabilities but thinking of the advantages she has as a white, heteronormative, cisgender woman brings her to a halt!

She is doing all she can to integrate how race matters and to slow down to pay more attention to stories of culture. She is moving away from "the habit of ignoring race [which had been] understood to be a graceful, even generous liberal gesture" (Morrison, 1992, pp. 9–10), to inviting and attending more carefully to how clients convey that culture is shaping their experience. She has explored explicitly the impacts of "racialism and its consequences upon the victim," as Morrison writes, but now is also delving into "the impact of racism on those who perpetuate it" (p. 11).

The central questions that Emily ponders while pursuing cultural humility are, "How do I recognize my whiteness without despairing? How do I continue to grow as an EFT therapist, attending both to attachment dynamics and to clients' social context? (Guillory, 2022; Hardy, 2022, 2023; Nightingale et al., 2019). How do I, as an EFT therapist, respond to the institutionalized discrimination and injustices of white supremacy? How do I embrace *a love ethic* (hooks, 2001) and make this part of my culturally humble EFT practice with couples and individuals?"

Emily struggles with the ethics of embracing a model developed by white people and validated primarily by white researchers with white clients, for all her clients. She is pleased that EFT research is expanding across cultures and around the globe. She ponders the essence of EFT's collaborative, egalitarian values and its goal to make therapy *a safe haven, secure base context*. Fervently concluding that EFT, by its very principles, must expand and grow to embrace the world's non-white majority and all groups experiencing oppression in a world of systemic racism and hetero-dominance, she begins a *commitments-for-inclusion* list as she continues to explore and expand her grasp of EFT. "Emily's Commitments for Inclusion" are in the Chapter 5 Support Material (routledge.com/9781032151335).

6 Emotion as Target and Agent of Change

> Emotion is a verb – a rapidly unfolding cascade beginning with an external trigger, followed by
> limbic perception, bodily arousal, meaning making and behavioral responses.

EFT focuses upon emotion as the target and agent of change. In this chapter, you are introduced to emotion as verb. We first examine emotion as an active process, involving a cascade of elements: A trigger and immediate perception; bodily arousal; meaning-making; and impulse to action. Second, we look at a simple view of basic emotions, their embedded needs, and their adaptive action tendencies. Third, we explore how an EFT therapist distinguishes between core, implicit, visceral emotions (formerly called *primary* emotions) and reactive, surface emotions (previously called *secondary* emotions), noting that core emotions, with their reliable source of information and adaptive action tendencies, are frequently disregarded during moments of threat and reactivity. Fourth, we review (from Chapter 2) the EFT Tango Move 2 that equips EFT therapists to engage clients in formulating their emotional experience and using newly discovered and expressed emotion to shape new ways of interacting (internally and interpersonally). Fifth, we review several emotions that typically challenge EFT therapists – hurt, shame, and anger. Sixth, we note the growing awareness in EFT of the cultural nuances of emotional experience and expression, and the need to use EFT interventions in culturally sensitive ways. Finally, we emphasize distilling emotion in concrete, vivid, and specific ways, as part of deepening emotional engagement, a fundamental part of creating change in EFT.

Emotion as an Active Unfolding Process of Distinct Elements

Emotion is more than feelings or affective experience. It is an unfolding interpersonal process that motivates behavior and influences meaning. It contains adaptive guidance for survival. "Emotion" is from the Latin *emovere*, meaning to "move out," and from the twelfth century French word, *emouvoir*, meaning to "stir up" (Harper, 2001–2016). "Emotion is not a noun, but rather a verb" (Siegel, 2009, p. 148) – a rapid unfolding of various elements, beginning with a preconscious appraisal of an environmental cue as good or bad, followed by a bodily felt sense of arousal or calmness, meaning-making, and action tendencies (M. Arnold, 1960; Ekman, 2007). The first core feature of the process of emotion has to do with *when* it occurs (Gross, 2014). *When* refers to the specific external cue that is perceived as safe or dangerous and which propels the emotion process into action.

The second core feature of emotion is that it is a multi-step, rapidly unfolding, dynamic process (M. Arnold, 1960; Barrett, 2017; Gross, 2014; see Figure 6.1) involving perception of a cue followed by an immediate, preverbal limbic appraisal of whether the cue has a feel of good or bad, safe or dangerous; bodily arousal readying for action; a compelling action tendency or behavioral

DOI: 10.4324/9781003242673-7

Action Impulses and Behaviors
↑
Meaning Making/Attributions about Self and Other and the World
↑
Bodily Response
↑
Danger Cue or Trigger → Immediate Perception (Safe or dangerous? Good or bad?)

Figure 6.1 The Dynamic Process of the Elements of Emotion.

response; and conscious neocortical reappraisal or meaning-making regarding the view of self and the reliability of the other. Emotions, as a multi-faceted process, make us feel, they prepare the body for fight or flight, they compel us to act, they activate thoughts about self, other, and the context, and they color perceptions (Johnson, 2020).

Ledoux (1996) gives a simple example of this rapidly unfolding emotional process. When coming upon a curvy shape on the forest path, instantaneously, before there is time to think, the limbic brain does a *felt-sense* non-verbal assessment: Good or bad? Safe or threatening? If the body senses safety, it relaxes. If the body senses threat, it readies for fight or flight. After the compelling action tendency of running in the other direction, the person might consciously reflect, "That was a snake!" and, shuddering in fright, have more disgusting thoughts about the encounter.

The appraisal/information-processing view of emotion (M. Arnold, 1960) fits with Bowlby's (1973) claim that there are triggering situations in intimate relationships that humans are genetically wired to respond to with fear and avoidance. In effect, these situations are like an air-raid siren or a red light. These danger cues include "noise, strangeness, rapid approach, isolation, and for many species, darkness" (p. 110). We are predisposed during times of danger to approach and seek comfort and protection from a trusted attachment figure, and when received, this safety is a "sanctuary on sacred ground" (p. 168). Bowlby maintained that a hint that one may be unwillingly separated from an attachment figure is a danger cue throughout the life cycle.

Replace the curvy shape on the forest floor with a disparaging look or tone from your partner or a significant other and you can imagine how the process could unfold (Brubacher & Lee, 2014). Bowlby claimed that the attachment system is activated in moments of perceived threat, covering the entire range of physical or emotional threats, from fears of rejection or abandonment to dire situations of life-threatening attack. The two worst things for a mammal, claims neuroscientist Porges (2016), are isolation and restraint. This complements the attachment perspective that the greatest threats are experienced when an individual in need has no available secure base attachment figure to reach to in order to regulate fears, stress, and uncertainty.

In EFCT, therapists identify that emotion is set in motion in a distressed relationship when a cue is perceived to threaten the loss of an attachment figure or when threat is experienced and the attachment figure is unreachable. In EFIT, since attachment as a developmental theory holds that the self is constantly under construction in relationship, emotion is similarly set in motion when interpersonal security is threatened. Attachment threats exist for all human beings as survival threats. For survivors of intergenerational trauma and present-day discrimination, danger cues are pervasive! These triggers must be recognized for their undeniable impact on the emotional experience of clients experiencing minority stressors of any kind.

Basic Emotional Responses and Their Adaptive Action Tendencies

Therapists search with clients for words to accurately formulate understanding of their emotional experience (Martin, 2016), knowing emotion is never as static as one word. Considering emotions

---

Box 6.1   Core Emotions Contain Messages of Needs and Motivation to Act

Emotions, like an internal GPS, orientate individuals to their world and tell them what they need and long for to survive and to thrive. Implicitly embedded in core emotions are messages of needs and adaptive action tendencies of what to do to meet these needs.

Emotion	*Embedded Need*	*Adaptive Action Tendency*
Anger	Safety and limits	Assert oneself, move towards
Surprise/curiosity	Engage	Move towards, explore
Joy	Engage	Relax, move towards, be open
Disgust/shame/guilt	Disappear/expel	Hide, become invisible
Sadness	Comfort	Seek solace or retreat when comfort not forthcoming
Fear	Protection	Seek safety and support, flee from danger, freeze/shut down

---

as six basic *feeling words* can help EFT therapists to be focused, while at the same time, to continually seek more granular expressions to capture clients' nuanced, present-moment experience.

EFT draws on Ekman's (2007) succinct categories of emotional responses, each with a unique and adaptive motivation towards different actions (Johnson, 2019). Approach emotions are anger, which, in couple therapy, is frequently reactive anger at a partner's unresponsiveness; non-reactive, core anger, which, motivates a person towards assertiveness and achieving goals; surprise, which motivates one to move towards with curiosity; and joy, which motivates one to be open and to engage. Avoidance emotions include a category for disgust/shame/guilt, which motivates towards expelling, hiding or withdrawing; sadness, which motivates one to withdraw, or as an approach emotion, to seek comfort from another; and fear, which motivates one to flee from danger or to shut down and freeze in the face of danger (see Box 6.1).

Each of these categories can be differentiated with granular specificity. Panksepp (2003) defined a special kind of fear or "primal panic" that is triggered at the loss, or threat of loss, of a significant other. In attachment relationships, fear is the central emotion (Johnson, 2019). It has a primary survival instinct that motivates individuals to seek proximity to another when they detect a threat of loss or social rejection (Bowlby, 1973). Fear is mitigated by maintaining the availability of a secure attachment figure for comfort and safety (Johnson, 2013, 2015). Without social connection, we live in pain and isolation (Eisenberger, 2016).

Hurt, or emotional pain and anguish, is found to be a complex mixture of anger, sadness (grief), and fear of relational loss. Typically, the fear of loss has to do with a sense of devaluing the importance of the relationship or the worth of self (Vangelisti, 2009). The pain of social rejection has been found to activate some of the same parts of the brain as physical pain (Eisenberger, 2016). The brain sends a survival message, "Don't stray too far from your loved ones." It hurts to be separated. A broken heart is a reality. Social exclusion hurts (Jordan, 2018).

Secure individuals can listen to the needs embedded in emotion and can congruently seek support from others in times of need. Having had repeated experiences of attachment figures being available to support them in times of threat and stress, they have enough internal calming that they are less likely to be overwhelmed. "Believing that support will be available if needed, secure people can creatively explore a challenging situation while tolerating ambiguity and uncertainty"

(Mikulincer & Shaver, 2016, p. 189). Secure people can recognize the adaptive messages of need embedded in core emotions (as distinguished from reactive emotions described in the next section) and can send clear messages of need to safe others for support or engagement.

Without a secure base of emotional responsivity, the adaptive action tendencies of emotion frequently get distorted. Instead of responding with adaptive action tendencies, partners and individual clients can become caught in emotional cascades. In a split second and outside of conscious awareness, they are held in the grips of an emotion (Ekman, 2007). A cue, such as a tense look on a partner's face, is perceived and rapidly leads to changes in bodily responses, action impulses, interpretations of what is happening within oneself and the partner, and changes in facial and vocal signals and behaviors. When feeling threatened and flooded with emotion, partners experience increasingly negative felt senses and make more rigid interpretations of their partner's signals. Reactive emotional responses and fiercely self-protective behaviors obscure core emotions and needs and communicate mixed messages.

In attachment relationships, such as that of Jessica and Wayne, Wayne's turning away alerts Jessica's limbic brain to sense threat; her body prepares to fight, underlying attachment panic plays out on the surface as an angry protest, and her thoughts are that he does not care. Caught in the emotional throes of a distressed cycle, partners rarely have words for the underlying sense of attachment panic playing out in the cycle. In the withdraw–withdraw cycle of Julia and Phil (Figure 7.2), two trauma survivors, they both use suppression and numbing as a survival strategy, with little awareness of underlying fears and attachment needs.

Sahra is triggered into rapid cascades of overwhelm and panic at hearing loud voices. "It's irrational," she insists. "I know I am not in danger. Half the time the loud voices that frighten me are not even angry, but I am suddenly transported back to the room with my raging ex-partner. I freeze or crumble in tears. I hear, 'Run, run, you must get out'." What was once an adaptive action tendency – to get away from an abusive partner – is no longer adaptive in a setting where no one is about to hurt her but she is swept up in rapid reactivity.

Sophie and Ella are overjoyed at expecting their first child. Sophie looks at Ella's growing belly with pride and joy. Ella exclaims, "My family is so excited about our baby!" and a cloud of panic suddenly crosses Sophie's face as she blurts out:

Ella's family is thrilled, yes, but I am jealous of that! Jake, my homophobic brother won't even talk with us anymore. He would have been the most fantastic uncle but ever since Sophie and I got married, he has rejected us and won't speak to me. I'm terrified we will never reconcile!

Sophie feels herself pulling away from Ella in a stew of confusing emotion. Rapid cascades of emotional reactivity have control precedence. Core emotions with their adaptive action tendencies are out of reach. When Sophie and Ella stabilize their pattern, Sophie will not be swept up by her panicky cascade of emotional reactivity. She will be able to feel her core emotion of sorrow over her family's homophobic rejection and to reach to Ella for comfort.

Distinctions between Core Emotions and Surface, Reactive Emotional Responses

Core emotions are immediate, visceral, typically non-conscious (Stern, 2004) responses to an environmental cue, such as a partner's look of disapproval or a distancing move. The external cue may be almost imperceptible but if it stirs some bodily sensation, then the brain gives it meaning. This is part of the theory of emotion construction, beginning in the body (M. Arnold, 1960; Barrett, 2017; Kailanko et al., 2022). In fact, inner body movements, known as interoception, are found to be one of the core ingredients of emotion and to be highly influential to perception (Barrett, 2017).

For this reason, EFT therapists are finely tuned to track external bodily shifts as signs of inner movements of implicit emotional experiencing. Core emotion disappears from awareness when clients are caught in cyclic, reactive emotional cascades.

Reactive emotions are explicit responses or emotional behaviors, such as partners getting angry at each other, or turning away in coldness or numbing out in front of a screen when a partner asks for comfort. They are typically responses to an unacknowledged threatening core emotion that begins with bodily arousal (such as a tightening chest) and are accompanied by attributions about self or other, such as, "I am unlikeable," or, "You don't care about me."

Reactive emotions frequently conceal the initial core, bodily emotional response. Sophie's emotional stew laced with jealousy, described above, is a reactive emotional response covering her core fears of abandonment by her brother, and ultimately, by Ella as well. Unlike implicit, underlying, core emotions that contain messages of unmet needs, reactive emotions contain no such guidance. If her core fear was clear, it would tell Sophie that she needs contact comfort and assurance that she is loved.

Sahra's sudden freeze or flood of tears is a core trauma response. The reactivity is her dismissal of the gravity of the abuse she endured and minimizing of how frightened and injured she still is from the pain she did not deserve! When caught in reactive anger at self or in numbness, Sahra does not have clarity of what she needs. She is caught in an incoherent spin or soup of emotion. Her core pain (a mix of anger, sadness, and fear) when it can be assembled, will contain clear messages of need: Her core anger will validate that the abuse was wrong and that she needs protection and needs her voice to be heard; her core sadness will tell her she needs comfort and soothing; her core fears of being devalued, blamed or shamed will tell her she needs the physical and emotional safety of being valued and treasured.

Reactive emotional responses reinforce the negative appraisals and interpretations that are fueled by unacknowledged core emotions and bodily felt sensations. When one is caught in the throes of reactive emotion, no cognitive thoughts are powerful enough to contradict the emotion-fueled interpretations one has made. "Affect [core emotion] is in the driver's seat and rationality is a passenger" (Barrett, 2017, p. 80; see Figure 6.2).

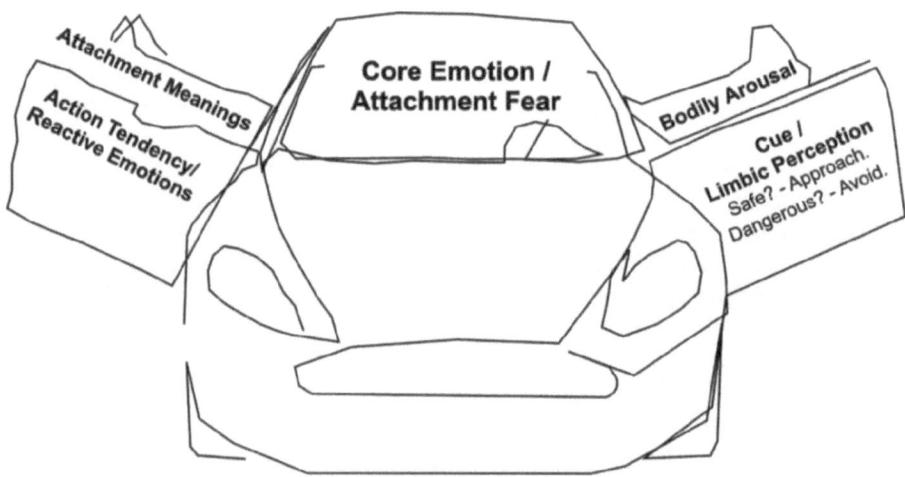

M. Arnold's (1960) Appraisal / Information Processing Theory of Emotion

Figure 6.2 Elements of Emotion.

It is important for an EFT therapist to attend to and validate both core and surface emotions. What matters most is that we begin with where a client is. "*It is the primary core emotional responses that are unattended to, undifferentiated, or disowned that the EFT therapist focuses upon most. However, therapy often begins with the therapist reflecting and validating the most obvious surface emotional responses*" (italics in original; Johnson, 2020, p. 63). This is equally true for EFIT. Reflecting and validating the obvious, surface emotions in a client's current imprisoning pattern of distress is the most respectful and expeditious way towards forming a trusting alliance and moving towards the first change event of stabilization. The importance of starting with where a client is emotionally will become clearer in the discussion of non-distilled emotions of hurt, shame, and anger that follows.

Metaphors to Access/Assemble Core, Underlying Emotion

Images of doorways can be helpful metaphors for EFT therapists to get a felt sense of emotion as an active process which comprises a series of elements, all of which may conceal and also open to the core underlying emotional surge. Imagine a four-door car (Figure 6.2), the interior of which represents withdrawer Ella's unacknowledged core emotional surge when she angrily storms out of the room upon seeing a look of disappointment on her pursuing partner Sophie's face. The driver's door represents the perceived trigger (the look on Sophie's face) and Ella's immediate, non-conscious, perceived sense of danger. It is significant that this is the driver's door, since this immediate sense of danger is the part of emotion that *drives* the process. The passenger door behind that represents Ella's bodily arousal in fight or flight mode (tensing jaw, clenching stomach, internal physiological arousal). The third door represents the meaning she makes ("I'm failing her again!"), and the fourth door represents Ella's action tendency of throwing up her hands and storming across the room, expressing reactive anger. Therapist Emily can see the doorways to open to reflect, evoke, and linger with each acknowledged element of Ella's emotion process. This will make it possible for Ella to incrementally discover the coherent whole of these fragmented elements of emotion. After she has been helped to assemble these elements, she can then share with Sophie her vulnerable, deeply hidden fear of ultimately losing her beloved wife because she cannot seem to get it right with her.

Another metaphor to focus a therapist on this multi-faceted process of unpacking emotion is that of opening doors along a corridor to gain access to the center of the house – the core, vulnerable, carefully guarded source of heat and energy, representing underlying core emotion. An EFT therapist will open the doors of:

1. The trigger or cue that is (preconsciously) perceived as dangerous.
2. The bodily sensations experienced when that cue is perceived (sensations in the stomach, heart rate, breathing, muscles – wherever one experiences bodily arousal).
3. The meanings made of that cue.
4. The automatic action tendencies and explicit emotional reactions in response to perceiving the cue.

Each door opens a path into discovering and formulating the core attachment fear which has been hiding behind closed doors. (Metaphors of the emotion process as opening doors along a hallway, from E. Katz and A. Lee, personal communications, n.d.)

Doorways to Sahra's core emotion can be seen in the example of how she is rapidly triggered into hypervigilance by loud voices. The loud voices are a present-moment danger cue. The hypervigilance is her immediate bodily response of physiological arousal. She becomes overwhelmed with a flurry of memories and questions about what she did wrong that caused her father to leave and her ex-partner to become abusive (meaning-making; view of self and other). She shrinks, feeling small and insignificant (bodily arousal and meaning-making), and goes silent (automatic action tendency). Sometimes in her silence she detaches so well that she is transported in her mind to a fantasy place (more action tendency and meaning-making), jolted back to reality at the sound of her daughter's sweet voice (a cue of safety), and face-to-face with frustration at herself (reactive action tendency and meaning-making) for "disappearing from her daughter." Her fearful avoidant pattern of hyperactivating and then shutting down repeats itself across relational contexts. The core fear in her rapid cascade of emotion is fear of being hurt, devalued, and abandoned.

Interventions for Assembling Elements of Emotion

Emotion, which is always *in motion*, is carefully assembled – discovered, distilled, and deepened – with EFT Tango Move 2 to access the more vulnerable, unspoken emotions and attachment fears that are fueling the pattern of reactivity. These core unacknowledged emotions are beacons for transformation.

Move 2 is the crux of how EFT therapists help clients gain stability and then harness the life-giving energy of core emotion. The simple poem (Box 6.2) first presented in Chapter 3 captures all the elements of Tango Move 2, illustrating evocative questions that open doorways to core emotion. These evocative questions, which can take varied forms, are not asked one after the other; rather, they are integrated with reflections and validations, linking them together into a coherent whole. First, the interpersonal trigger (What is the cue?) and the immediate, preconscious limbic appraisal of safety or danger (How does it touch you?) is evoked, followed by the bodily arousal (What does your body do?), the meaning made (What does it say to you?), the action impulse (What do you do?), and all the while, attuning to hints of core emotion so that when the fragmented emotional experience is distilled into a coherent whole, the client can be helped to "Now own what's true." *Owning what is true* alludes to the distilling and deepening of core emotion in the second part of Tango Move 2.

Emotions that Can Challenge EFT Therapists

EFT is essentially about harnessing core emotion as the beacon and fuel for transformation. Assembling and deepening emotion with Move 2 in preparation for shaping engaged encounters becomes particularly challenging for EFT therapists when working with the complex emotion of hurt, or with the uniquely *disappearing emotion* of shame, or working with anger, which can frighten a therapist with the possibility it will get out of control. Looking specifically at each of

---

Box 6.2   EFT Tango Move 2

What is the cue?
How does it touch you?
What does your body do?
What does it say to you?
What do you do?
Now own what's true.
This is Tango Move 2.

– Adapted from B. Goettle

these emotions can help regulate an EFT therapist as they seek to help a client work at an optimum level of emotional arousal – engaged but not overwhelmed. This is also known as staying within the *window of tolerance,* a maximum level of emotional intensity that a client can tolerate without becoming numb or overwhelmed. An EFT therapist seeks to work at this manageable level of emotional depth while they order chaotic emotional experience into coherence that is emblematic of secure attachment. Although attachment science prioritizes fear as a survival emotional response, an EFT therapist begins with whatever emotion a client is presently experiencing.

Hurt

Hurt or pain, defined earlier as a mix of sadness, anger, and fear of loss, is a complex emotional experience for a clinician to distill. "Feeling hurt" is too complex to capture precise experience. An EFT therapist takes time to attune fully and help a hurting client explore the leading edge of the experience of hurt to discover if the person is closer to the angry part of hurt ("Why don't you respond to me!" or, "How dare you treat me that way!"), or the sadness aspect. ("Feeling all alone, as if I could weep for years.") Or perhaps the experience of hurt or pain is more the fearful part of dreading that one has already lost a significant other ("The sharp pain piercing through my heart that says, 'They are gone—I'm afraid I've lost them forever!'") Alternately, the fear could be a fear of loss of value. ("After that experience, I'm afraid I've lost all respect and likeability! I feel disgusting and want to disappear in shame!").

This framework of the complexity of emotional pain or hurt is helpful to EFT clinicians in that it illuminates the inner experience of some very extreme emotional action tendencies. It helps us to understand and assemble the embedded anguish and pain hiding in reactive rage, disappearing shame, and unstoppable weeping (Johnson, 2012). When Max gains enough emotional balance to explore his hatred, his feelings of "badness," and befriend his core anger towards the perpetrators of his childhood sexual abuse, he discovers grief for the childhood he lost and new, life-giving energy. His core anger does not run amok and become aggressive. He uncovers an important message that needs to be heard, "What they did was wrong!" In discovering and disclosing his anger and grief, his shame and fears lift and he discovers new motivation to engage in life.

Shame

Underlying vulnerable, core emotions have the power to create change; however, the one core emotion that an EFT therapist does not heighten is shame. Rather, shame is validated for its action tendency of hiding or disappearing. Other core emotions embedded in shame are discovered, distilled, and deepened. These emotions – core anger, fear, and sadness at loss – are safe to experience, heighten, and express. Emily validates Phil's and Julie's impulses to hide: "It feels safer to hide than to risk getting close when your survival has depended upon staying distant from others. Counting on someone else has always been hurtful, yes?" It takes a long while before Phil and Julie are able to acknowledge the pain – anger, fear, and grief – hidden within their shame. When these core emotions are discovered amidst the chaos of reactivity, they are tasted, savored, and heightened. When the anger, grief, and fear are reprocessed, shame is transformed. New core emotions, meanings, and adaptive actions emerge, replacing shame and its negative views of self and its action tendency to hide, with clarity and agency.

Max's shame and down-regulating patterns hide anger towards his childhood abuser and towards the guards in jail; they hide his fear of facing what the street-racing crash did to his friend's body; they hide his grief at how his time in jail *broke* him. Emily helps Max to face his fears, his loses, and his responsibility and in so doing, to reprocess his emotions. Encounters with imaginal others lifts his shame and gives him access to the resources of his full emotional experience. He discovers others' love and acceptance and a worthy sense of self, capable of loving others in return. Facing his fears, remorse, and responsibility for how badly his friend Léo was damaged, Max says aloud to an image of him, "What I did was wrong! I have tried to justify my actions. I've lived with this internal conflict. I was wrong. I am responsible for your death! I am so sorry!" Engaging this core emotion is an interpersonally healing experience and shame no longer mutes him nor causes him to hide.

Anger

Anger is an important emotion to befriend in EFT. "Attachment science tells us who we are and shows us how to *befriend our client's emotions* and use the power of corrective emotional experience" (italics added; Johnson & Campbell, 2022, p. 2). This is as true for anger as any emotion. Given that fear and vulnerability are often the most useful foci in creating change in EFT, EFT therapists are at risk of missing the powerful messages in clients' core anger and rushing too quickly to reframe the anger as a different, softer underlying emotion.

Following are various examples of the value of befriending anger. Attachment science normalizes reactive angry protests as an attempt to get a response from a nonresponsive attachment figure. Validating angry responses can help clients to take their own experience more seriously, to access more coherence about what is clearly wrong, and then to formulate a clear message of what they need another to hear.

EFT therapists need to attune carefully to hints of core, assertive anger. Core anger appears as part of the complex emotion of hurt and as a resource to transform shame. The value of core anger becomes very clear in EFIT, where holding others, and not self, responsible for abusive and neglectful behaviors is fundamentally important. Accessing core assertive anger takes the shape of assertive expression of needs and wants in the EFT engagement change event, such as when a withdrawn partner asserts, "Tone down your yelling and give me a chance to talk with you." Expressing core anger, while assertive, is also a vulnerable experience. (See Training Videos at www. steppingintoeft.com with Ted and Jed (pseudonyms), also available with German, Spanish and Italian subtitles; and video titled *After an Affair* with an interracial couple).

Core anger is also an important element of experiencing and reprocessing grief. Monique (pseudonym), stuck in lethargic grief and depression, is able to access life-giving grief and recover the warm connection with her deceased mother after she risks accessing and expressing her core anger at her beloved mother for dying. (Training video available at www.steppingintoeft.com.)

Therapists sometimes become anxious or judgmental when what they hear from marginalized or historically marginalized clients is not gentle or soft. In order to deeply understand our clients, we need to befriend anger and hear its message. Culturally sensitive, empathic therapists understand that when people who have had to *accommodate to survive* risk speaking up, their messages and stories have every reason to contain anger that needs to be listened to, honored, and validated, before searching for softer underlying emotions. When Wayne quotes James Baldwin, "To be a black man in America is to live in constant rage," Emily initially feels she understands that he is referring to the discrimination and injustice he lives with daily, but she quickly recognizes a huge opportunity to understand him more deeply. She pauses, "Ah, please tell me more about how that quote speaks to you…and how containing all this legitimate rage plays out in your relationship at home." EFT therapists seek to attune to hear the whole person and their entire range of reactive and core emotions. Core anger has a key message which needs to be heard if the entire person is to be deeply known and their survival strategies and patterns of emotion regulation are to be delineated.

Trauma survival strategies are far too often misrepresented as a cultural trait or as personality (Menakem, 2017) and core emotion can be missed. Hints of core anger in particular can be disregarded. P. Muhwati (2022, personal communication), born in Zimbabwe at the height of the 1970 war for liberation, describes how his people are mischaracterized as friendly, very welcoming, and very accommodating. That is not the full story, he explains. *Accommodation* in Muhwati's experience is what has been necessary for survival. He recalls his father speaking of being forced to sit at the back of the class so the white students wouldn't notice there was a black person in the class. Survival was at stake if he were to show anger for this discrimination.

Whether hearing anger from clients or warm agreement to their interventions, therapists working with people from any marginalized group need to attune carefully and check for client confirmation about the accuracy of their understanding. Therapists from dominant groups can inadvertently bypass the full story that their clients are conveying, unless they deliberately slow their pace and refrain from making assumptions and conjectures from their own personal, cultural frame of reference. "Take just a little more time to listen and to check for confirmation. Find emotional and cultural handles to invite more disclosure. Stay as close to a client's present-moment verbal and nonverbal expressions as possible," Emily reminds herself repeatedly.

Reviewing her videos, Emily is reminded of the value of listening with an open and courageous heart to validate anger. She notices her tendency to move past anger to conjecture at core fear or sadness underlying a client's anger. She sees, however, that at times she is sidestepping a client's anger for the sake of her own comfort when she might actually be disrespecting or minimizing the felt experience of the client. "If I sidestep a key part of their core experience, how can I hope to keep them coherently engaged with their experience to fully process their emotion?"

Emily recognizes that Phil has every reason to be angry, for example, that Julie is losing her eyesight. She acknowledges:

> Yes, he feels grief for her loss, and yes, he feels fear at the prospects of the future with a wife who can no longer see, but he also needs me to validate his anger when he finds himself stomping off in exasperation over the many additional tasks he now has. Anger is not his entire story, but it is a part of his present moment experience.

When each emotion within a conglomerate is named and validated, and the actions are linked to the triggers and meanings of the trigger, then the overwhelming emotional chaos *makes sense* and thus is contained and regulated. Clients "who have been violated by the very people they loved and depended on may access terror, shame, grief, and rage almost in the same moment" (Johnson, 2020, p. 205). Emily ponders:

> Phil needs me to validate his anger and his helplessness. While I may be tempted to attribute these emotions to his experience with his abusive father, he also needs me to help assemble and validate how all these emotions are also alive in his present interactions with Julie as they cope with her health crises and failing eyesight. When I am not afraid to validate his core anger in this experience of enormous loss, I help him own his anger and express it coherently.

Emily is struck with the empowerment of clear expressions and engaged encounters. Instead of getting aggressive towards Julie or withdrawing from her, Phil is able to disclose:

> Yes, I am angry about you losing your eyesight. I care a lot about you but it is a big loss for me, too. This is really making life difficult. We are not who we used to be as a couple.

Inside Emily feels herself gulping. "Is this a bullet I need to catch," she asks herself. "Do I need to protect Julie?" Before she can finish the thought, Julie sighs a huge sigh, saying:

> I am so glad you can say this Phil. I have heard you trying so hard to be stoic —heard you get frustrated —and every time I've said you seem angry at me you've denied it, yet the next moment growled with irritation. I am so relieved you can tell me you are angry about all this. I am angry, too! We can be angry together at what my failing eyesight is doing to us!

After processing the encounter with Phil and Julie, Emily celebrates with them the growing safety of being able to share their anger and grief. Her courage to listen deeply to befriend anger is bolstered. She recalls a phrase from a colleague who specializes in working with anger and aggression, "Anger is the gatekeeper to the broken heart" (J. Slootmaekers, personal communication, March, 2023). Anger definitely has adaptive action tendencies and Emily is eager to listen for them and to heighten their messages.

The more distressed a client is, the more chaotic and diffuse their emotional responses may be. Just as hurt is a complex emotion with anger in the mix, so too, do many overwhelming emotional conglomerates contain a whisper of anger that needs to be heard. When Emily validates Phil's reactive anger (stomping off in anger or raging at Julie's requests) and links these reactions to the cue of Julie's failing eyesight, his churning stomach, his meanings ("her extra demands will be endless; I am helpless to stop this from happening; I am overwhelmed and afraid I can never do enough,") they are on a path towards Phil owning his core anger and to their Stage 2 change events. "Making sense out of compelling experience makes it easier to deal with" (Johnson, 2020, p. 205). Emily is pleased to be discovering, again and again, that listening to emotion, including anger, is a reliable guide toward meeting attachment needs and creating lasting change.

In EFIT, Sahra discovers anger at her father for leaving the family – anger that she had fought to suppress for her entire life. Accessing this anger lifts her shame and sense of having somehow failed him and her mother. She is also safe with Emily to explore and distill the silent resentment she feels towards her father for the exclusion she experiences as a result of her darker-toned skin.

Culturally Sensitive EFT Interventions with Emotion

EFT therapists need to be mindful of culturally sensitive ways to use EFT interventions to assemble and deepen emotion. One of the aspects of working respectively and responsively with clients with different social locations from their therapist is to be mindful that we cannot expect to understand people's stories and life experiences until we hear their stories. It is very important not to make assumptions but to pause to invite clients to share from their perspective.

Given the wide range of intersectionalities which result in therapists and clients having many different social locations, one of the aspects of providing culturally sensitive therapy is having the humility to invite descriptions from clients before paraphrasing, reflecting or validating (F. Villodas, personal communication, October, 2022). Marginalized and historically oppressed persons live with pervasive stress alarms from experiences of discrimination. These alarms are a core part of accurately assembling their emotional experience.

Emily is overwhelmed at times with the limitless different cultural experiences she feels she needs to discover to better understand her clients, yet she is also learning that regardless of what she learns, each client is unique and she needs to hear *their* stories *from them*. Her discovery that clients frequently do not have words to describe their own experience until they engage in sharing it is giving her increasing courage to show empathic curiosity. This adds a tone of the sacred and calms her pace, as she holds the privilege of forming relationships with her clients. She is becoming gentler with her self-expectations that she should understand her clients before fully engaging with them. For example, in the past with Wayne and Jessica she would venture a reflection of what she thought they meant. She is learning that she might unintentionally be communicating a white-dominant assumption that she understands and has the words to capture their experience. Previously she felt that to be a good therapist she "ought to understand." Now she is pausing to invite clients to share more. For example, she says to Wayne, "Tell me more about what you mean when you say you pull back to avoid triggering a harm response in Jessica and getting *hit in the crossfire*." On another occasion, she says to Wayne, "Tell me more about what it means *for you* when you say you need to 'perform blackness' all day at work."

Distilling Emotion to a Coherent Core

EFT has always emphasized the importance of moving from the general to the more specific and from discussions of the past to present-moment experience (Johnson, 2004, 2020). Clients' emotional chaos becomes clearer and more manageable when we evoke, reflect, and validate, making what is vague concrete, vivid, specific and alive in the present moment, and what is external, personal. This movement from impersonal, abstract, general, external descriptions towards present-moment specificity and personal ownership is precisely what the Experiencing Scale (EXP) (Klein et al., 1969, 1986), described in Chapter 2, has shown contributes to lasting change. Specificity is also captured in Barrett's (2017) term *granularity*. She points to research showing that during times of intense distress, highly specific, granular descriptions of experience reduce neural activity, depression, anxiety, self-injury, and substance abuse. Johnson (2020) suggests that EFT therapists are *granularity experts*, noting that "the concrete and specific seems to lose its power to overwhelm or intimidate" (p. 65). The acronym RISSSSSC (Repetition, Images, Simple, Soft, Slow, Specific, Somatic, Client's words) captures how EFT therapists distill emotional experience to facilitate deeper engagement with increasingly specific, precisely formulated experience.

The therapist helps clients to deepen their level of emotional experiencing to Level 4 or 5 on the EXP (a scale measuring levels of emotional depth; Klein et al., 1969, 1986). At Level 4, clients engage with the felt flow of affective, bodily, cognitive, urge-to-action inner experience. At Level 5, new emotional depths begin to emerge, and vague, emotional experience becomes clearer, and clients appear eager to explore more. In the depths of coherent engagement with emotion at Levels 6 and 7, *felt shifts* and an increasing trust of inner experience emerge. Process of change studies in EFT (Greenman & Johnson, 2013) have found that clients who attend to their inner felt flow, experience the most change and that the change is lasting.

Cultural differences carry different rules for emotional expression that also impact information processing (Keller, 2021, 2022). Thus, it is an ever-present concern of EFT therapists to capture the specificity that accurately matches each client's experience.

Conclusion

In summary, emotion is far more than a *feeling word*. It is an active, rapidly unfolding process of distinct elements. Considering six basic emotional responses helps EFT therapists to work with emotion in a focused way, while also listening to evoke more of each client's granular emotional experience. Distinguishing between surface and core emotions helps EFT therapists to join with clients where they are. It also provides guidance on which emotions to linger with and to assemble and deepen. EFT therapists are continually sensitive to cultural differences in display and expression of emotion and are ever mindful that each client needs to be afforded the time and respect to elicit the specific image, word, and/or bodily sense to capture their unique experience of that emotion. Moving from emotional conglomerates or numbness to finer-grained emotional construc-tions empowers clients to draw upon emotion as a beacon of transformation – a reliable guide and agent of change. This overview of emotion provides the foundation for understanding how emo-tion is the target and agent of change in EFT. The positive, growth-oriented model of EFT helps clients discover how to trust core emotion as a reliable guide for creating safe relationships and reaching their therapeutic goals.

While brushing wisps of snow off her car windows after a long day of work, Emily thinks of how far she has come since she began learning EFT. As the car windows clear, she is happy to notice that her own window into emotion is also clearing:

> I've come a long way since I thought emotion equals *feelings,* and that to do EFT, I needed, most of all, to *get people to talk about feelings*. We don't *discuss* emotions, rather, we experi-ence and expand emotion in order to revise it.

Her confidence in using emotion as the target and agent of change is growing, as she is integrat-ing that emotion is a multi-faceted trigger/perception-feeling-meaning-action process. This rapid process consists of limbic perception of an external cue of safety or danger, sensing bodily arousal, cognitively assessing, and being motivated to act. She is feeling empowered and more confident to patiently assemble this process with her couple and individual clients, validating and respecting the cues which signal danger, until each client finds words for their nuanced version of attachment panic and cultural danger.

Part II
Stabilizing in Stage 1

Introduction to Part II

Stabilizing in Stage 1

[W]hen we define [love] with precision and clarity it brings us face to face with our lacks – with terrible alienation. The truth is, far too many people in our culture do not know what love is. And this not knowing feels like a terrible secret, a lack that we have to cover up. (hooks, 2001, p. 11)

With the attachment theoretical answers to, "*What is this territory called love?*" (Johnson, 2013) and "*What is optimal dependence?*" (Feeney et al., 2015), mental health professionals are afforded the clarity and acuity needed to be facilitators of lasting emotional and relational change. Love defined as *secure connection* (hooks, 2001; Johnson, 2019) is the EFT pathway out of relationship distress, depression, anxiety, and post-trauma reactions. With EFT, we have an attachment-based model, grounded in empathic understanding and responding that can shape optimal dependence and connection as the antidote to alienation and despair.

As the decade of the twenties unfolds and awareness of intersectionality and oppression abounds, the world is awakening to the need to add a caveat to our confidence in this model. The qualifier which we are adding to this reliably effective model is an empathically curious commitment to invite exploration of the racial, ethnic, and cultural (REC) impacts on clients' lives. Culturally humble invitations to explore racial-sociocultural experiences are included in Part II.

In Chapter 7, we explore the interplay between building a safe haven, secure base alliance and engaging in assessment of clients' core issues and interaction patterns. Alliance building and assessment are both needed for creating therapeutic safety and case conceptualization. This lays the groundwork for shaping the first change event – de-escalation/stabilization – discussed in Chapter 8.

To collaborate *with a couple* in Stage 1 alliance building, assessment, and de-escalation of their imprisoning pattern, a therapist needs to have their own solid felt sense of how romantic love is an attachment dance and how emotion, like music playing in the background, is an active dynamic that is both the target and agent of change. In addition, the therapist needs to be curious about how a romantic relationship is impacted by sociocultural context(s). Similarly, to collaborate *with an individual client* in early EFT sessions, a therapist needs to be grounded in an attachment view of humans as innately co-regulated with survival needs for dependency on reliable others, and to take an active interest in how each client is impacted by their sociocultural identities.

Couples and individuals discover through EFT, in an immediate and vivid way, that the real problem contributing to their distress is their present-day strategies and patterns for coping with emotional experience (Johnson, 2019). EFT therapists do not focus on historical explanations for current distress, rather, on the *circular causality* of contextual and interpersonal interactions that impact and are impacted by internal emotional experience. The systemic approach of circular causality acknowledges that clients' manner of encoding present-day experience and the strategies they develop to regulate emotion and interact with others are influenced by early experiences. The

DOI: 10.4324/9781003242673-9

availability of childhood safety and nurturance and experiences of generational oppression and trauma all impact clients' present-day patterns for interacting with selves, others, and the world.

In early sessions, an EFT therapist engages with each client to form a collaborative secure base alliance from which to explore stories of distress, lack of safety, resources, and strengths, and to formulate unmet longings and goals for therapy. The initial assessment includes delineating explicitly, the key patterns of clients' coping. From there, clients are helped to discover the deeper emotions driving these patterns and to stabilize the patterns enough to enter Stage 2 transformative change.

EFT therapists seek to befriend and become familiar with clients' patterns and strategies rather than merely label them. They want to welcome and become fully acquainted with clients' forms of engagement and patterns of anxious pursuit or avoidant withdrawal/defense or survival-necessitated down-regulation of emotions and needs that are active in the present moment with clients. Culturally sensitive EFT therapists listen to the impact of clients' contexts and seek to understand the survival nature of clients' strategies for engagement. For example, down-regulation of emotions and needs is a survival necessity for many in contexts of minority stress and marginalization. It would be unsafe to send clear messages in a social context likely to return degradation and humiliation (Hardy, 2023).

The task of an EFT therapist is not to attach finite labels such as *anxious pursuer* or *avoidant withdrawer*. It is to engage with clients in deep listening and to validate their strategies and positions in the present context. While referring to withdrawers and pursuers in EFCT, it is important to remember that these are fluid terms that represent partners' typical self-protective strategies in a particular relationship under stress but are not unchangeable styles. One is not stamped a pursuer or a withdrawer for life. The term *attachment strategies*, used in much of the adult attachment literature, implies behaviors that are specific to context; that is, in some contexts, an individual may use a secure strategy of clear reaching for support, and in other contexts may use more avoidant or anxious strategies. Repeated strategies in relationships become habitual and form self-reinforcing patterns. The term *habitual forms of engagement* (Sroufe, 1996) conveys the interpersonal nature of these strategies and patterns. "These forms of engagement can and do change when relationships [and context] change and are best thought of as continuous, not absolute (one can be more secure or less secure)" (Johnson, 2020, p. 32). EFT therapists seek to validate the strengths in all strategies – secure, anxious, avoidant, and fearful avoidant – while also guiding clients to explore "unimaginable and unthinkable…strong emotions and urges to action" and to discover the core, "frightening and/or alien and unacceptable emotions (Bowlby, 1988, p. 139) that underlie and drive these patterns.

Assessment of patterns, described in Chapter 7, is the underpinning for the deeper exploration of the core emotions driving these patterns, described in Chapter 8. Emily is coming to value, more and more, the powerful start to lasting change that happens with the first change event of stabilization (*de-escalating negative cycles of interaction*; Johnson, 2020). The main goal of Stage 1, described in the following two chapters, is to shape less reactivity and numbing so that clients stabilize their problematic patterns and attain greater emotional balance. Stage 1 sessions become a secure base where clients can explore internal and interpersonal patterns and the core, unacknowledged emotions driving these patterns. This exploration builds a secure foundation for the deeper adventures of Stage 2. Clients begin, in Stage 1, to recognize their distress as created and exacerbated by the repetitive patterns of their best attempts to manage emotions and protect important relationships. As they gradually come to accept and own their emotional experience, they are ready for Stage 2 corrective emotional experiences that reshape rigid habits and patterns into more flexible, effective ways of engaging interpersonally, internally, and with life challenges.

Emily sees, time and again, how crucial it is to have this solid foundation of Stage 1 change to make Stage 2 change possible. She appreciates how very empowering and hopeful Stage 1 stabilization can be. Valuing what she and her clients do in Stage 1, she is learning patience and trust in the model.

7 Alliance Building and Assessment as an Attachment Experience

[E]mpathic therapist responses encourage ... the wider exploration of, and closer acquaintance with, the visceral experiencing going on within. (Rogers, 1980, p. 158)

In experiential therapies, one map is the therapist's own sense of empathy...The therapist allows him- or herself to engage in the client's experience, to taste it and process it further, using his or her own emotional responses and empathy as a guide to the client's experience. The second map is the drama of positions that [clients take] in the interaction... Emotional realities are often connected with particular positions... We can then often predict a relationship stance from emotions, and inner emotions from relationship stances. (Johnson, 2020, p. 210)

In this chapter, I hold up an attachment lens for you to see and experience how attachment sculpts and forms the EFT Tango moves with which EFT therapists build a secure therapeutic alliance and begin the assessment process. Empathic exploration of clients' experiences builds alliance with respect to a trusting bond and agreement on tasks and goals. At the same time, it pulls a therapist to experientially engage with the self-protective pattern in which a couple or individual client is caught. In attempting to offer engaged, respectful, responsive presence, it is paramount that EFT therapists find the skills and comfort to mindfully acknowledge when clients' socio-racial-cultural differences or experiences of persistent oppression are beyond the therapist's empathic imagination. Empathically responsive EFT therapists need humility to invite stories of client's lived experiences before assuming they understand. They seek to offer empathic curiosity that makes it safe for clients to explore the impacts that racial, religious, and sexual-orientation oppressions are having on their emotional and relational functioning (Nightingale et al., 2019).

Alliance building and assessment are prerequisites to de-escalation/stabilization, the first change event of EFT. They are, however, active, overlapping processes that continue throughout all of therapy. In experiential therapy, change is seen to happen in session and thus treatment and assessment intertwine. Like building blocks of a secure structure, the importance of initial alliance building and assessment never wanes.

This chapter and the following four chapters have a similar format: Examining particular steps and stages of client change from the perspectives of (1) what EFT therapists see and hear during each step of clients' change process; (2) what EFT therapists do to guide clients through that step of change; and (3) *how* – the manner by which – EFT therapists interact with clients to guide them through this part of the therapeutic change process.

What EFT Therapists See and Hear in Alliance Building and Early Assessment

When joining with a couple in distress, an EFT therapist sees a dynamic of romantic love as an insecure attachment dance. The attachment lens reveals two good people caught in a negative

DOI: 10.4324/9781003242673-10

interaction cycle that is blocking them from secure connection. Joining with an individual in distress, in EFIT, a therapist similarly sees and hears longings and potential for growth and secure connection that are blocked by imprisoning patterns of protection. Through a culturally sensitive attachment lens, an EFT therapist perceives all clients' reactive behaviors and extreme emotional responses as understandable and legitimate in their relational and broader cultural context.

Bonding Mammals in Need of Connection

An attachment lens in relationship therapy reveals an insecure bond of individuals doing their best to be safe and secure with each other. It reveals partners with good intentions for the relationship inadvertently triggering one another's attachment insecurities and becoming stuck in a negative feedback loop of unclear signals and fears of loss and rejection. This view normalizes and respects seeking closeness through angry, desperate demands for a response. It also normalizes dismissively avoiding closeness when in distress or at a loss for how to respond. An attachment perspective shifts a deficit orientation regarding "neediness" or "problems with intimacy," to one of validating and normalizing human experience and longings and needs for connection.

In individual therapy as well, the attachment lens heightens the positive view of individuals as relational beings, needing others upon whom they can depend (Bowlby, 1979, 1988). *Within and between* emotional dynamics are seen to shape and be shaped by each other. Individuals are seen as continually evolving in the dramas of their intimate connections and in their larger socio-cultural context. Given the inevitable impacts of oppressive racial-socio-cultural contexts and adverse childhood trauma on the construction of self and relationships, it is especially important for EFT therapists to attend to *cultural handles* (Box 12.2) and stories of clients' unique lived experiences.

Emily notices the attachment frame has shifted her internal dialogue from implicitly asking herself, "What diagnostic factors do I see in my clients?" to viewing the context and needs for emotional and relational safety as most important in both individual therapy and couple therapy. This view sets her on a trajectory of listening with attachment-orientated, contextually sensitive curiosity to discover, for example:

> How is the relationship distress a protest against the sense of having already lost one's most important person? How is a client's depression a story of survival and resilience in the face of loss or fear of loss? How can I sensitively invite further exploration of hints of trauma, oppression, and resilience?

Different Attachment Strategies in Action

Some of the first things an EFT therapist sees and hears are markers of the different attachment strategies of anxious pursuit or avoidant withdrawal, used when a signal from a partner threatens a couple's attachment bond or when an external cue signals danger to an individual. (Box 7.1 summarizes basic strategies.) The therapist attends carefully to discern signals that trigger reactive strategies. Harsh criticism from Sophie is likely to be triggered by a signal from Ella, such as shrugging her shoulders, that Sophie perceives as indifference. Ella's shrug is likely to be triggered by a signal from Sophie that she is unhappy or annoyed. Recognizing that both strategies suggest a partner is experiencing their own form of attachment panic helps a therapist to attune with genuine, unconditional acceptance and empathy.

Markers that a partner, such as Ella, is using an avoidant attachment strategy are her dismissive tone and comments such as, "I don't see what the problem is," and, "There is no point in talking with you. All I hear is a litany of complaints!" Markers of Sophie's anxious attachment strategy are complaining statements like, "Why can't we ever sit and talk like we used to?" or more accusatory, "You never show any feelings! You are as cold as an iceberg!"

Box 7.1   Typical Attachment Strategies

An EFT therapist sees and hears characteristic signs of anxious hyperactivating or avoidant suppression of emotion. As described in Chapter 5, these are the *secondary attachment strategies* that individuals develop in the absence of a safe context or reliable "other" for co-regulation. It is important across modalities of therapy that therapists tune into these signs of hyperactivating or deactivating, as each client's strategy helps a therapist to choose interventions to heighten or to contain emotional experience. Each strategy is also validated for its strengths and costs in a client's socio-cultural context.

Anxious/Hyperactivating Strategies

A client employing a hyperactivating strategy:

- is highly aroused, agitated, vigilant for rejection or abandonment by others;
- shows high needs for support, reassurance, and contact comfort;
- is demanding, critical, readily lapsing into despair in response to others' lack of response;
- may interrupt narrative with sighs, tears;
- hyperactivates attachment fears and needs.

Examples: "No one understands me, no one is there for me." "I'll never survive this disaster!" "I am in pain all the time, crying out for help at every turn and nobody notices." "Everyone has better things to do than be my friend." "My heart is breaking... no one listens." "No one has ever been there for me."

Avoidant/Deactivating Strategies

A client using a deactivating strategy:

- displays a sense of stoicism and independence;
- is concerned with performance and success;
- shows little affect, with speech distant from their experience, not alive or fresh;
- has a robust voice quality and appears resilient, confident, and strong;
- dismisses, suppresses, minimizes, and disregards their own and others' attachment needs and fears;
- avoids close relationships.

Examples: "I'm fine. There is no problem. I don't need anyone or anything." "I've gotten by this far, and I can manage on my own." "I don't need anyone's help!" "Why bother? All I ever hear is that I am not good enough" (individually or culturally). "I don't feel anything at all, really. Just numb."

Fearful-avoidant Strategies

A client applying a fearful-avoidant strategy:

- shows a mixture of anxious hyperactivating and avoidant deactivating;

- is using a strategy common in trauma survivors where others have been both a source of hurt and comfort;
- conveys a sense of push-pull, flipping between wanting interpersonal closeness and loathing or mistrusting it;
- may have a fragile voice, with an externalizing quality, interrupted by tears, numbing, and detachment.

Examples: "I'll never get a promotion – everyone is against me so I'll just settle for this damn job." "I may as well give up – no one cares." "What does it matter anyway? Nobody gets it." "Nobody cares, and if they act like they do, they always hurt me in the end anyway, but I'm fine." "Everyone kicks me when I'm down. I keep looking for someone to recognize my accomplishments, but I don't trust them."

Noticing different strategies in couple and individual clients, Emily ponders two elements that cast all attachment strategies in a welcome, positive light. Instead of perceiving anxiety and avoidance as pathological, she appreciates that the secure attachment strategy of reaching clearly to another when in need is not the only valuable strategy. She recalls Bowlby (1980) highlighting that the *secondary strategies* – anxious, avoidant, and fearful-avoidant – can also be useful at times and that flexibility with strategies to fit the context is valuable. Second, she pauses to attend with humility and curiosity to the contexts where clients have needed survival strategies that became their default survival patterns across contexts. She is learning from black and brown colleagues and attachment scholars that, "historically, Black people have been expected to suppress their emotions as a survival tool during various articulations of White terrorism (e.g., the transatlantic slave trade, Jim Crow, and even presently as White supremacists and police target them)" (Causadias et al., 2021, p. 3). She recognizes the strength and resilience, as well as the personal and relational costs, for example, in the *strong black woman* stereotype and in the immigrant experience that leaves no room for grieving the homeland, but pressures people to *put the past aside and appreciate their new home.*

The Real Problem as a Self-Reinforcing Pattern

In early sessions of alliance building and assessment Emily sees and hears bonding mammals in need of connection, employing different attachment strategies that have both utility and personal and relational costs. The third element she sees and hears is that the clients' real problem is their self-reinforcing pattern of interaction.

EFT therapists witness the real problem in client distress to be not in a person, but in a feedback loop of distress that then creates more distress. Various examples of the cyclical dynamic appear in couples: The more avoidant, dismissive or defensive one partner appears, the more anxious and desperate for response the other partner becomes, and *vice versa*, in a continuous feedback loop. Understanding this dynamic gives Emily a clear picture of how each partner's reactions are legitimate responses to a sense that his or her primary relationship is under threat. Additionally, there is an interplay between self-reinforcing patterns of attachment strategies for survival and differing survival responses to racial and cultural danger cues. For example, what emerges for Wayne and Jessica is that the code switching and accommodating that Wayne needs to do to be safe in the business world carries over into their relationship. He continues to hold himself back with Jessica, as well as in his work relationships, and the more Jessica complains about his holding back, the more his marriage starts to feel unsafe like the rest of the world. The complexity of clients' self-reinforcing interaction patterns is intensified by contextual variables. Identifying the survival patterns *in context* is the first step toward change in EFT.

Each of Emily's couples have their own identifiable cycle: Wayne and Jessica are caught in a pursue–withdraw cycle. Parents of an eight-year-old son and two preschool-age daughters, Wayne identifies as black with Ethiopian descent and Jessica, with very light skin, as Hispanic, a child of a white father and a mother of Indigenous-African heritage from Argentina. Jessica anxiously, and sometimes angrily, seeks Wayne's response when he seems emotionally unavailable. Wayne then puts up a wall of silence and hides from what he perceives to be her criticisms and demands. The added complexity in their pursue–withdraw cycle is that Jessica *turtles* when Wayne appears agitated. He becomes frustrated when Jessica becomes non-responsive to him in her self-protective turtle shell (see Figure 7.1).

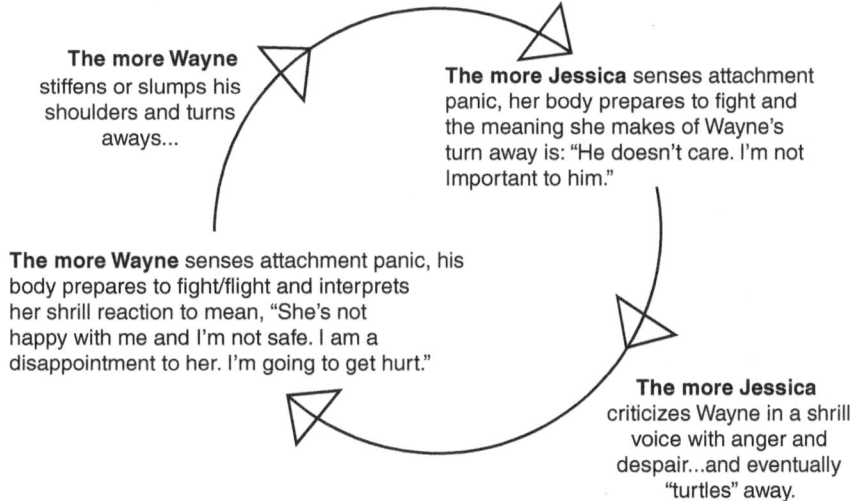

Figure 7.1 Emily's Visualization of Wayne and Jessica's Pursue/Withdraw Pattern.

Sophie and Ella, cisgender women, identifying as Caucasian and Chinese, respectfully, are caught in attack–attack sequences they call the *raging storm*, where the more panicked and desperate for connection Sophie becomes, the louder she gets. Ella becomes explosive in self-defense, ready to fire back as soon as she senses more demands from Sophie that suggest to her that she is a totally disappointing partner. She frequently storms out of the room. They experience homophobic judgment, particularly from Sophie's conservative, white family. Despite their attack–attack sequences, Sophie's pursuit and Ella's defensive withdrawal are becoming clearer to Emily.

The *frozen lake* cycle of Julie and Phil, dissatisfying to both of them, is also understandable and legitimate when viewed through Emily's attachment glasses. She sees a withdraw–withdraw cycle of two abuse survivors. Both were raised in poor, working-class, white families where alcohol abuse and violence were the norm. Julie, on hyper-alert for signals from Phil that he is about to distance emotionally or be angry with her, freezes, hoping not to make any moves that will send him away. Phil, sensing her caution as disinterest in him, throws up his hands in silent frustration

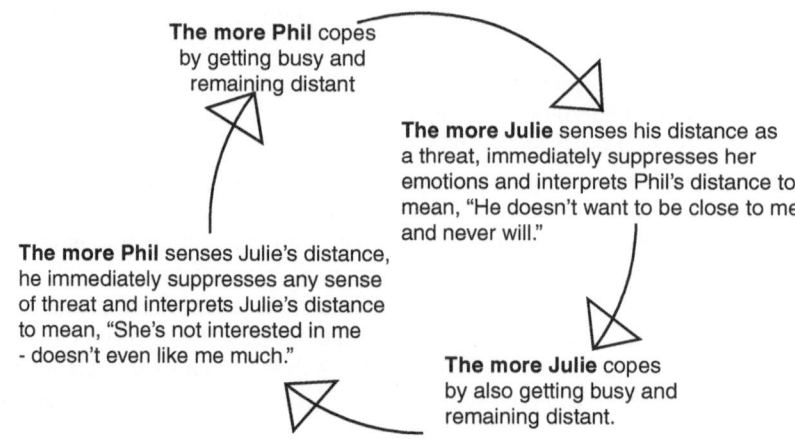

The more Phil copes by getting busy and remaining distant

The more Julie senses his distance as a threat, immediately suppresses her emotions and interprets Phil's distance to mean, "He doesn't want to be close to me and never will."

The more Phil senses Julie's distance, he immediately suppresses any sense of threat and interprets Julie's distance to mean, "She's not interested in me - doesn't even like me much."

The more Julie copes by also getting busy and remaining distant.

Figure 7.2 Emily's Visualization of Phil and Julie's Withdraw/Withdraw Pattern.

and busies himself with his solitary activities. Both live in terror of being hurt by closeness, and at the same time, fear they might lose the other. Withdrawal is the position each one takes in their interactive cycle. See Figure 7.2

Box 7.2 describes the typical patterns traditionally considered to be the problem in EFCT. With the growing awareness of the significant impacts of race and cultural marginalization, expanded attention is being paid to the interplay between regulation patterns and racial/cultural cues of threat (Guillory, 2022). Working with Jessica and Wayne, and consulting regularly with an expert on cultural competence in therapy, Emily is learning that it is not enough to simply identify a couple's repetitive "the more you… the more I…" pattern. She must also attend to how Jessica's lighter skin allows her to dismiss the discrimination that Wayne regularly experiences out in the world. It is not uncommon for Jessica to downplay the threats he experiences at every turn in the *world.* Wayne's bowing his head in defeat at never being safely understood happens outside in the world at large and it also happens with his wife. "Don't let it get to you so much!" says Jessica in a session as Wayne describes a moment of racial aggression in the office. Emily slows down the process and helps Jessica to discover that her outbursts at Wayne for more closeness and intimacy feel similar to threats he lives with every moment in the outside world. With this discovery, Jessica is mortified and motivated to do everything she can to change her step in their repetitive pattern.

Emily's individual clients also have identifiable recurring patterns of emotion regulation (see Box 7.3). Max, self-identifying as neurodiverse, grew up in Spain until his early teens, at which time he moved back to the United States. He calls his pattern *cognitive dissonance* and describes a lifetime of avoiding and pushing bothersome things into the background. He also carries many regrets for his outbursts of anger that he has dismissed from memory, but which family members recall vividly, recounting stories of turbulence that he created on family vacations. He describes having packed much of his life into a box, so that he feels he is a *monster in a box.* Emily's visualization of Max's pattern is seen in Figure 7.3. She honors that within Max's pattern of avoidance are some very adaptive survival strategies and that some of these strategies are shared by others on the autistic spectrum. She sees how this pattern reinforces his internal working model (IWM) of self as a damaged, harmful person. The "nugget" of gold in the center of her diagram, represents Max's difficult and frightening emotions, which Emily also sees as valuable core emotions that will be reprocessed and transformed, later, in Stage 2.

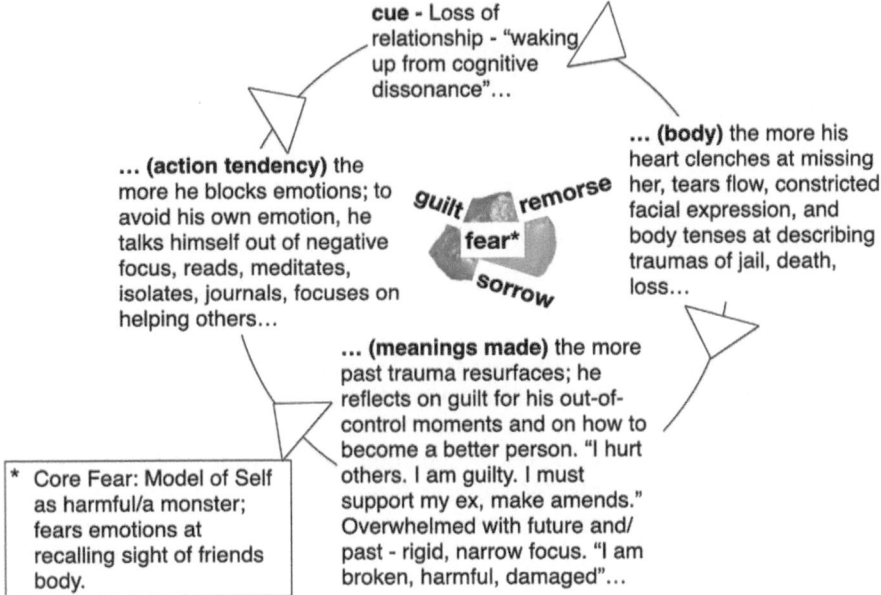

Figure 7.3 Emily's Visualization of Max's Repetitive Pattern.

Box 7.2   Typical Rigidly Recurring Patterns between Partners in EFCT

Pursue–withdraw. The critical, demanding pursuits of a more anxious pursuer trigger avoidance and distancing in the other partner. Distancing and avoidance trigger more anxious and critical pursuit. In a typical pursue–withdraw cycle, a critical pursuer (using an anxious attachment strategy) may say, "Even when they are home, they can't be found. I can never reach them or get them to really listen to me at all." A typical withdrawer (using an avoidant strategy) is likely to say, "I wish we could just have peace and get along, but they are always upset about something."

Attack–attack sequences. In what appears to be an attack–attack cycle, there is most likely to be an attack that is code for pursuing for connection and an attack that is a more defensive avoidance of intimacy and protection against criticism and demands. In spite of vocal protests from both partners, there is likely to be one partner who tends to use a more anxious attachment strategy, hyperactivating and exaggerating their attachment needs and relentlessly pursuing connection. This can then trigger the more avoidant partner to turn and fight back in self-protection mode. The more avoidant partner, although fighting in defense, continues to minimize and dismiss their own and others' attachment needs.

Withdraw–withdraw. Typically, one avoidant partner is slightly less avoidant than the other. Both partners default to avoidant positions of not counting on or trusting the other to be there for them. Withdraw–withdraw couples seldom argue and seldom get close. Some have occasional blow-ups when an emotionally raw spot is touched – one partner hears criticism or discontent from the partner and reacts in self-defense.

Reactive cycle. Positions of pursuit and withdrawal can morph over time. Following a long history of pursue–withdraw, a pursuer could burn out from desperately seeking response and step back, prompting the former withdrawer to become alarmed at the change and to begin pursuing to keep from losing their partner. Tracking the present cycle will make it possible to discover if these positions shift as the safety increases.

Complex cycles are common with trauma survivors where both anxiety and avoidance are high. The positions of pursuit and withdrawal flip back and forth. With fearful avoidance as a survival strategy, one fears that the very one on whom they rely for comfort and support is also the one who is likely to hurt them the most. In these complicated cycles, the pursuer and withdrawer appear to randomly shift positions. Pursuers might withdraw when connection is offered because it is not trusted. Withdrawers can become anxious and demanding when the other partner does not respond. Here, we see multi-move cycles and complicated sequences.

Box 7.3   Typical Emotion Regulation Patterns in Individuals: Depathologizing Anxiety and Depression as *Patterns for Emotion Regulation*

Attachment theory as a theory of emotion regulation recognizes three basic strategies for regulating emotion when in distress (Mikulincer & Shaver, 2016). The primary and considered to be the most effective pattern is the secure strategy of clear reaching to an accessible and responsive attachment figure. Our mammalian nervous systems are wired for safe and secure interpersonal connection; however, unfortunately for many, this is not available. The secondary strategies typically used in the contextual and interpersonal absence of a secure base of support and caring are anxious hyperactivating and avoidant deactivation.

Sahra is caught in a fearful-avoidant cycle. "What's the point in noticing my pain?" she wonders. "It will just hurt more, and no one cares to listen anyway!" she exclaims. She pushes for responses from friends and family, then retreats in frustration and fear of getting hurt or being disappointed. Becoming familiar with key figures that populate a client's world helps Emily to see similar patterns across relationships. There is no clear, reliable other for Sahra. Repeated attempts for response from her attachment figures – father, mother, brother, and ex-partner – have been disappointing at best and blatantly hurtful at worst. Her attempts to get respect and kindness from her graduate advisor have also been to no avail. Every day she fights against the impacts of colorism: "the allocation of privilege and disadvantage according to the lightness or darkness of one's skin" (Burke & Embrich, 2008, p. 17). In response to racial discrimination and colorism distress cues that she faces daily in the medical school and in her work at the hospital, she *wears the mask of a smile* (Angelou, 1987; Harrell, 2010) and shudders with the weariness of racial battle fatigue in private – tension headaches, jumpiness, and elevated blood pressure (Burton et al., 2010; Smith et al., 2011).

The expansion of EFT to explicitly honor the rainbows of racial-socio-cultural diversity, throws wide open any tendency to categorize the primary attachment strategy of secure reaching and responding as superior to the secondary strategies. Hyperactivation and deactivation for emotion regulation and interpersonal functioning are honored as survival necessities in unsafe contexts of oppression and discrimination and in the absence of an interpersonal secure base of support and caring. It is never a therapist's role to try to remove self-protective strategies. For survivors of trauma, including all forms of socio-racial-cultural discrimination (historical and present-day), it is a very sobering reality that one's survival depended upon, and may still require deactivation and suppression. EFT therapists are committed to attuning and evoking the unique stories and experiences of each client with deep respect that the coping strategies they are using have validity and value. At the same time, they are willing to collaboratively explore with their clients the costs of their default self-protective survival patterns, within and between, and to help them explore safe contexts and relationships to reshape these patterns. Chapter 7 Support Material (routledge.com/9781032151335) contains several clinical examples of individual clients' nuanced versions of these secondary attachment strategies and patterns, vividly portrayed with their spontaneous, poignant images and emotional handles.

The Depathologizing Attachment View of Emotional Distress

In the scenario of what an EFT therapist sees and hears in assessment and alliance building, there are bonding mammals in need of connection, different attachment strategies in action, and repetitive interaction patterns as the real problem. The depathologizing attachment view of emotional distress adds a refreshing hue to this picture. Anxiety, depression, post trauma reactions and relational distress are de-stigmatized within an attachment orientation. Bowlby (1980) claimed that all manners of coping with life events and the resulting frightening and/or alien and unacceptable emotions have their merits but can become problematic when a client gets stuck in rigid applications that are no longer relevant to the context. He writes that "loss and disappointment are the central features of most events bringing about clinical depression" (p. 254), suggesting that "hope, fear, anger, satisfaction, frustration or any combination of these may be experienced" (p. 246), but that it is when supportive interactions with others have ceased that depression, disorganization, helplessness, loneliness, and a sense of being unwanted and unloved occurs and continues until new patterns of interacting have been created.

An EFT therapist is more focused on validating clients' evolving personhoods and attuning to within-between patterns and views of self and other, than on specific diagnostic categories (Johnson, 2019). With this focus in mind, Johnson discovered a close companion for EFT's growth-oriented attachment frame of depression and anxiety in Barlow's Unified Protocol of Emotional Disorders (UP) (Barlow et al., 2018). UP stands in contrast to the traditional symptom-focused psychotherapeutic diagnoses of mental disorders in the DSM-5-TR (American Psychiatric Association, 2022), suggesting there are many features (or symptoms) common across diagnoses, and that overwhelming negative experiences and a sense of the world as dangerous and threatening are at the core of all disorders. Barlow's emotional-process-perspective on emotional distress has become a staple of EFIT assessment and case formulation (Johnson, 2019) (see Box 7.4).

Box 7.4   Key Elements of Emotional Disorders

EFIT draws upon elements identified in the Unified Protocol of Emotional Disorders (UP) (Barlow et al., 2018) to be common across emotional disorders:

- Frequent strong, intense, unwanted, unclear emotions, e.g., fear, loneliness, sense of isolation, loss, fear of death.
- Intensifying negative reactions and attributions to strong, unwanted emotions, e.g., critical of self, negative views of self as unwanted, helpless, unlovable, a failure; isolate selves, experience vigilance, fear of fear itself; fears intensify to panic proportions.
- Efforts to dampen down, suppress, or control these emotions tend to backfire, making symptoms worse.
- Socio-cultural context impacts the presentation and client experience of all the above, e.g., somatic complaints, appropriateness of being assertive.

Impacts of the Socio-cultural Context

The final element to consider in the scenario of what an EFT therapist sees and hears in alliance building and assessment is the frame in which the picture is held and the canvas on which is it painted. The frame represents the racial-socio-cultural context and the canvas, the lived experience of each couple and each individual.

When an EFT therapist engages with cultural sensitivity, they see and hear resourceful survivors telling finely nuanced stories of their lived experiences. A culturally humble lens reveals impacts of intergenerational trauma and marginalization on clients' emotional and relational safety. Therapists attune to times when clients downplay the acts of exclusion and aggression. When they detect subtle doorways or hints of oppression, they invite a client to explore how this may be part of an imprisoning pattern.

In summary, what an EFT therapist sees and hears from an attachment perspective in early sessions of couple and individual therapy are bonding mammals needing secure connection; different attachment strategies for emotion regulation in increasingly rigid, recursive patterns; the real problem as an iatrogenic pattern, causing and being caused by emotional distress; a strength-based attachment view of emotionally distressed individuals; and various contextual impacts on emotional and relational experiences.

In early EFCT sessions, a therapist sees partners unwittingly caught in a repetitive cycle that intensifies problematic behaviors and underlying fears of loss. Partners are sending unclear signals to each other about their needs for connection and support. Signals are mistaken to mean, "You will leave me," or, "You will reject me." A therapist sees different self-protective attachment strategies of pursuing and withdrawing as indications that each partner must be perceiving a threat to their bond, while remaining mostly unaware of attachment needs and fears within self and in the other. Critical pursuit is seen as code for an underlying desperation to obtain a response. Numbness and apparent nonchalance are seen to be concealing a sense of being overwhelmed, at a loss for how to respond and protect self, other, and the relationship.

Similarly, in early EFIT sessions, therapists notice that individuals' suffering is shaped by their strategies of anxious hyperactivating or/and deactivating suppression to regulate difficult, unfamiliar, or unacceptable emotions in the absence of contextual safety and interpersonal support and connection. With the depathologizing focus of attachment theory, a struggling individual is seen in a positive light, with strengths and growth-oriented potential, not as deficient or to blame for their distress.

What EFT Therapists Do to Build Alliance and Begin Assessment

The simple answer to what EFT therapists do in early sessions is that they use all moves of the Tango; however, Move 1, reflecting present process, is especially important for alliance formation and for shaping the therapy process as a collaborative endeavor where clients experience agency and feel valued and respected for who they are. An EFT therapist leads and follows clients with Move 1 as they form a collaborative alliance, share their story, identify goals for therapy, and put words to the repetitive pattern that is blocking them from their longings. In addition to micro-interventions of empathic reflection, tracking, validation, and some evocative questions, there are occasions that a therapist will contain escalation by *catching bullets*.

Reflecting present process (EFT Tango Move 1), EFT therapists seek to enter the experience of each client, to help them formulate their understanding and experience of their relationship (couples) or of their emotional distress (individuals). The story telling or dialogue facilitated by Move 1 is a powerful process because it gives clients an opportunity to formulate their chaotic or rigid moment-to-moment experience in a way that makes sense and feels understandable and relevant to their socio-cultural context. EFT therapists explicitly track with clients the recurring sequences of interactions that perpetuate their distress. They also identify positive patterns of interaction where clients reach for and respond to another's need for support and comfort. Reflection, validation, and tracking are used more than questions.

EFT interventions, beginning with the empathic attunement, reflection, validation, and evocative responding of Move 1, can be a consistently reliable guide. Move 1 has the flexibility to deliberately welcome racial and cultural diversity (Nightingale et al., 2019). Curiosity of how experiences of marginalization or privilege affect the therapeutic relationship and clients' survival strategies and patterns of interacting and regulating distress keeps the within/between dynamic consciously embedded in the client's socio-cultural context.

Building and maintaining a therapeutic alliance and collaborating with clients for assessment and treatment are continuous and overlapping processes. The first concerns are to help clients to feel safe and to guide them to clearly formulate their hopes and goals for therapy. In early EFT sessions, therapists draw on the acronym of C.A.R.E. (Furrow et al., 2022) to guide their use of Move 1. They attune to and evoke experience regarding the overlapping aspects of **C**ontextual impacts on emotional and interpersonal experience (traditions, values, trauma), **A**ttachment strategies and patterns, **R**elationships (including the therapeutic alliance) and the nuanced experience and expression of **E**motion. This is similar to the E.A.R. of empathic attunement in Box 1.3.

Emily was initially overwhelmed by the many factors she needs to consider for building and strengthening the alliance and doing assessment in EFT: Broach social-cultural-racial identities; explicate engagement strategies and the within/between patterns; pinpoint strengths and competencies in relationship bonds and coping strategies; take note of factors that can interfere with a working alliance or contraindicate therapy; consider a host of different areas for assessment, such as sources of comfort, addictive processes, sex, violence, and more; form an informal therapy agreement; balance process and content and identify the basic repetitive pattern as the problem! "OMG!" Emily says, over and over to herself on an exceptionally slow drive home with multiple detours through street construction sites. Catching her breath, she recalls several new couples and individuals with whom she is forming alliances and beginning assessment. "I haven't discussed nearly all these topics for assessment with everyone yet!" she gasps. She takes comfort, however, in her attuned engagement and deliberate slow pacing with clients through the EFT Tango. "Some of the elements they have responded to on their intake forms; some I will revisit or introduce as we move along."

Emily slows with the traffic. Typically impatient with congested traffic, she takes a deep inhale. *Slowing down:* This is an essential element of culturally humble, collaborative therapy. "Slowing down is what I need to *level the power dynamic* (Seiff-Haron & Calamur, 2022) to truly work collaboratively with my clients." *Slowing down is a process of decolonization* (Guillory et al., 2022). With growing confidence, Emily ponders:

> The humanity and flexibility of the EFT model encourages me to trust my interactions with my clients, including persistent and patient pacing for broaching topics along the way. We are unfolding this assessment/treatment process together, and with Tango Moves 4 and 5, I am getting client feedback that can strengthen our working relationship. We validate their resilience and summarize their experiences at the end of each session.

The following activities in the alliance/assessment interplay are not administered chronologically but are woven into conversations as needed. As this overview attests, alliance building, assessment and treatment are inextricably intertwined in EFT. Emily repeats a little mantra to herself, "Attunement is foundational to forming a safe haven alliance of comfort and trust and a secure base for exploring clients' most vulnerable emotions that drive their ways of engaging and interacting in life."

Build a Safe-Haven, Secure-Base Alliance

The first concern in early EFT sessions is to help people feel safe and to guide them to clearly formulate their hopes and desired outcomes (goals) for therapy. From the first moment of meeting a couple or an individual, EFT therapists seek to create safety and to set the stage for a working alliance and ongoing collaborative assessment. Near the opening of Emily's first sessions with couple or individual clients, she is transparent in stating that she wants to hear the clients' hopes for therapy, acknowledging that, of course with couples, they may have different hopes and perspectives and that it will be important to hear from each of them. She is focused on building a trusting relationship where clients feel heard and seen and valued for who they are.

EFT clinicians are particularly attuned to how an attachment lens with culturally attuned humility can help to normalize and make order out of a distressed drama of hostility and shutting down that couples frequently demonstrate. Likewise, the attachment lens, which validates all coping strategies, can help a therapist to normalize and bring relief to individual clients' emotional distress and disorders. A culturally humble attachment frame guides the therapist in alliance formation and treatment planning in a way that is consonant with Rogerian unconditional acceptance and positive view of human nature. It depathologizes the assessment process and creates a safe haven of support and a secure base to explore and reshape individual and relationship distress. "I am afraid if I tell Wayne about my pain and loss, it will push him away," says Jessica, stoically determined not to show her vulnerabilities. Emily attunes to *racial stress cues* from outside the relationship that bleed into the cycle as Wayne sighs, "At work I have to perform blackness all day. When I come home, I brace for more tension. I don't burden her with my workday but if I make the wrong move, she overreacts and shuts me out."

When Sahra, in EFIT, describes "keeping many stories of exclusion boxed up and out of sight," Emily respects Sahra's way of coping with experiences of exclusion and discrimination. She stays close to Sahra and as much of her story that she is willing to share, while also expressing empathic curiosity to hear the struggles of immigrating and living in a society that mistreats people of color. Underlying emotions frequently seem too dangerous or unacceptable, to explore (Bowlby, 1988). To help Sahra to feel safe to explore her experiences of exclusion when she is ready, Emily shares:

> You found ways to pack up those unfair experiences of being excluded (adding "unfair" to heighten respect and validation). I know something of living with exclusion with neurodiversity in my family, and I want to offer you a safe place to share your stories when you are ready. Your experiences, though undoubtedly very different from mine, are something I am very open to hearing about anytime.

Broach Different Social Identities

Broaching racial issues in therapy can begin in the first session but it is never too late to start the conversation, suggests Williams (2020). Guillory (2022) and Guillory et al. (2022) do not recommend leading with these discussions but may add something in their descriptions of the therapy process and will respond openly throughout therapy as issues arise. Williams makes the following suggestions for broaching that are respectful, gentle, and forthright. [My comments follow in parentheses.]

- Ask clients to share something about their cultural heritage that they want us to know. [Optionally, ask clients to share about what makes them unique.]
- Invite them to share about experiences with racism – inquire, for example, about how much racism they have to deal with in the workplace. [A potentially less intrusive invitation could be to inquire about experiences of exclusion or mistreatment.]

- Acknowledge and apologize for microaggressions you may commit. For example, "I don't understand your culture as much as I'd like to. If I have said things that were insensitive or even hurtful without realizing it, please let me know and if it happens in the future, I'd appreciate if you'd let me know." [This is a kind sentiment. At the same time, a therapist needs to attune sensitively to each client, knowing they may be very reluctant to talk about a hurtful moment or a *subtle act of exclusion* (Jana & Baran, 2020).]
- Open the door for a client to share about their experiences of mistreatment by describing one's own experience of feeling ignored or dismissed, even if it is not related to race. [Draw on personal experiences of exclusion if available.]
- Check at the end of the session about client satisfaction and their sense of feeling understood, including their experience of your cultural sensitivity to difference. [Invite clients' perspective when summarizing in Move 5.]

Much multi-cultural literature (Davis et al., 2018) suggests that key elements to being a culturally humble therapist are, first, having the skills and openness to welcome and invite discussions of racial-socio-cultural influences and second, being comfortable and ready to be transparent with one's own social identities and experiences as are relevant to the clients. Day-Vines et al. (2020) suggest that broaching REC differences is an important element throughout therapy in order to maintain or repair the therapeutic alliance. It is a way to continually acknowledge the impact of socio-cultural minority stressors on relational and emotional health and to acknowledge the "reality that many have experienced hate-based discrimination and violence" (Allan et al., 2022, p. 66).

Emily realizes that she and her clients may have some very different life experiences and identities that can limit her understanding of their experiences. She also recognizes that racial identity development is dynamic and shifts across time and relationships. She is eager to create enough safety and sufficiently explicit invitations for her clients to help her fully understand what is important to them. Having repeated conversations and consultations with colleagues from different socio-cultural identities and attending ongoing *diversity, equity, and inclusion* (DEI) trainings are ways Emily seeks to become a more culturally humble, sensitive EFT therapist.

Hinson and James (October 2022) suggest a therapist explicitly acknowledge that given different lived experiences and different racial identities, we are likely to see the world through different lenses and to be treated differently in the outside world. They emphasize making an open invitation that any exploration of different lived experiences and different racial identity experiences are welcome any time. This open invitation can be given clearly many times throughout therapy, whenever the therapist sees hints of cultural impacts. Whether or not clients respond to the invitation, the significance of the therapist noticing cannot be overstated. Clients will hear the invitation and will feel seen and thus safer to be themselves with a therapist who continues to hear hints of cultural handles and gently taps on the door. In fact, Hinson and James suggest that failure to acknowledge difference can be experienced as a microaggression. "All people of color experience microaggressions – whether or not they recognize it – and as a good therapist you want to understand how your clients have been managing them" (Williams, 2020, p. 101). Williams suggests that clients' harmful coping with microaggressions can range from "denial, substance-abuse, aggression, self-blame, self-harm, and even suicide attempts" (p. 101).

On her life history intake form and in early EFT sessions, Emily invites clients to share the identities they feel are important for her to know about them. She discloses a welcome and eagerness to hear how their identities and life experiences may be different from hers, and in couple therapy, how they may also be different from each other. Emily notices a tinge of appreciation from her clients when she acknowledges a difference of sexual orientation or racial background, "I want you to know I'm comfortable discussing our differences and hope you feel free to tell me if I don't seem to fully understand your experience."

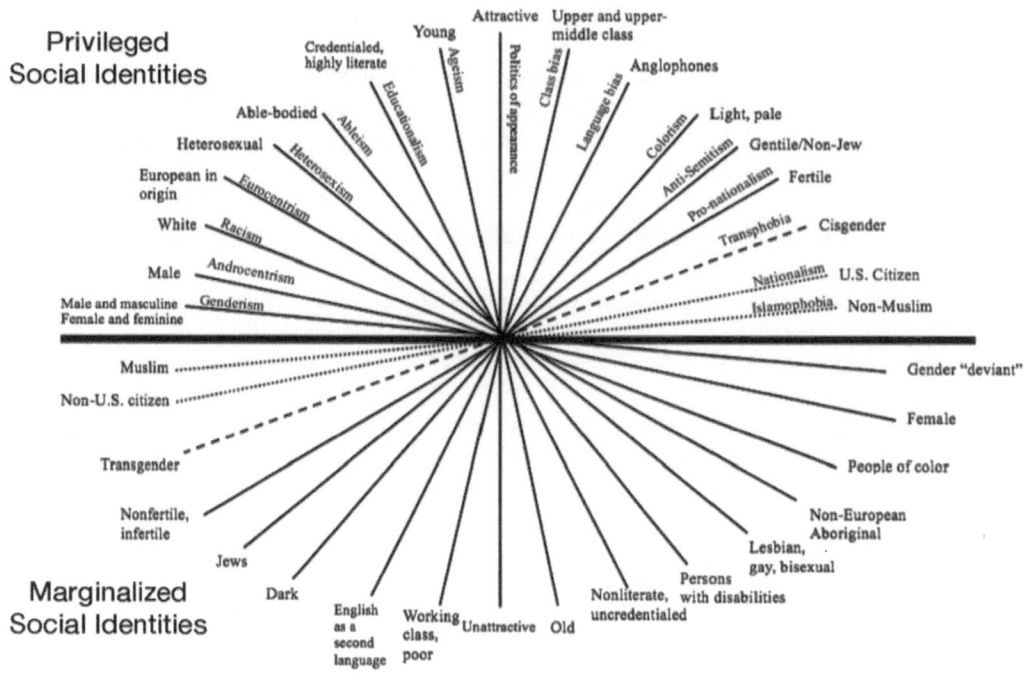

Figure 7.4 Intersecting Axes of Privilege, Domination, and Oppression.

Examine One's Own Identities

Emily is well aware that intersections of therapist and client identities can impact the therapeutic alliance, and the way differing identities are addressed or avoided in therapy can open or block the conversations clients need to have. She spends time reflecting upon and discussing with colleagues the intersecting identities of privilege, domination, and oppression as portrayed in PettyJohn et al. (2020) (see Figure 7.4).

Awareness of one's own identities of privilege and marginalization is imperative to finding the courage and comfort to broach social identities in therapy. As EFT therapists seek to create welcoming spaces for clients to explore emotional expression and attachment behaviors that are fitting to their culture, it behooves every EFT therapist to examine their own social locations and identities that shape how they engage internally and interpersonally.

To be culturally humble and sensitive, EFT therapists make room for key stories of clients' lived experiences. They are mindful that experiences of difference or marginalization are not always obvious. They invite clients to share their identities and experiences that are important to them and are willing to provide their own social locations as relevant to client's situation and interest. For example, in seeking to be transparent and to validate the silent grief Emily senses in some immigrant clients, she says:

> I have lived in North America all my life so I have no lived experience of leaving my home country to make a foreign country my home. I know a tiny bit about feeling excluded as a parent of special needs children who were not included by their peers, but I have no experience of fleeing danger, coming to a new country and never finding a safe place to discuss how much I miss my homeland.

Identify Attachment Strategies for Engaging

EFT therapists listen for client's manner of engaging with the therapist and their descriptions of how they engage with key figures in their world (as described in Box 7.1). In couple therapy, they witness the strategies in action between partners and with the therapist. In EFIT, they experience the strategies while interacting *with* the client and hear strategies in how they speak about others.

The manner in which a client tells their story can inform the therapist about clients' strategies for engaging. A therapist can get a felt sense of whether the client is hyperactivating their emotions to cope, dismissing them to "get over them," or flipping between the two attachment strategies of anxious hyperactivation or avoidant deactivation. Coherent organized narratives with specific details, where the storyteller shows emotion in the telling, is a sign of security and strength. Clients who are experiencing overwhelming anxiety and hyperactivation are likely to tell extremely fragmented stories, fast-paced, jumping from topic to topic, with bursts of emotion. Clients who tell robotic, almost impersonal narratives, skimming the surface and recounting what sound like painful events without reflection or engagement are likely to be coping by deactivating and avoiding emotion.

Identifying attachment strategies for engaging helps an EFT therapist in several ways. It helps them choose whether to heighten or contain emotion. Clients who default to anxious, hyperactivation need to be calmed and contained to access coherent emotional experience; clients who default to avoidant over-regulating, or deactivating need acceptance and validation to awaken and heighten awareness of their emotional experience.

Anxious, avoidant, and fearful-avoidant coping strategies all serve to maintain a person's distance from their core, inner experience. Thus, identifying each person's typical attachment strategy helps a therapist more fully empathize with clients' experience and their working models of self, other, and the world and to identify their recurring behavioral patterns.

Grasping Sahra's fearful-avoidant strategy, Emily says in an early session:

> Before you turn away and buckle down in isolation, you make great efforts to get the kind of responses you long for and deserve from each of them – your mother, your brother, your ex-partner, and your graduate advisor, yes? Internally you are crushed. Each time it confirms a sense that there is no one you can depend on. No one who simply sees your goodness and seems to care, yes? Pushing, moving towards them. Backing away in defeat. Just safer on my own, yes?

"That's it. Yes, that's it!" Sahra says with a deep sigh. "You make it sound like it actually makes sense. Like you understand my losing battle!"

Interpersonal strategies tend to mirror the internal strategies a client uses to engage with their own emotions. Strategies reveal how clients deal with vulnerability, fears, unmet needs, longings, and sense of attachment threat. Do they heighten the sense of threat, or do they do their best to ignore it? Sophie engages with hyperactivation and increasing panic about getting Ella's love and care; internally a similar flood of worries about her competence and worth spirals out of control. In contrast, Ella, suffers from persistent stomach aches, but when it comes to Sophie's demands and her own worries, she pushes them aside. "Can't do much about it so I'll just ignore it and move on."

Attuning to clients' narratives gives a therapist a window into the client's IWMs of self and other, including how they experience their socio-cultural world. Client's stories are very likely to convey the dominant models of self ("Am I loveable, worthy and competent?") and of other ("Are others reliable, trustworthy, and responsive?"). The model of other extends beyond relationships to the broader context ("Is my context culturally safe for me?"). Anxious strategies are usually associated with a positive view of other, ("If you respond to me, I will be fine,") and a negative view of self, ("I am unworthy, unlovable, and incompetent without you.") Avoidant strategies are associated with a pseudo positive sense of self, ("I'm fine on my own, thank you – though I need to keep producing to prove I am this great,") and negative view of other, ("Others are unreliable and hurtful.") Fearful avoidance is associated with a negative view of self and a confused model of other, ("Sometimes good, yet unreliable and sometimes hurtful and abandoning.") (Mikulincer & Shaver, 2016).

Repeated survival strategies form recurring patterns. Recurring patterns of well-intentioned strategies ironically form tighter and tighter restraints, blocking the path toward relationship longings and deepest yearnings. More detail of how to track the patterns is provided later in the chapter. It is important, however, to pause and notice that from the moment of meeting clients you can detect signs of their typical strategies for engaging with life. When you notice a typical strategy, you are already stepping into normalizing the client's problem as a recursive strategy. You are beginning to recognize the pattern that is imprisoning the couple or individual, and thus are on the way toward shaping the first change event of stabilizing this pattern. In the stabilizing change event, clients own their emotional triggers and actions in the pattern, and find hope and empowerment in naming this pattern as the problem.

The better sense a therapist has of the clients' typical strategies for regulating emotion and their recurring within/between patterns, the more empathically attuned they can be, and the more able they are to validate and reframe action tendencies for their positive underlying attachment intentions, in spite of their costly or shameful consequences. Having an affair, caring for multiple dependents, isolating, or persistently badgering another are all examples of patterns that can be seen for their positive attachment intentions and for their enormous costs to a relationship or an individual. A therapist's initial assessment of clients' patterns may change as they get to know each other. That is ok. This is not about assessing to be correct. It is about tracking explicitly what is observed and linking it to the emotional processes as revealed by the client. Considering "Attachment strategies as *positions* of pursuit or withdrawal in EFCT," can help therapists make sense of the patterns they see occurring in sessions (see textbox in Chapter 7 Support Material at routledge. com/9781032151335).

Identify Strengths and Resources

Attachment theory implies the following three kinds of client resources to which an EFT therapist attends:

Emotion Regulation Patterns. Strategies and patterns of emotion regulation have strengths as well as liabilities. They have both protective and imprisoning impacts. Of course, any examples of secure attachment relationships, where a client reaches to another in distress, receives a supportive response and is strengthened to carry on, will be noted as a strength and a resource to draw upon throughout therapy. EFT therapists validate clients' strategies with a view that the strategy of deactivating or hyperactivating is not the problem; it is only a problem when it becomes a rigid pattern, employed across all situations. For example, deactivating her emotions helped Sahra, a black immigrant woman, to survive medical school in the United States. Now, in a potentially safer, friendlier environment with several young moms from her daughter's daycare, her automatic deactivating pattern is holding her back from reaching for support when she needs it.

Attachment Bonds. Stories of positive attachment bonds are a resource. This can include times of experiencing another as a source of safe-haven comfort and secure-base encouragement. Having survived mistreatment and dismissal from his childhood caregivers, in addition to his current partner's choice to leave the relationship, Max is struggling to trust anyone. He can however, recall the strong bond he shared with his grandmother. From her imagined presence, Max experiences a wave of confidence and empowerment, and a few seeds of hope to begin to trust his intuition.

Success and Competence. Achievements and stories of success and personal competence provide markers of client resilience that can be drawn on throughout therapy. Phil and Julie have grown extremely distanced and mistrusting. While recounting the stories of what drew them to one another initially, they are both flooded with tender feelings toward each other. This resourceful experience restores their determination to heal their ruptures and restore trust.

Monitor for Impeding Factors

It is important to check for the following factors that could interfere with the alliance or contraindicate therapy:

Cultural Misattunement. A culturally insensitive therapist who neglects to consider the role of contextual stressors on clients' emotional and relational experiences jeopardizes the safe alliance. Emily recognizes that she lives with many positions of privilege. To create safety in therapy, she needs to continually expand her cultural sensitivities and to respect how little or how much her clients want her to share. (See Emily's Commitments-for-Inclusion in the online support material for Chapter 5.)

Cultural values and impacts of client's socio-cultural trauma must be validated. An EFT therapist is continually listening for the contextual and attachment significant elements of clients' frustration and distress. Emily remembers Adrah, a recent Syrian immigrant getting annoyed with her when she said, "You seem exhausted over the enormity of caring for your disabled brother while also working full time." Emily's cheeks tinge with regret as she recalls the look of hurt on Adrah's face. She had an alliance rupture to repair, since in that moment she had implicitly minimized the cultural context of family loyalty and depth of pride that Adrah feels at having successfully brought her brother, her only surviving family member, to safety.

Emily is discovering in her work with Wayne and Jessica that listening deeply to clients' stories may be the deepest form of respect a therapist can show, particularly to bridge contextual, power differences. At times when Wayne begins a rather long story, she initially perceives it to be an exit. She discovers, however, that his stories invariably convey his experience in his marriage and the dangers of racial trauma that play out in their relationship. Wayne cannot yet be vulnerable with Jessica, given his strategy for surviving the racial trauma he faces daily.

Factors That Can Contraindicate EFCT. Johnson and Talitman (1997) found that the degree of distress at the beginning of therapy is not a significant predictor of success for couples in EFT. When safety can be established, highly distressed couples can repair their relationships with EFT. There are, however, factors that block the creation of safety. For example, one partner's rigid blaming of the other partner as being entirely responsible for the problem, such as attributing mental illness, might become an indication that safety cannot be created. Some partners start out with a rigid position and become more flexible and open as the alliance with the therapist strengthens. However, if the rigid refusal to engage in the process of tracking a joint cycle continues, safety might not be possible.

Other factors to consider in creating safety and assessing the appropriateness of couple therapy include an active affair, unacknowledged addictive behaviors, and some types of aggression, intimidation, and physical abuse.

An Active Affair. An active affair interferes with establishing a safe working alliance. One partner's acknowledgment that they are unwilling to discontinue an active affair is a clear marker that safety cannot be created in-session, and the bond cannot be restored. The competing attachment of an active affair is different from consensual nonmonogamy where it is possible to create safety (Edwards et al., 2023).

Addictive Processes. Addictive processes, such as alcohol, drugs, pornography, and gambling can interfere with creating safety and forming shared goals for therapy in EFCT. The impact of one or both partners' active involvement in various addictive processes can be explored openly in the relationship to collaboratively determine whether the relationship is enough of a priority to make therapy feasible. Most often, addictive processes can be worked with in the early stage of EFT if the using partner acknowledges the addiction and is willing to seek help for the habit. Alternatively, if one partner is in denial that his or her addictive process is affecting the relationship, EFT therapists can explore with partners how the addictive behavior is part of their recurring pattern of turning to a substance for comfort and support, instead of turning toward the partner. This exploration can become the motivation to seek addiction treatment or to relinquish the addictive pattern through strengthening the relationship. See Chapter 15 to examine treating addictive processes in EFT.

Violence and Aggression. Unacknowledged physical violence and intimidation with a lack of remorse and responsibility for the aggression, blocks creating safety in session. If the abused partner expresses fear or intimidation or if the couple cannot create a safety net outside of sessions, it is likely not safe to do couple therapy. Jacobson and Gottman (2007) suggest not all batterers are alike, distinguishing between what they call *pitbulls* and *cobras*. Pitbulls use desperate, aggressive attempts to take control in an abusive way when anxiety is triggered by a partner's perceived distance, whereas cobras use a more cold, calculating, unpredictable sort of aggression that uses intimidation to control. It is definitely unsafe to do therapy with cobras. With remorse from the offending partner and sufficient lack of fear on the part of the injured partner, however, it may be possible with pitbulls to create enough safety to do EFT with the couple (Bograd & Mederos, 1999; Brubacher & Johnson, 2017). "Viewed from an attachment perspective, [the pitbull type of] couple violence is an exaggerated form of protest against perceived partner unavailability and lack of responsiveness" (Mikulincer & Shaver, 2016, p. 338).

Recent years have seen an expansion of EFT therapists working with domestic violence and aggression. Slootmaeckers and Migerode (2018, 2020) propose that situational couple violence (SCV), frequently bi-directional aggression, can be safely treated with EFCT. The path toward reducing violence in EFCT begins with empathic attunement and genuine acceptance to build a safe haven and secure base with the violent couple so that the partners can take responsibility for their behavior. The EFT therapist needs to feel safe enough to work with domestic violence to slow the process down and place the aggression in the interaction cycle. Violence is framed in the cycle, not as a power dynamic, but as either proximity-seeking or distance-seeking efforts to meet attachment needs. Partners are helped to craft therapeutic goals that are in line with their underlying attachment needs. Hope is promoted for the relationship. As described in Chapter 6, EFT therapists also befriend anger in EFIT, drawing upon the adaptive tendencies of core emotion.

EFIT Contraindications. In EFIT, the most obvious contraindication to building a safe working alliance is psychosis or an anti-social personality disorder that blocks engagement with the therapist and the therapy process. EFIT clients need to be able to safely tolerate engagement in the therapy process and to maintain some focus. When risk factors are high, for example with addictive processes, chronic depression or high suicide risk, EFT therapists seek to maintain safety by working in tandem with other professionals with expertise in specialized treatment and medication (Johnson, 2019).

Assess for Compatible Agendas: Turn Hopes and Longings into Concrete Goals

With a couple, EFT therapists assess whether partners have compatible and appropriate agendas. They use Move 1 reflecting present process, to assess the degree to which partners share the goal of reshaping their attachment bond, and whether safety can be created in session between these two distressed individuals caught in a problematic pattern.

At times, partners express uncertainty and mixed feelings. An EFT therapist needs to be comfortable with ambiguity and curious to explore whether one partner has actually detached emotionally from the relationship or is expressing distancing or hostility simply as part of the self-protective pattern of interaction. With further exploration, it may become clear that both partners do want to repair their relationship. If one partner confirms an agenda to end the relationship, the therapist can facilitate clarity and support the partners in terminating their relationship.

Compelling content and different perspectives can distract a therapist while assessing for compatible agendas and safety. For example, Tyrrell and Dexter present with different views on polyamory. An EFT therapist might be tempted to narrow their perspective and lose the collaborative tone at this point, determining that the partners do not have compatible agendas, and thus, conclude that couple therapy is contraindicated, or digress into teaching or problem solving. However, the EFT therapist who can tolerate ambiguity can explore such questions as, "Can you discuss these differences together? What is it about polyamory that you value/do not value? How does it go when you discuss it?" This latter question also opens the door for the couple to clarify their negative cycle and to explore how the pattern takes over when they attempt to discuss their differences.

Frequently, partners' complaints and desire for change seem very different and it can be challenging for a therapist to find a compatible goal that is relevant for both partners. However, an EFT therapist tunes into the attachment channel to hear how the different complaints are actually related and then weaves the complaints into a goal that fits for both (Johnson, 2015). Jessica and Wayne seem to have totally different complaints and goals. Jessica is angry that Wayne walls her out when their discussions get a little heated, and Wayne is extremely uncomfortable having discussions with Jessica when she gets emotional and asks rapid-fire questions. He is left with a sense of futility that whatever he says or does just seems to upset Jessica, and he loathes hearing her get upset. Emily hears attachment themes, "Don't leave me. Don't shut me out" from Jessica, and "Don't rush me and judge me. Give me a chance to think!" from Wayne. She offers a starting point, "It seems that what you'd both like is to get through your conflicts and differences in a way that is comfortable for you both to remain in conversation and where you both feel accepted and important to the other." This encompasses Jessica's surface wish to talk more with Wayne, and her core attachment longing to know she is important to him and will not be abandoned. It also reflects Wayne's surface wish for less pressure to talk more, and his core attachment longing to feel accepted and wanted. Framing a compatible goal to create a relationship where they feel accepted and important to one another is an example of creating a mutually desired picture of their desired outcome or seeding a picture of secure attachment.

In EFIT, after it is clear there can be compatible agendas between client and therapist, specific goals targeted at the client's longings and unmet needs are set. Goal setting, like all of EFT therapy is a collaborative, fluid conversation focused on formulating goals for therapy that are achievable and relevant to client's concerns. Emily finds that being grounded in the basic goals of EFIT helps keep her focused on shaping a few clear, realistic goals for therapy that individual clients, in their initial chaos or distress, can imagine themselves achieving. Specifically, the goals of EFIT are:

- To create optimal (Feeney et al., 2015) or effective dependency (Bowlby, 1988) to cope with distress and effectively regulate emotions.
- To help clients move from defensiveness and rigidity to being more open to their experience, more able to explore and transform foreign, frightening and unacceptable emotions, and to create coherent, meaningful narratives about self and key relationships.
- To shape corrective emotional experiences that shift IWMs to a competent, loveable, worthy, sense of self, and a reliable, trustworthy, responsive and emotionally engaged sense of at least some others. Differentiating safe, dependable others from unreliable, dangerous others is part of forming a positive working model of other.
- To move into accessibility, responsiveness, and affiliative engagement with others that typifies secure attachment and bolsters emotional fitness (flexibility and resilience) and zest for living (Johnson, 2009a, 2019).

This vision of the powerfully transformative potential of EFIT equips a therapist with empathic imagination to collaborate with a client in formulating specific therapy goals that are relevant to their concerns. EFT therapists listen to clients' longings and unmet needs as the means from which to shape concrete, achievable goals.

To seed hope of secure connection, EFT therapists focus on articulating specific, realistic goals. Rather than focusing on "ending depression" or "stopping the fights," for example, Emily works with her clients to reframe their longed-for alternative. An achievable goal needs to be stated in a positive, imaginable format. For example, for Wayne and Jessica, a goal to "stop fighting" is not a concrete goal, nor is it one they agree on. From Jessica's perspective, there is little fighting; there is not enough conversation and too many walls. From Wayne's perspective, conversations are futile because she gets too worked up and loses all perspective. Together, they imagine a collaborative goal of "staying in meaningfully engaged conversations when they have differences of opinion."

Max begins therapy saying he wants to get over negative impacts of traumas from the past. He wants help to stop the biggest fear still haunting him far in the background – that one day he will have a conscious memory of a horrific scene from the past. Although these expressed longings are vague and not imaginable as final outcomes, they are great starting points from which to collaboratively shape more concrete, specific, realistic goals. Emily hears that Max wants to find the resources and the courage to safely walk into his present experience and his past memories with his eyes wide open. He is eager to embrace that goal. Together, they shape these goals for therapy:

- To become more aware of his own emotions as they unfold and to listen to them.
- To clearly face the traumas he has survived.
- To restore relationships and repair damage.
- To face his constant ache of grief.
- To process the guilt and responsibility for the death of his friend.

When Ella and Sophie talk about wanting to stop their fights, Emily helps them develop an imaginable picture of this longed-for outcome, in place "stopping the fighting." They create a goal of "being able to count on each other in spite of differences; to know you like and want me, and to feel safe to be in this for the long haul."

Sahra says she is getting weary of the highs of anxiety and the lethargy of depression. Her hopes for therapy are to stabilize the highs and lows, to process her flashbacks of her ex's violence, to heal her broken heart from the harsh men in her life, to touch her untouchable grief over her mother, and to come to trust her emotions as a guide.

With the depathologizing attachment frame, EFT therapists help clients feel acceptable and safe to identify their strengths and vulnerabilities, and to formulate concrete, specific, imaginable, achievable, goals for therapy that are relevant to their longings.

Review Areas for Assessment

Judiciously selected evocative questions can be *interspersed with reflections and validations* to evoke discussions for alliance building and early assessment. Evocative questions can elicit strengths in the relationship bond, in EFCT: "Are there times you can reach to one another when you are struggling or to reconnect after an argument?" Questions can help partners identify their typical negative cycle of distress: "How does it go when you have differences of opinion? Who tends to start an argument? Who typically walks away first? Who is likely to be the first to reconnect after an argument?"

Typically, an EFT therapist engages with a couple in exploring how their relationship evolved, what attracted them to one another, what prompted coming for therapy at this time, and what historical, pivotal events might have changed the course of their relationship. A brief attachment history can also help to make the attachment frame of love explicitly alive. This can include questions such as: "Whom did you go to for comfort as a child? Who held you when you cried?" Evocative questions elicit engaged, concrete responses. Any of these questions are then followed with reflections to validate, slow the processing, and encourage sustained engagement.

Frequently, it is new for clients to discover that adults have survival needs for comfort. Giving clients life history forms to complete helps to lay the foundation for an attachment perspective, normalizing the universal needs for support and respecting contextual impacts that have shaped their life. See www.SteppingintoEFT.com for a sample EFT compatible life history form.

While assessment is more of a dialogue than a series of questions and answers, questions can be asked to open conversations, in areas, including expectations for therapy; racial, social, cultural, ethnic identities; sources of comfort; chemical use; current emotional distress patterns; leisure; childhood family; religion or spirituality; sexuality; abuse and violence; current relationship; and relationship history. EFT therapists intersperse questions with empathic attunement and curiosity, making empathic reflections, validations, and evocative responses to invite expansion while listening and responding to clients, in an *accessible, responsive, emotionally engaged* manner. An extensive list of areas for assessment and sample questions covering the 12 areas above are available in Chapter 7 Support Material (routledge.com/9781032151335).

Forming a Therapy Agreement

An informal therapy agreement is often initiated by the therapist's transparency about therapy. Clarity about the therapy process is important for creating safety and for helping clients to embrace goals. For clients new to therapy or those with previous negative therapy experiences, a therapist's openness about how they will work together is particularly important to build confidence that the therapist is competent and trustworthy. Liu, an Asian EFT trainer and therapist, describes how this transparency is of particular importance to create safety and trust with her Asian clients (Dockett, 2022). It is good practice, as an EFT therapist, to know how to describe the model, in a succinct, manner that conveys hope and clarity about the therapy process. Examples of how to describe EFCT and EFIT to clients or prospective clients are available in Chapter 7 Support Material (routledge.com/9781032151335).

A therapy agreement is reached in a collaborative manner. A therapist will check for client agreement to work together, offering 8–20 sessions as a realistic expectation, with longer options available if needed. The therapist's collaborative position is reiterated. This might be presented as follows:

> I will be working with you as a process consultant. This means I will not always be right, and I want to be corrected if I don't seem to understand correctly. You are the expert(s) on your relationship and on your life experience(s).

If the therapy is being done online, part of the therapy agreement will include discussions of how to maximize the experience and ensure that it feels safe and respectful for all parties. EFT is well suited for online therapy across modalities (Brubacher & Liu, 2023). Demonstrations of online EFT with couples and individuals can be found at www.steppingintoeft.com and with a Chinese Canadian family at https://tceft.ca/product/canada-talks-series/

Balance Process and Content

Much of the EFT literature refers to *privileging process over content*, however, this does not mean that content is unimportant. It means that EFT therapists attend to the emotional process of discussing that content, rather than get distracted by clients' content as a problem to be solved. There are several ways in which content *is* important. It may be best to describe an EFT therapist's task as that of balancing process and content.

When a couple presents a conflict over household responsibilities or differences about sex or finances, an EFT therapist will avoid getting pulled into this content as something to fix. Instead, they will explore the process that takes place between partners around these issues. Emily feels relief as she discovers how to embrace clients' content as a way to engage with the process between them. She tracks who pushes the topic and who moves away from it in the present moment in session. She also invites partners to describe how their content and contextual differences play out between them, "Are you able to talk about this on your own? How does it go between you when you attempt to discuss this? Who is likely to initiate the discussion about this? Who is likely to walk away first?"

Similarly, in EFIT, when a client presents a specific problem, the EFT therapist will engage with the client in exploring their current strategies of emotion regulation and patterns of coping (process) in their lived experiences (content). Dimitri presents with wanting help to stop his "random rageful outbursts." Before getting pulled into problem solving and anger management, Emily listens to his stories of trauma that he thought he had "put behind him" but are now "eating away inside" and seeming to trigger random outbursts of rage. She validates his coping strategy as having been an effective survival strategy for the traumatic events he endured and together they explore his hidden core emotions that need to be heard and processed in his content of "surviving horror."

Content of particular importance to explore are the larger contextual stories and experiences of socio-cultural values, traditions, trauma, and *subtle acts of exclusion* (Jana & Baran, 2020). EFT therapists invite couple and individual clients to explore how their emotional and relational experiences of self and other are impacted by these contextual factors.

The other content which is important is that of naming pivotal events that have had a life-altering impact, particularly specific events of relationship trauma which shattered assumptions of safety and views of self and other. These crucial events are known as *attachment injuries* (see Chapter 16). An important aspect of assessment in EFCT is to invite each partner to reflect on their history and to identify relationship-specific attachment injuries by asking, "Are there any pivotal events that changed everything between you?" Likewise, in EFIT, invitations are given to name and explore pivotal events that have shattered a client's sense of safety and positive view of self and other.

Story telling can be a way to balance process and content. Engaging with clients' stories is a path toward forming a safe, collaborative alliance and assessing the key problem and goals for therapy. Attentive listening to clients' stories of their lived experiences, told in their own way, may be the deepest form of respect a therapist can show, particularly to bridge contextual, power differences. Nightingale et al. (2019) suggest, "Attentive listening may be the most powerful tool a therapist has to build trust with African Americans" (p. 237). To be immersed in *culturally humble, deep listening* (Guillory, 2022) is an important goal for EFT therapists with clients of all races and cultures. Using Move 1, with respectfully paced, attentive reflective listening, an EFT therapist builds an alliance with clients while also helping them to discover how they actively create their own experience. With Move 2, therapists help clients deepen their connection with their own experience (Johnson, 2019). Clients gain agency and empowerment as they experience this balancing of their process of engaging with the content they are living.

Individual Sessions in Couple Therapy

It is standard practice in EFCT to have individual sessions with each partner following the initial one or two couple sessions. The basic function of the individual sessions is to deepen the alliance with each partner and to allow each partner to freely elaborate on perceptions and experiences of self, of the other partner, and of the relationship in general. Individual sessions provide an opportunity, unhampered by the presence of the partner, to further explore ambivalence or uncertainty about investment in the relationship, and to explore issues of safety, fears of intimidation, or violent or abusive behaviors that might have been hinted at or even dismissed in the couple sessions. Finally, disclosure about involvement in secret affairs or addictive processes can be invited during individual sessions.

At the beginning of the individual sessions, an EFT therapist will share that in order to work as a team with the couple, they do not want to be in possession of a secret, and thus, will communicate:

> If you share something that you or I feel could threaten your relationship, I will encourage you to also share it with your partner on your own, or I will support you to share it when we meet together.

In the face of one partner's reluctance to share a secret, the therapist can explore with them how keeping secrets undermines everyone's goals for therapy and can revisit the kind of relationship they want to have. (See www.SteppingintoEFT.com for a guide to individual sessions.)

Identifying Patterns of Protection

From the moment of meeting a couple or individual client, the EFT therapist observes closely to identify the attachment drama or pattern that has taken over their life. The repetitive interactive pattern is identified as some variation of a dance between anxious pursuit and avoidant (dismissive or defensive) withdrawal in a couple, and in EFIT, a within – between stuck pattern and prison of hyperactivating or deactivating emotions for self-protection. All survival strategies have their strengths and costs, depending on the context.

The repetitive pattern is identified as the problem that is blocking longings and needs from being met. In order to reach a chosen destination, travelers need to know their starting point and their chosen endpoint. Having articulated the goal for change in language that is relevant for them, couple and individual clients can visualize their targeted destination. With the therapist's help, they can also track how their default survival pattern may be keeping them stuck at the starting point, holding them back from fulfilling their longings and needs.

It is the therapist's job to validate the client's so-called defenses and self-limiting responses as protective strategies that have now become prisons, and to respectfully lead clients out of these prisons, much as a good parent does with a child. (Johnson, 2019, p. 225)

Leading our clients out of prisons begins with helping them to discover the recursive pattern that imprisons them. That discovery is clients' Step 2 of EFT, as described in the EFT Steps of Client Change delineated in Boxes 1.1 and 1.2.

Couples are on a journey toward a safe and secure connection, a harmonious dance of reaching and responding. Analogously, EFIT clients are on a path to fuller engagement in life with secure attachment with others and a newly confident, worthy sense of self.

Using Move 1, tracking and reflecting, and the beginning of Move 2, linking triggers and action tendencies, therapists help couples to name how they get caught in one of several typical patterns (Box 7.2), seeing no exit routes and blocked from reaching the destination of secure connection. EFT therapists help partners to identify each one's position in this dance as either an anxious pursuer fighting for connection and pushing for response, or an avoidant withdrawer defending against criticism and avoiding closeness that feels dangerous or suffocating.

Jessica and Wayne's moves and positions in the cycle are quite clear. The dynamic of one partner's behaviors triggering the other into the cycle are readily observable. Jessica hyperactivates the attachment system to push Wayne to respond, pouring forth a tirade of questions tinged with complaint, or turtling into a steely silence and stolid independence. In response, Wayne appears increasingly rigid and calm, a deactivating strategy, which, in turn, triggers more desperation in Jessica which sometimes shows up as angry protest, and other times as indifference. From a story that Wayne related about his childhood, Jessica and Wayne soon come to name their negative cycle the *spilled milk tango*. The more she pushes him with specific details about housework, the more he defends himself, internally burning with the sense of shame he felt as a five-year-old, chastised for spilling the milk. He sullenly retreats to his computer, leaving all the tasks he had promised to do unfinished, after which Jessica puts up a wall of anger against her loneliness and against Wayne. Then they do not talk for days.

Identifying EFIT clients' *pattern as the problem*, gives individual clients an increased sense of agency. The therapist tracks the moves of hyperactivating or deactivating survival strategies to help clients take ownership for what triggers them and how they reflexively react. EFIT client Sahra makes moves that are as evident as those of Wayne and Jessica. She is rapidly triggered into hypervigilance by loud voices. She becomes overwhelmed with a flurry of memories and questions about what she did wrong that her ex-partner became abusive. She shrinks, feeling small and insignificant, goes silent, and becomes numb. More details and case examples about tracking patterns in EFCT and in EFIT are available in Chapter 7 Support Material (routledge.com/9781032151335).

Tracking the recursive, imprisoning pattern with couples or individuals can be broken down into a series of mini steps to make the process simpler and more natural for a new EFT therapist. Chapter 7 Support Material also includes "Mini-Steps for Tracking Patterns of Protection."

Attachment Reframes for the Problematic Patterns of Emily's Clients

Simple, validating reframes from an attachment perspective can be made for each of Emily's clients' recurring patterns. Let us examine the attachment reframes for each couple and individual.

Wayne and Jessica. The attachment frame for the basic moves and positions in the cycle for the pursue–withdraw couple, Wayne and Jessica, is: The more Jessica turns up the volume, the more Wayne steps further away. The more Wayne steps away, the more Jessica turtles for days and the more Wayne explains to Jessica how she needs to change. Both are trapped in pain and isolation as they seek to keep from hurting the other and to preserve the relationship.

Phil and Julie. For Phil and Julie, a withdraw/withdraw couple, the attachment frame of the endless loop of their cycle is: The more Julie walks away, looking unhappy, "*with me,*" Phil assumes, the more Phil walks away and makes himself busy, to numb the pain of sensing rejection. The more Phil stays busy and distant "abandoning me," Julie senses, the more she also distances to cope with the pain of isolation. Both are thus trapped in pain and isolation as they seek to protect themselves and their relationship.

Sophie and Ella. The more volatile couple, Sophie and Ella, caught in a heated attack/attack drama, can be seen in an attachment frame, as follows: The more Sophie complains about Ella's distance and tries to pull her close, the more Ella hears that she's letting Sophie down. In self-protection, she reacts by angrily shutting Sophie out. When Ella shuts down, Sophie becomes frantic and aggressive. Underneath, she is lonely and afraid she'll lose Ella at any moment, and Ella is afraid Sophie doesn't really love and accept her. When this cycle takes over, they are both caught in pain and loneliness, all the while fighting to save the relationship!

Max. Attachment reframes can also be made for Emily's EFIT clients. Emily reframes Max's pattern as follows:

> You are longing for safety and good relationships between people yet feeling so far away from being the *kind gardener of people* you have always wanted to be. It seems the more you attempt to lock away your fears and anger and stories of loss and trauma, the more you end up blurting out accusations to others who do not seem to hear you or see how much you are struggling inside. When others walk away from you, it confirms your sense that you are a *monster in a box,* even as you are wanting them to see good in you. Together, we will listen to your fears and angry messages that feel monster-like now and we will listen to their good intentions and needs.

Sahra. The attachment reframe that Emily describes for Sahra's pattern is as follows:

> You tell me how much you long to "feel anything – or to have a simple good cry," feeling like everything is numb and far away yet eating away silently inside of you as you navigate from one set of rapids to the next. You've honed your skills at keeping busy and numbing your emotions to cope with the unfairness the world hurls at you, with your harsh father before he disappeared, with your overwhelmed mother after that, and several turbulent friendships and betrayals. Spinning between dangerous contexts and one unsafe relationship to the next keeps you from feeling the pain, and also leaves you so alone and distant from others and yourself. When we quiet the spin together, we can create the safety to listen to your deep needs and longings within your painso you are no longer alone in this chaos.

HOW EFT Therapists Interact while Building Alliance and Beginning Assessment

An EFT therapist's *way of being* (Rogers, 1980) makes all the difference as to whether early sessions become a collaborative engagement with clients' emotional experiencing in the present moment, or a non-engaged insight conversation, unlikely to influence lasting change. The manner in which assessment questions are asked and responded to can limit or enhance the growing safety in the alliance.

The Rogerian therapeutic stance of empathic responsiveness, unconditional acceptance, and genuine engagement (Bowlby, 1988; Rogers, 1980) provides a reliable and practical guide for *how* to move with the EFT Tango in early sessions, utilizing micro-interventions of moment-to-moment empathic reflection and tracking, validation, evocative questions, reframing in the attachment context, catching bullets, and shaping encounters. This stance parallels the attuned and emotionally engaged interactions seen in secure parent–infant interactions. An EFT therapist embodies this stance with empathic resonance to self and to clients, engaging in the here-and-now, and transparently attending to the task aspect of the therapeutic alliance by confirming with clients if the process of therapy continues to feel relevant to them.

Offer Attuned, Engaged Presence

The manner in which an EFT therapist collaboratively builds an alliance begins with offering an attuned, engaged presence. To be culturally humble, one needs to slow their pace to give space for clients' voices to be heard. A therapist needs to continually show empathic curiosity and to take time to check with the client that they are accurately understanding them. When threats to the alliance arise, EFT therapists seek to be fully present, self-aware, and ready to repair ruptures.

Therapists Stay Close to the Here-and-now

One can stand far away in a past event or in an intellectual explanation, or one can move "closer to the here-and-now and the real" (Stern, 2004, p. 211). Practicing experientially, EFT therapists step fully into the moment of their own and their clients' present moment experiencing. This helps clients to engage in exploring the emerging awareness of experience *within* self, and *between* self and other. It helps therapists to distinguish between lower levels of experiencing, where a client talks *about* events, ideas, or others from a personal distance, and the increasingly engaged levels of experiencing, where implicit feelings and meanings emerge and are distilled and integrated (Klein et al., 1969).

Promote task alliance

As mentioned in Chapter 2, it is critical to success in EFT that clients experience trust in the process of therapy, and that the tasks be seen as relevant and meaningful to them. Being transparent about the process and inviting client feedback throughout the process contributes to alliance around the tasks of therapy.

Speak Clients' Language

For some clients *feeling words* or the language of emotional intimacy is foreign or distasteful. Beginning with clients where they are and matching language that captures their present experience is important for building alliance and assessing collaboratively.

Give Tools?

Therapists new to EFT frequently dread the question, "Aren't you going to give us tools?" While EFT does not involve teaching tools, there are several congruent ways for an EFT therapist to respond this this question and to describe the type of tools clients will gain. This topic is included in the expansion of *how* an EFT therapist engages in alliance building and assessment in the Chapter 7 Support Material (routledge.com/9781032151335).

Nurture Relationships of Support

It is important for EFT therapists to be embedded in *broaden-and-build cycles* (Mikulincer & Shaver, 2016) with colleagues who validate them in their imperfections, and support and challenge them in their growth to be culturally humble EFT therapists. Internalized discrimination can easily remain outside of one's consciousness since "racism is embedded within societal structures" (Causadias et al., 2021, p. 4). EFT therapists' supportive cycles with colleagues can strengthen their courage and confidence to continue to monitor and invite client feedback on whether they feel understood, during alliance building and assessment processes.

Seek Cross-cultural Experiences

Consulting with colleagues from other cultures can help to make an EFT therapist more conscious about balancing empathic attunement with curiosity to evoke specifics about the clients' nuanced experience and being increasingly intentional to not assume understanding before eliciting specifics.

In the supplementary material for Chapter 7 (routledge.com/9781032151335) each of these elements of how EFT therapists engage to form an alliance and begin assessment are expanded.

Conclusion

The foundation for the first change event, *de-escalation or stabilization,* is laid in the early sessions. It begins to emerge from building an attachment-informed safe-haven, secure-base therapeutic alliance. This includes the safety and growth-orientation of a non-blaming, de-pathologizing orientation where clients formulate clear therapeutic goals, relevant to their concerns. The problem is framed as an automatic, self-reinforcing pattern of emotion regulation. Clients identify their fight-or-flight moves in some variation of a repetitive pattern that has taken over their most important relationship(s) and their life. After developing a trusting therapeutic alliance (Step 1) and identifying their basic pattern or way of engaging with self, other, and the world (Step 2) clients are ready to more deeply assemble the attachment emotions that are driving their interactions (Step 3).

Get Ready – The Clients Are Coming!

In the support material (routledge.com/9781032151335) there is an opportunity for you, at the end of each of Chapters 7–10, to review each of the five cases we are following in this book. There is a summary of the key ingredients of building alliance and beginning assessment, and you are invited to imagine that you are Emily reviewing each of your client cases at the beginning of your therapy day. There you are guided to identify key issues to focus on, including their basic pattern, emotional and cultural handles you want to explore, core underlying fears if you have discovered them, and finally, goals and longings you hear or have made explicit with the clients in each case.

8 Heeding Attachment Alarms to Shape Stabilization, the Stage 1 Change Event

> In EFT, we speak of an 'alarm being constantly on' … and the 'noise' blocking out other cues. (Johnson, 2015, p. 104)

Attuning to the emotional alarm bells that signal threat in our clients' worlds and becoming familiar with the repetitive loops that exacerbate the sounds of danger are two important features of helping clients to de-escalate their self-protective patterns. Understanding how emotion is conceptualized and engaged in EFT, as described in Chapter 6, is paramount to grasping what EFT therapists see and hear through de-escalation/stabilization and how they facilitate this first change event. Learning how to follow and assemble the active trigger-perception-feeling-meaning-action elements of emotion will become one of your greatest assets for helping clients to stabilize.

EFT therapists attune to the alarms of attachment threat that their clients – couples and individuals – are hearing. They work together to frame the real problem as lying not in self or other but in the self-reinforcing pattern of rapid reactivity to the alarms, which ironically intensifies the alarm.

Wayne says, "She can ask for all the reassurance she needs. What puts alarms in my system is her complaints, not her asking to be reassured of my love… When alarmed, I do step back." This of course sends alarms to Jessica's system, confirming her fear of abandonment and her sense that he must not love her.

Sahra, struggling with depression and anxiety, readily detaches from her emotions. At times, in and out of session, she suddenly has no feelings about her circumstances and has little interest in discussing her losses and traumas. "There is no time for it – it's too loud, too alarming, too much," she insists. She describes putting more and more effort into work and studies and parenting "just to stay afloat." "I'm working hard to be a better person…I have a lot of resentment…but I am losing motivation… and some days it is hard to get out of bed."

Max acknowledges:

> It's always in the background. I try to ignore it, to keep busy and to create alternative explanations, but for the last 28 years I hear this constant alarm bell ringing with my biggest fear that suddenly one day I will have a conscious memory of the accident – like a nightmare coming to get me.

"If I listen to every complaint, I'll be sucked dry," says Ella coldly. "I brace myself not to listen." Danger bells ring for Ella each time Sophie tries to reach her. She doesn't hear kind reaches – only demands and complaints.

DOI: 10.4324/9781003242673-11

Attachment Alarms

Clients come to therapy caught in patterns or cycles of repetitive responses that perpetuate their distress. Vaguely recognized emotional alarms and unclear fears trigger protective reactions, and the protective reactions heighten these cloudy attachment fears. Attachment fears are hazy and imprecise, in that they are of survival proportions and frequently too overwhelming to be noticed clearly. We don't have time to formulate the thought, "I am afraid" when we are running for our lives. We run, we fight, or we freeze. Similarly, in a moment of relational danger there is no time or space to pause and articulate a core fear. Our attachment fears of loss, loneliness, despair, and panic remain unexpressed in moments of threat. Unexpressed fears trigger reactions and reactions trigger fears in a continuous feedback loop.

Analogously, after owning their self-protective patterns, EFIT clients are ready to explore the core emotional surge within their bodies in response to external warning bells. The emotional surge is what pulls them into the pattern. Emotional music, playing in the background, compels them to repeat self-protective moves that weaken and destroy a relationship bond or reinforce depression, anxiety, and other forms of emotional distress (see Box 7.4).

Repetitive Feedback Loops

Danger bells activate the attachment system and reinforce feedback loops of internal experience and interpersonal interactions. When clients do not have a safe and secure context with an available attachment figure to turn to, they resort to hyperactivating or deactivating emotional behaviors that, in turn, form self-perpetuating patterns. The pattern is a negative cycle of interaction or loop of self-protection. Strategies for engaging with emotion, with self, and with others in one's socio-cultural context form self-perpetuating feedback loops. These loops of intensifying (pursuing) or deactivating (withdrawing) to regulate difficult, strong emotions tend to backfire, making symptoms worse (Barlow et al., 2018). Bowlby's image of mirroring processes – we do as we've been done to – conveys two feedback loops of inner experience and interpersonal interactions, each impacting and being impacted by the other. Adding a third ring of socio-cultural context to Bowlby's two interacting rings of inner experience and interpersonal interactions, as seen in Figure 1.1, emphasizes that threats from the larger context seep into internal processing and views of self and other. Internalized homophobia or internalized racism is bound to impact relational patterns as well.

An EFT therapist helps each couple and individual client to bring order to this chaos by becoming familiar with the pattern and the separate, interconnected elements in the cascade of emotional reactivity that happens mostly outside of clients' awareness. Together, they identify the trigger of attachment threat that pulls the client into the pattern, how this trigger is perceived as threatening, their typical emotional behaviors of intensifying or suppressing, what happens in their body, and their meanings and attributions about self and other. Assembling the rapid, repetitive emotional reactions helps clients to make *acceptable sense* out of what is happening and opens doorways into the core, underlying emotion that is frequently unheeded during reactivity.

What Is the First Change Event of De-escalation/Stabilization?

In contrast to strategies of hyperactivation and deactivation that entrench self-perpetuating patterns of distress and pain, the goal of EFT is to transform these limiting patterns into what Mikulincer and Shaver (2016) call *broaden-and-build cycles* of attachment security – a cascade of emotional, cognitive, and behavioral processes that enhance relational satisfaction, emotional stability, and personal growth. When clients acknowledge with a *felt-sense knowing* that the real problem in their relational or emotional distress is being caught in a repetitive pattern of trying to manage their deepest fears, they are taking Step 4 – the first change event of EFT. This change event is frequently referred to as *de-escalating the negative cycle* in EFCT or *stabilizing the self-protective pattern* in EFIT. For most of this book, as mentioned in the introduction, this change event is referred to as *stabilization*.

When a couple stabilizes, they de-escalate the speed of their reactivity to one another and thus have the capacity to explore the emotional intensity fueling their reactivity. Likewise, when EFIT clients stabilize, they reduce their rapidly reactive suppressing or intensifying of difficult emotion and have the emotional balance and awareness needed to begin Stage 2 change. The hallmark of completing Stage 1 change is that clients, individuals and couples have the emotional balance and safety that is needed for the deeper, more vulnerable emotional exploration of the Stage 2 transformative change events.

Stabilization entails a couple or individual gaining the clarity and acceptance that a well-intentioned, rigid, stuck pattern driven by emerging, newly expressed core fears is the real problem. The problem is the self-perpetuating pattern of emotional protection. "Self-protection becomes a prison; in fact, it becomes solitary confinement" (Johnson, 2019, p. 135), wherein the client is shut down, shut in and others are shut out (Johnson, February, 2021).

In stabilization, clients discover that it is this negative feedback loop that has "*condemned them to isolation*" (Jordan, 2018, p. 33), feeling unseen, underappreciated, and devoid of relational connections. They come to appreciate that their best attempts to protect their relationship and/or themselves are the very self-reinforcing strategies that are exacerbating their isolation, conflict, and discontent. The principles of Jordan's Relational-Cultural Therapy (RCT) (2018) support EFT's depathologizing attachment views that human connection is the foundation for survival and flourishing, and that strategies of separation distress or strategies of disconnection are the real problem. Interestingly, RCT also extends the need for human connection to the impacts of socio-cultural exclusion and marginalization as a major source of suffering. "The invisible and unearned privilege that supports the dominant groups in any culture is kept invisible" (Jordan, 2008, p. 3). Current-day EFT is responding to the need to integrate socio-cultural impacts into framing the *pattern as the problem*.

With a fresh perspective of the problem as a *context-specific within/between pattern*, clients discover how they are the architects of their present experience and how they can be the agents of change. A more pursuing partner in a biracial couple conveys hope, "In our best attempt to protect the relationship, we got caught in this pattern. Now that we have named each of our fears that pull us in – his fear that I'm out to destroy him and my fear that he will disappear –I already see hope for us in changing our pattern. I want to be his sanctuary of comfort even if the outside world continues to be dangerous!"

"In my best effort to manage my trauma, my guilt, my fear, I got caught in this pattern of dissonance – living in fear, feeling like a fraud. Now that I see it more clearly, I see the path forward. I feel hope," says Max, his voice trembling as he acknowledges how much courage it will take to move into and through his fears.

The transforming impact of the first change event is that clients experience a shift in framing what their true problem is. This is a move away from fault-finding to collaborative exploration. They discover the real problem to be their self-reinforcing pattern of rapid reactivity fueled by unheeded attachment emotions, and not a deficit in self or other. The cyclic nature of this problematic pattern becomes clear: Rapid reactivity ironically intensifies the signals of danger, which, in turn, trigger more reactivity. Couples discover, for example, "Neither one of us is at fault here, but we are caught in a pattern that is our problem. If we created this pattern, we can change it" (Johnson, 2020). Correspondingly, individual clients, with the therapist's Move 1 reflections, tracking, and validation grasp their struggle in a new way, and realize, for example, "My struggle really is this challenging! I am doing my best to manage overwhelming, threatening experience. If the problem is my pattern of coping with these newly discovered difficult emotions – I can find new strategies. Listening to my emotion motivates me to find options." Couples and individuals appreciate having their struggle validated and clearly understood for its good intentions. This frame of their *problem as the pattern* points to new meanings, new ways of coping and new-found hope. What an EFT therapist does to facilitate this first change event is described below, building on the description of emotion as target and agent of change, as detailed in Chapter 6.

What EFT Therapists See and Hear in Stabilization

Emily reflects on her current clients, many of whom are in Stage 1 and recognizes four commonalities:

1. "With each couple and individual in distress, I see signs of attachment danger cues and hear alarms ringing."
2. "I observe a cascade of elements of emotion, set in motion by that danger cue. The cascades look different in my varied clients. Some get triggered into highly aroused, reactivity with torrents of words and exasperation, and need to be supported and contained. Others close down and are much more difficult to engage."
3. "With each client, however, I see how any one of those elements of emotion can be a doorway into a deeper, more core, vulnerable emotional experience. Each time we distil or link fragments of emotion into a coherent whole, it's like we have struck gold. We find the emotional logic of the core fear that is keeping these cascades of emotion in motion."
4. "I see the order and logic in the repetitive patterns and the safe foundation we are creating in this exploration. I see the patterns of reactivity continuing to happen but with a change in tone. The pace of the emotional cascades is slowing. Partners are aware of what is happening and can sometimes interrupt the cascade midstream. Individuals are gaining emotional balance to explore their experience more deeply."

As Emily reflects on these aspects, she sees and hears signs of hope. She feels that hopefulness in her own body as well.

Danger Cues and Alarm Bells

An EFT therapist is always on the lookout for signs that romantic partners are seeing danger cues and hearing alarms signaling a threat to their sense of safe connection and acceptability in the other's eyes. Signs of perceived threat can be seen in facial expression, tone of voice, and other nonverbal gestures. The cue of a partner turning away or turning against can be as subtle as a partner's raised eyebrow or a very slight bodily movement. The therapist sees, hears, and senses the beginnings of a repetitive cycle of distress and detects signs of what might be the underlying attachment fears being triggered and triggering the cycle. Similarly, in EFIT, a therapist attunes for signs in clients' accounts and in their bodily movements that they are perceiving a threat that sets their self-protective pattern in motion. The perceived threats may be threats of loss, threats of judgment, or threats of experiencing emotions they want to avoid. Emily detects the following alarms of distress: Wayne stiffens in his chair and turns away *when* Jessica's voice rises. Jessica sighs with exasperation *when* Wayne's body stiffens, just before he turns away. Emily recognizes the importance of these momentary cues and intuits that attachment panic is activated.

One of the biggest triggers for pursuer Sophie's cascade of emotion is when she sees Ella on the phone with her sister. For withdrawer Ella, one of the biggest triggers is that look on Sophie's face that she describes as "just before the bee is going to sting."

Although Max has a partial smile, Emily notices the color drain from his face and his smile disappears as he says:

> I have been afraid of this my entire life… Given the amount of damage my body suffered, I am so afraid I will have a conscious memory of seeing Léo's body. I am terrified of feeling! The fear is there all the time. Now that my partner has left, I have even more fear of my future.

Emily notes Max has no specific alarm bell that warns of the decades-old fear that he works hard to suppress but that his current grief at the loss of his partner makes him more vulnerable to the background fears and guilt that he has spent decades avoiding.

Sahra pauses and her face flushes with emotion, as she utters slowly, "It's that blank look on his face." Emily recognizes Sahra's facial expression and repeated trigger of a "blank face" when she describes her supervising physician's dismissal of her expertise to be the same expression she has when she speaks of her father. The dreaded blank looks and actions of dismissal (cue) trigger a similar cascade of emotion for Sahra.

Cascades of Emotion

The EFT therapist sees and hears clients' cascades of emotional reactivity unfolding in-session. (The elements of emotion in these cascades are pictured in Figures 6.1 and 6.2.) The attachment lens helps therapists detect shifts on a client's face, sudden bodily movements, or indications in vocal tone that something has just alerted their amygdala (the fear center of the limbic brain) to pay attention and to make an immediate and rapid appraisal. The immediate appraisal or evaluation is made at a preconscious, preverbal level with an affective sense of "good or bad," or "safe or dangerous." Without necessarily knowing how the client is experiencing the process of emotion as it begins to unfold, the EFT therapist sees and attunes to bodily signs that the process of emotion has been initiated.

The following example of Sophie and Ella illustrates the immediate link between when emotion begins (the cue) and the impulse to action. Sophie recalls Ella on the phone with her sister. Immediately, Sophie reports that her blood boils, and she snaps, "See, there she is talking with her family again. After how badly they've treated me! I guess that says who is most important to her!" (conscious meaning-making). The action impulse for Sophie is to react with anger, criticism, and demands for Ella to step away from her family, and then to stomp out of the room.

To Ella, the look on Sophie's face (cue), just before she storms out of the room, says, "Once again, she is fed up with me. Nothing I do is ever acceptable and I am forever in trouble with her!" (conscious meaning-making). The action tendency for Ella is a typical withdrawer's twofold reaction: First, she goes numb, quiet, and appears to carry on as usual, but internally longs to please Sophie. Second, when she tires of Sophie's demands, she fires back in self-defense and blame, followed by lengthy, hostile silences.

Emily sees and hears a cascade of emotion unfold as Sahra recounts an incident of the lead doctor on her ward ignoring her and her expertise. "The doctor bypassed me and discussed a patient's illness with a junior colleague with much lighter skin and flowing shiny hair. I was incensed, Sahra bristles, "That child's illness is my specialty!" She looks directly at Emily and with a smile says, "But I'm used to it…bypassed again!" The trigger for Sahra is the doctor bypassing her to talk with a lighter-skinned junior colleague. Sahra's cascade of emotion:

Trigger (perceived as dangerous): The lead doctor bypasses Sahra and turns instead to someone with less knowledge but with lighter skin.

Bodily response: A rush of adrenalin courses through her and she is incensed and disgusted!

Meaning made: I have much more to offer than this junior colleague! I am being bypassed because of the color of my skin. There is no point in my protesting!

Action Tendency: Dismiss my rage and pain. Put on a smile and act like it doesn't bother me. Ignore my experience. Let it roll off my back.

Hint of Core Emotion: Rage at this unfairness!

A different cascade of emotion unfolds in the present moment between Sahra and Emily. It begins with the visible shift in Sahra's face as she moves from disgust at the doctor for bypassing her, to a smile as she speaks her words of resignation, "But I am used to it." Sahra's automatic strategy of coping by dismissing her own rage at the injustice she experiences as a person of color, masking it with a smile, and carrying on, is disrupted by Emily's response.

Emily offers a tracking reflection of Sahra's rapid process of dismissing her own anguish with a resigned smile, and conjectures, "It must burn to the core." Sahra pauses to notice her own survival strategy in motion, and Emily continues, "You touched such an unjust moment and your face bristled as you said, 'That child's illness is my specialty!' and then you smiled as you said, 'But I am used to it!' You are used to these moments of unfair treatment and you cope by smiling, when inside it must burn to the core," adds Emily, again conjecturing to heighten the injustice and colorism (Burton et al., 2010) that Sahra has just recounted.

Sahra is silent, then exhales slowly "Thank you for noticing!" She pauses for a long time and then adds, "It is exhausting. I don't let myself feel the pain or the rage – but it's there. Thank you for noticing! Thank you for noticing how I cope with anguish I cannot control!" This example of therapist-client dialogue is a different cascade of emotion:

Trigger (perceived as safe): Emily reflects Sahra's present moment survival pattern of experiencing injustice and then dismissing it. She validates the injustice and conjectures at Sahra's anguish.

Bodily response: Silence, long exhale.

Meaning made: She notices me. She sees my pain and my rage behind my smile. I do cope that way – always have had to. It is exhausting!

Action Tendency: Catches her breath and appreciates being noticed and respected.

Hint of Core Emotion: A brief flicker of joy and comfort at being seen and valued.

Doorways into Leading Edge, Underlying, Unacknowledged Emotions

In Stage 1, EFT therapists see that core emotions are typically excluded from clients' awareness. The cascades of emotion in clients' typical patterns unfold so rapidly that the core emotions are unheeded. In the growing safety of the therapeutic alliance, the therapist hears hints and whispers of clients' emotional handles that can be grasped to open doors into discovering and assembling more vulnerable depths. Each of the elements of emotion – danger cue and rapid, unconscious, limbic perception of this cue; bodily sensations; meanings and attributions of self and other; action impulses, behaviors, and reactive emotions – can be a doorway to reach the core, vulnerable interior and to befriend the unacknowledged core emotion driving the repetitive, escalating pattern of emotional reactivity.

The attachment map guides the EFT clinician to "see and hear" beyond the surface and to detect alarm bells that may be sounding danger. Each client – a more avoidant partner, a more anxious partner, an anxious, depressed, trauma survivor – will have their own unique warning bell that activates the self-protective attachment system. An EFT therapist sees that clients caught in rigid, repetitive patterns are operating in emergency response mode, fighting for their lives (or their relationship) with little conscious awareness of the underlying panic of losing another's love or their sense of self. The attachment map shows the therapist in EFCT that reactive critical pursuit and defensive withdrawal are driven by fears of loss and rejection and anguished loneliness. The same attachment map shows a therapist in EFIT that anxiety, depression, and post trauma reactions are driven by perceived danger, a sense of uncontrollability, and a sense of disconnection from relational safety. Reactive emotions of numbness, frustration, angry outbursts, anxious perseveration, and flashbacks are seen by the therapist as code for as yet unexpressed core attachment emotions, such as vulnerable fears of rejection, annihilation, abandonment or isolation.

On the surface, the therapist in EFCT sees the signals each partner sends to the other partner and the typical reactions they evoke. The therapist also hears the threatening interpretations each partner makes about their partner's actions from within their heightened states of attachment panic. Correspondingly, in EFIT the therapist sees and hears individual stories of how clients prime and maintain their anxiety or depression. The therapist sees that while clients are beginning to recognize their automatic internal and interpersonal patterns (turning toward, away from, or against), they remain too caught up in the automatic self-protective dance to recognize and send clear signals about their core fears and needs. For example, Sahra describes her disappointment in her father and her daughter's father for not taking her seriously or responding with support. "There was no point in asking them," she sighs. Then, illustrating Bowlby's position that *we do as we've been done to*, she goes on to demonstrate a similar internal *turn away* pattern. She describes her fatigue and her anxieties, moving from tears to sudden dismissal and says, "It's not so bad…I'm fine." It is obvious to Emily that Sahra, like all her clients, needs a process consultant to help her to follow her dance and to listen to the core emotional music that is moving her feet in rigid self-protective patterns that exacerbate her distress.

Safety and Hope in Framing the Pattern as the Problem

By the end of Stage 1 stabilization (clients' Step 4), an EFT therapist sees the emergence of a new level of safety and hope, even though the protective pattern reappears at times. Sophie and Ella begin to find words for their newly accessed fears that underlie their volatile attack–attack cycle: Sophie describes it as a fear of never being precious to Ella and Ella describes it as a fear of Sophie giving up on her as a partner. They name their cycle "the raging storm." Phil and Julie name their cycle "the frozen lake," and they begin to access vulnerable fears of being rejected (Julie) and being destroyed (Phil) underlying their numbness and suppression.

Jessica and Wayne recognize with warm smiles how they automatically get pulled into their "spilled milk tango" and get glimpses of each other's underlying vulnerable emotions that endear them to each other.

Wayne says, "It means a lot to me that she understands my need to get away when she is overreacting. It feels crazy to me, you know." Jessica chimes in, "I do go crazy when he seems so far away. My first husband always felt far away, but Wayne can be so different. I freak out when he is far away, and I do go crazy." Wayne adds, "I also understand how she gets livid when I disappear and sink to the basement to get away from her."

Jessica continues, "And I'm getting, too, that when I get loud and pushy with him, he gets that awful knot in his gut." She tears up as she says:

I hate that I can make him feel so badly just trying to get him to *be with me!* I hate that my anger or my turtling away in silence makes him feel as badly as his mother's scolding did. And the really exciting thing is that I can see now that I do make a difference to him, and he is willing to discuss plans with me. We stepped out of our cycle last week. I don't fire up so fast anymore. I don't get afraid so quickly that he is about to disappear. And he's not disappearing so much either.

"True! It's a whole lot easier to stay near her now!" Wayne admits as he flashes her one of his magnetic smiles.

Emily also sees and hears signs of more emotional balance in her EFIT clients. She notices indications that they have stabilized in their increased awareness and acceptance of their emotional experience. She sees that they are more balanced emotionally, with less reactivity or numbness, and are more able to focus and outline key patterns. They show more curiosity and openness to explore inner experience and interpersonal encounters. Their stories have more coherence and clarity, and there is a new sense of hope, efficacy, and direction.

Emily validates how courageously Sahra is identifying her survival strategies to manage the impacts of the enormous losses and traumas of childhood, the stresses of immigration, the weight of grief for her mother who remained in Ukraine, the current demands of medical school and the countless incidents of racial aggression, all without a clear support network and with no current romantic partner. Sahra integrates:

Ignoring my own losses and grief has been helpful but it's come at too great a cost. Now I recognize I carry a lot of grief and anger – like immense pieces of locked luggage. It is exciting and frightening to be discovering that I don't need to keep my grief and traumas packed up and out of sight anymore. It is definitely scary but relieving to imagine opening that luggage! That I couldn't bring my mother to America has left me so angry and so lost!

Several Stage 1 encounters with her *imaginal mother* are helping Sahra to stabilize. Initially her mother looked terrified when Sahra told her how difficult it was caring for her from a distance and how disappointed she was that she refused to immigrate with her. She imagines terror on her mother's face, signaling a fear that Sahra might abandon her. She appreciates that vulnerable sense of terror from her mom because she longs for a felt sense of softness in her mother that she'd known as a young girl. It helps to soothe the reality that her mother, until her death, remained guarded, critical and full of complaints. These explorations are helping Sahra to stabilize and recognize her pattern of ignoring and minimizing her struggles. This is opening new fields of possibilities for her to safely explore her "packed up" stories. New meanings and new action tendencies are emerging.

What EFT Therapists *Do* to Shape the First Change Event of Stabilization

The stabilizing change event of Stage 1 takes shape with all moves of the EFT Tango, but Tango Move 2 assembly and deepening is central to engaging the client – couple or individual – to more deeply explore and stabilize their pattern of rapid reactivity to signals of alarm (see Summary in Box 8.1).

In her early days of using EFT, there were times that Emily felt such urgency to improve a couple's distressed relationship or to get an individual client to stop their self-deprecation or rigid faulting of others, that she lost focus and tried teaching them how to change. When she slips off track and begins to teach her clients about the pattern or to question her clients about *why* they think are getting caught in these patterns, she pauses to notice she is losing her own emotional balance and her attunement with the clients. She finds her balance and regains attunement through the moves of the EFT Tango. "Simply put, to guide my couple and individual clients through the first change event of stabilization, the moves of the EFT Tango are my guide":

Box 8.1   Summary of Shaping Stabilization – The First Change Event

What EFT Therapists and Clients Do

1. **Review the pattern of protection and explore the elements of emotion in that pattern:**
   Therapists outline, in early sessions, what Bowlby referred to as the mirroring patterns of "the inner ring of emotional processing and the outer ring of interpersonal responses" (Johnson, 2019, p. 88). With Move 1 tracking and reflecting present process and some Moves 3 and 4 shaping and processing encounters, therapists help clients to own their self-protective action tendencies.
   Clients Identify triggers and own action tendencies in their self-protective pattern (aka they take Step 2).
   Therapists invite further exploration of the impacts of the third ring of the socio-cultural context, using Move 1 present process tracking and reflecting and facilitating Move 3 encounters and Move 4 processing.
   Clients explore more deeply the attachment and contextual triggers and self-protective action tendencies (they continue to take Step 2).

2. **Distill the elements of emotion driving the pattern into a coherently expressed and tangibly felt core emotion:**
   Therapists, with Move 2 assembly and deepening and through encounters with Moves 3 and 4, help clients to discover, distill, and deepen their ownership of and engagement with the specific core attachment fear that was mostly outside of their awareness in the cacophony of rapid emotional reactivity.
   Clients access and express the core, underlying emotion driving their pattern (aka they take Step 3).

3. **Integrate, summarize, and celebrate stabilization:**
   Therapists, with Move 5 integrate, validate, and summarize the specifics of the new frame for the problem as the self-protective patterns of love gone wrong, or of the survival needs for human connection gone awry.
   Clients grasp *how their pattern*, not personal deficiencies in self or other, *is the problem*. With this stabilization and more engagement with core emotion, they have hope, more clarity, emotional balance, and a new sense of agency (aka they take Step 4).

---

1. Review the basic pattern with Move 1, sometimes followed by Moves 3 and 4 encounters to engage clients in experientially owning their action tendencies.
2. Assemble and order their *trigger/perception–feeling–meaning–action* responses with Move 2, until the core driving emotion is accessed. Discover, distill, and deepen. Create deeper levels of awareness with various intimate interpersonal encounters, using Moves 3 and 4.
3. Integrate the new frame of *problem as pattern* with Move 5, while also summarizing, specifically, how the clients have stabilized. Celebrate the empowerment and hope they are creating.

Review Basic Pattern with Tango Move 1

With Move 1 reflecting, Emily finds her balance. By reflecting clients' present moment experience and tracking what they identify as their action tendencies to difficult triggers (relationship-specific and socio-cultural context-specific), she maintains attunement. Clients are calmed and focused with her replay of their current pattern and her validation of how challenging this is. Move 1 settles and focuses. Many times she will *mine these moments* with Move 3, shaping a simple encounter to engage clients in the emotional impact of owning their default positions and their self-protective strategies, and with Move 4, processing the impact of this sharing.

Move 1 sets the trajectory for affect assembly and deeper emotional discovery. EFT therapists begin ordering emotion when they identify the basic self-protective pattern. Since emotion is first about a readiness to act (Frijda, 2007), the assembly begins with linking *when* emotion begins (the trigger or cue) to the impulse to action (e.g., "*When* Jessica's voice sounds loud and angry, Wayne turns away; *when* Wayne turns away, Jessica gets loud and angry"). When both partners in a couple (or an individual client in EFIT) recognize and *own* the link between the danger cue from their partner in EFCT (or the specific trigger in EFIT) and their typical behavioral response, they will have taken Step 2 of client change.

Owning the link between trigger and response essentially means helping clients acknowledge, "This is what I do in a moment of threat," and, "This is one of the triggers which I find most likely to pull me into doing that." Couples identify what Johnson (2008) calls their *Demon Dialogue* or their distancing dance. The more withdrawn client of the couple Ted and Jed (pseudonyms; training video at www.steppingintoeft.com) capture this link, as Jed says, "The more I sleep with one leg out of the covers to be ready to escape in case Ted explodes, the more he fears I will disappear; and the more upset he gets with me for being distant and ready to flee, the more I prepare to flee. Hence - - the dance."

Individuals in EFIT also own the link between the trigger and response. Max says, "It makes sense, the more I downplay my own emotions, the more others seem oblivious to what is happening for me; the more others appear distant and uncaring, the more I downplay my experience." Sahra notices the link between a trigger of receiving praise and her habit of isolating, "The more credit I get from colleagues, the more I mistrust it and feel lost and depressed and the more I isolate; the more I isolate and doubt myself, the more I mistrust others' compliments. I see how this pattern feeds my anxiety and depression."

Discover, Distill, and Deepen with Tango Move 2

Emily notices time and time again how Move 1 flows organically into Move 2 assembly. With empathic engagement, she repeats the danger cue to evoke other elements of emotion: Bodily reactions, meanings, and attributions about self and other. Hints of core emotion emerge. From some clients, she hears subtle whispers of underlying emotion and from others she hears adamantly declared meanings ("She just doesn't care! I'm a total loser!") and troubling attributions ("Maybe I'm too much? What if he doesn't love me anymore?"). She also sees nonverbal displays of somatic reactions (head dropping, face twisting, muscles tensing). Linking these pieces together into core, distilled emotion is the first part of Move 2.

Unformulated emotional experience, which is on the leading edge of client awareness but has not yet been put into words, is what an EFT therapist helps clients to discover, distill, and once formulated into a coherent whole, to deepen with the second part of Move 2. Opening doorways of the elements of emotion grants gradual access to the underlying core emotion. Emily repeatedly discovers the significance of the "driver's door" – the trigger or the emotional alarm bell of danger, which sets the process of emotion in motion. In helping clients to enter into core emotional experience, it is helpful for her to repeat the cue, to bring alive the initial felt sense of good or bad, safe or dangerous, and to open all the doors of the process of emotion until, together with her clients, they can formulate the core attachment emotion, typically expressed as some form of fearing that one is not precious, loved, wanted, accepted, capable, or worthwhile, or that significant others are not reliable.

What If My Client Has No Emotions? An amazing resource in the EFT model is that harnessing the power of emotion is possible with all clients, including those who claim they have no emotional awareness or words for emotional experience. At times, the action tendency part of emotion ("What I do," or, "What I feel like doing") or the surface, reactive emotional behaviors (getting angry, going numb) seems to be the only part of emotion of which a more avoidant client is aware. Thus, the doorway of action tendency and reactive emotional behaviors is a very helpful way to begin to assemble emotion in an avoidant client.

Wayne, for example, might say, "I don't actually feel anything. I just want to shut down." Here, the therapist can explore what triggers his desire to shut down. It might be seeing a look of disappointment on Jessica's face that moves him to shut down and go numb. From having identified the trigger (Jessica's disappointed look) and his immediate action impulse (to shut down and disappear), the therapist can open the door for him to describe the meaning he makes of her look. ("That's it! I had my last chance. She'll never accept me.")

Emily can, thus, distill Wayne's core emotion down to his dread of disappointing Jessica and losing her entirely or getting hurt by her harsh reaction. Emily intentionally stops herself from using the word *fear* and replaces it with *dread*. She senses that the word fear is too far on the leading edge for Wayne and it would not feel at all accurate. As a black man in America, he has let her know he cannot afford to feel fear but he can certainly identify with dreading the outcome of letting Jessica down. Emily seeks to titrate emotional exploration and naming of core attachment emotion to retain a respectful match for clients' present moment experience.

She evokes the felt sense of underlying emotion by replaying (tracking) the process, in an empathically engaged, slow, low, tone, "So you see that look on her face, and you say, 'Uh oh!! Here goes—I've just blown my last chance… and this is it, and she'll give up on me forever.' Is that it?" (checking for confirmation). After Wayne agrees it really is this bad, Emily validates and heightens with repetition:

> Wow—you see that look and hear her sigh, and immediately you're sent into this dangerous spin, this dreadful sense you have already lost her, and you go numb. Outside you may look rather blank, yet inside you feel cold and lonely. So full of dread that you will never get her warmth and acceptance, yes?

Sahra maintains, rather matter-of-factly, that she has no feelings about her circumstances and has little interest in discussing her losses and traumas. Emily recalls Sahra's earlier words, "I'm working hard to be a better person… just to keep afloat… but I am losing motivation." Emily remembers several emotional handles from Sahra that she can access to assemble more of Sahra's emotional experience:

- *Having no feeling about past traumas.* Emily validates Sahra's clever, adaptive strategy to distance from the emotional impacts of the trauma she has endured so as not to be overwhelmed.
- *Requiring more and more effort to stay afloat.* Emily empathically engages with Sahra's action tendency to put more and more effort into her work and parenting, and links it to her poignant emotional image of trying to stay afloat.
- *Working to be a better person.* Emily hears this negative attribution of self as needing to be better and links this to Sahra's action tendency of *working hard to be better*.
- *Losing motivation.* This bodily felt experience of lethargy is another emotional handle that Emily can explore with Sahra. "Working so hard to be safe and to keep afloat. It makes sense your body is saying, 'Stop. Slow down! This all seems like too much!'"

- *Every piece of clutter in my home sends my system on alert that there is something I must do.* As Emily repeats those words from Sahra, Sahra gradually acknowledges, "I guess it's safer to focus on immaculate tidiness and cleanliness than on how lost I feel without my people in Ukraine, especially since the ongoing war … wanting to help my country." After a long pause, she begins, "And now," her voice freezes, then in a whisper she says, "My African roots. I want to know my family. I want to see family members who look like me! My mom loved my dad – I know. When I was little, she'd look at me with love and say, 'You look like him – so strong and beautiful!'"

Validating Reactive Emotions as a Doorway to Discover Core Emotion. When partners are expressing reactive anger or describing a sense of "feeling nothing," an EFT therapist validates these emotions. Anger and numbing are typical reactive, protective emotions in response to an unresponsive or unsafe attachment figure or context. Validating reactive emotion is a doorway into core emotion. Clients discover, when feeling uncertain, that the vulnerable core emotion "slips right by" and disappears into the background and they "go straight to anger or to numbness." EFT therapists' validation of reactive emotions creates safety and conveys that the therapist understands what they are so angry about, or what is so difficult about another person's behavior that they simply feel lost or numb.

Emily opens a doorway to some of Wayne's core emotion by validating the numbness he feels when Jessica describes her disappointment in him, "It makes sense you feel numb and sink to the basement when what you hear is that Jessica is nearly giving up on you!"

Emily validates Jessica's eruptions in the "spilled milk tango," "It makes sense that you feel angry when you can get very little response." She links Jessica's reactive anger to the trigger of Wayne's abrupt disappearance to the basement. As she assembles Jessica's emotions, they gradually access the core, unexpressed, softer emotions. First, she accesses the core sadness that the man she fell in love with is rarely *within reach.* Then, she accesses her fear that he no longer wants her as his partner.

Paradoxically, Sahra, who is overwhelmed as she describes to Emily her fears of speaking to a group of colleagues about her refugee and immigration experiences, discovers that fear is not her core emotion. As Emily validates her fears, linked to her expectations of touching her deep traumas, "appearing pathetic," collapsing in tears, and receiving sympathy and compassion, Sahra shakes her head, accessing core anger with an adaptive action tendency to be assertive:

I agreed to speak, knowing I will relive my trauma and face things I have remained detached from. But I am not doing it for sympathy. I am doing it because I want my colleagues to know about what my people are living through!

Her voice strengthens and her clarity increases:

I want them to know my tears, if I shed some, are not only my tears. They are the tears of all my people. I want the audience to be moved to care and to take action for my people! I want them to see and hear how urgent the needs of my people are!

Her core anger, strength, and power, with its action tendency to move out, move close, and be seen and heard, empower her and transform her sense of being overwhelmed, to one of courage and determination.

Shaping Stage 1 Change with Tango Moves 2, 3, and 4

The assembly and expansion of emotion continue until each client's elements of emotion have been linked in a coherent manner to the other elements of emotion, and the underlying core emotion has been discovered and deepened. With Moves 3 and 4, shaping and processing encounters, therapists help clients to disclose their newly discovered coherent emotion. This empowers them to further deepen and expand their awareness of how their default manner of engaging is what is constructing their distress.

Interventions in Tango Move 2. Many tracking reflections are made in Move 2, particularly repeating the cue that sets the cascade of emotional responses in motion. Linking the cue (*he turns away*) to the terrifying attachment meanings made (*he must not care about me*), frequently evokes a felt sense of underling core pain and fear. Surface, reactive emotions and actions are validated in the context of the recurring pattern. ("Of course you react with rapid anger, when his shoulders stiffen and to you this usually means he is about to turn away and leave you all alone, thinking, 'See he doesn't care about me!'" Or, "Of course you avoid people from your past if seeing them tells you that you are somehow a bad person.") Evocative questions (what, when, where, and how, but *not why*) are used to assemble the elements of emotion and to access the unacknowledged fleeting emotions underlying positions of pursuit and withdrawal ("What did you feel *just before* you turned away?" or, "...*just before* you exploded with rage?") Evocative questions are also used to invite more of the story when a hint of emotion related to a contextual trigger appears. ("Tell me more about what it means when you say, 'But I'm used to being ignored.'" Or, "Say more about what it says to you when you get 'these looks' in the bookstore with your baby because of your different skin tone.") Empathic conjectures (empathically attuned hunches on the leading edge of the attachment experience) are also used to access underlying emotion. ("Under all that numbness you feel after she stomps off, I wonder if you might feel fear that she is disappointed in you as her partner?" Or, "When you say, 'I don't want to feel anything about that injustice,' and your jaw tightens, I wonder if you're almost feeling some anger about what you have had to endure?") Validations function to normalize these emotions and reactions and make "attachment sense" out of them. Tracking reflections are made of the steps in the repetitive pattern. Validating the links between cues, bodily arousal, attachment meanings, and action tendencies, brings the newly emerging core emotion to the surface. When a core emotion is accessed, the therapist lingers with it and heightens it. Heightening, or deepening clients' experience is the second part of Move 2, where emotion that was assembled and distilled in the first part of Move 2 is repeated and heightened with the RISSSSSC manner.

Interventions in Tango Moves 3 and 4. Once partners have discovered a felt sense of their core underlying emotion, with Move 3, therapists shape encounters to heighten ownership of this experience and to create a new experience of more vulnerable contact between partners (Tilley & Palmer, 2013). The therapist choreographs encounters for each partner to disclose the link between their step in the dance (action tendencies of demand–pursue or defend–withdraw) and the underlying attachment fear or anguish.

Therapist: Sophie, can you turn and tell Ella about this fear underneath your outbursts – fear that you say, "never shows it's face?"

Sophie: I know I go straight to anger and start tearing you down. When I can't get you to respond to me, I get terrified that you don't care about me at all, and I go ballistic!

Following the encounter, Emily processes with Sophie how it feels to be letting Ella know that she does tear her down with anger and that her outbursts are code for her fear that Ella doesn't care about her – a fear that she tries to hide at all times. Then she checks with Ella how it is to hear Sophie owning that she does "go ballistic," when inside she is "terrified you don't care about her."

Similarly, in EFIT Stage 1 Emily assembles Sahra's emotions to a core fear of unworthiness and guilt for having left Ukraine to study medicine in North America. The responsibility she feels for having left her mother, suffering ill health and in danger as the war began, weighs heavily on her soul. In EFIT, when clients have distilled their core emotion, a therapist will use Moves 3 and 4 to help them engage more fully with disclosing how the core emotion is linked to their actions in their recurring pattern. But before using Move 3 to SHAPE an encounter, Emily uses Move 2 to help Sahra shape a coherent message to share with an image of her mother. The emotional elements which they assemble are:

Trigger: Mother refused to come to the US where Sahra could have supported her.
Body: Tension, stomach ache.
Meaning: "I feel I have never been a good enough daughter for you since *Aabo* (her father) left us. I wanted to help you – I wanted to protect you and you never allowed me to make a difference for you!" And, "I feel guilty for leaving her in Ukraine where she died without me."
Action tendency/reactive emotion: "I am so angry at you for not coming to the US where I could have taken better care of you… and where I could have been a better daughter for you!"
Hints of core emotion: Exhausted – tired of feeling guilty and angry; deep sadness; fear that her mother stopped loving her.

Then with Move 3, Emily helps Sahra to *SHAPE* a message to her imaginal mother. Emily **S**harpens and **H**eightens a message about Sahra's core fear that her mother had stopped loving her. She helps Sahra to **A**nticipate the encounter by picturing her mother ready to listen to her share how the refusal to come to the United States held her in the grips of fear that she had turned her back on her mother and that her mother had stopped loving her. Emily directs Sahra to **P**resent the message to an image of her mother. When Sahra becomes distracted, Emily **E**ngages her, refocusing on her core emotion – fear her mother has stopped loving her.

After Sahra speaks to her imaginal mother, Emily progresses to Move 4.

Emily: How was it to share this very alive fear with an image of your mother?
Sahra: (Weeping through her words.) It feels so good to cry – I am so sad that I lost you. (Continuing to talk to this image of her mother.) I lost my sweet kind mother when I was a child. I was still trying to get you back!
Emily: How do you picture your mother as you speak to this image of her?
Sahra: She looks stunned. It's like she never knew I lost her as a child… and like she didn't know how much I truly longed to help her. She is just listening. Listening to me –amazing!

Sahra is exploring new territory as she opens to depths of emotion that she has packed away for years. She is beginning to get glimpses of a new view of self and other. Most importantly, she is beginning to discover that it is safe and hopeful to experience emotions that she has blocked for decades. "Packing everything away is no longer what I want to do! It is just too difficult and too costly!" she says with a brightening smile.

Flowing with Tango Moves 2, 3, and 4 toward Stabilization in EFCT. The goal of stabilization is for clients to get a felt sense of their self-protective pattern in response to a core underlying fear that has not yet been explored. Thus, therapists use Moves 2, 3, and 4 to help clients gain a coherent story of the links in the process of emotion and their two-person pattern or dance. The goal is not only to access and deepen engagement with the core vulnerable fear and distress that they habitually avoid. It is also to help them get a felt sense of the links between what they perceive, what they process in their body, how they make meaning, and their behavioral strategies which ironically heighten and reinforce the problematic feedback loops of inner processing and interpersonal interacting.

In EFCT, a therapist uses Move 1 with the couple to track and validate the present process *within and between.* Then, using Move 2, a therapist assembles and deepens emotions with one partner at a time, while maintaining connection with the observing partner. In Stage 1, there is no need to engage a more avoidant or a more anxious partner first. It is simply important to fully assemble with each partner, one at a time. The choice of whom to begin with is a matter of attunement to the clients and attunement to the emotion in the room. In the moment, who is most willing to explore, or who most needs to feel understood? Emotion offers various guides to EFT therapists as they choose which emotion and with which partner to focus. In Stage 1, EFT therapists are guided to focus on (1) emotion that is most poignant; (2) emotion that is conspicuous by its absence; (3) emotion that seems most relevant to attachment needs and fears; or (4) emotion which seems likely to initiate cascades of difficult interactions (Furrow et al., 2022; Johnson, 2020). These are all viable options for which emotion to choose. Emily notices as she reviews her videos and identifies the principles that are guiding her choices that her confidence and clarity are strengthening.

EFT Tango Move 2. Emily chooses to use Move 2 with Jessica because her reactivity in the face of Wayne's subtle shrug seems closely connected to urgently felt attachment fears and needs. She wants to help Jessica get a felt sense of her inner and outer moves in their imprisoning pattern as part of shaping Wayne and Jessica's stabilization. She tracks, with genuine curiosity, how Jessica ramps up and increases the volume immediately after Wayne shrugs and turns away. To evoke Jessica's meaning of the trigger of Wayne's shrug and turn away, she asks, "What did it say to you when Wayne shrugged and turned toward the window?" Jessica clarifies that she took his move to mean he is not interested in her. "It proves he doesn't care one bit!" sighs Jessica. Emily validates, "Of course, if his shrug tells you that he is not interested in you, it makes sense you'd get alarmed and want to go after him to pull him back, yes?" Here, Emily is adding an attachment element, reframing Jessica's critical pursuit as having a positive attachment intention – to pull her loved one close when she is afraid that he is turning away from her. Presuming an attachment frame shines a warm and accepting light on even the most hostile or cold behaviors. Emily continues to replay this trigger of Wayne's shrug and turn away as she opens doorways of the emotion process. Assembling the elements of Jessica's emotional experience, Emily links and lingers with Jessica's attachment meaning that she is not important or precious to Wayne, her action tendency of turning up the volume and pushing hard, and her bodily arousal of "a stab in my heart." Emily expands the emotion until Jessica is able to access a felt sense of her underlying fear of being alone, without Wayne.

EFT Tango Moves 3 and 4. To help Jessica and Wayne make intimate contact with each other while disclosing and receiving this expanded view of their dance, Emily uses Moves 3 and 4. After lingering with Jessica's fear and the stabbing in her heart at the image of being without Wayne, Emily uses Move 3 to SHAPE an encounter, to help Jessica own her action tendency in their negative cycle, and to link her reactivity to her core fear. She repeats the *within experience* of panic stabbing her heart, and the *between images* of Wayne's shrug and being without Wayne. Then she asks Jessica to link this trigger and her core fear to her actions in the cycle:

Can you turn and tell Wayne, "When I see you turn away or make the tiniest shrug, my heart stabs with panic that I have lost you, and I do get loud and pushy to make you talk to me"?

After Jessica's disclosure, Emily uses Move 4 to elicit Jessica's experience in making this disclosure, followed by inviting Wayne to reflect on how he experienced hearing this from her.

When Core Emotion Slips by Unnoticed! With Sophie and Ella, Emily uses Moves 2, 3, and 4 to identify the underlying, core emotion and heighten awareness of how rapidly the core emotion slips by unnoticed, only to be replaced by reactive, triggering responses. Emily uses Move 2 to lead Ella and Sophie to stabilization. She begins with Ella by repeating what pulls her into their pattern – the look of disappointment on Sophie's face (perceived cue). Slowly she links this trigger to the other elements, expanding awareness until the underlying sense of danger is felt, and the primary core attachment fear is revealed:

> You see that look on Sophie's face, "Uh oh!" (limbic perceived danger); for one second your heart sinks (bodily arousal) and says (meaning made), "I'm failing her again. I'm never enough to make her happy." You throw up your hands in exasperation, storming out of the room in anger (action tendency and reactive emotion).

Again repeating the cue perceived as dangerous, Emily reiterates:

> It makes sense you would get frustrated each time Sophie looks disappointed, when you long to be enough for her (validating the surface reactive emotion, linked to the cue and meaning made). Can we go back to the moment when you saw that unhappy look on her face? (driver's door opening; repeating the cue of limbic danger).

As Emily slowly unpacks the moment with her, Ella's inner experience of the alarming danger comes to life. She begins to recognize how she rapidly sidesteps her core fear of disappointing Sophie with surface reactions of frustration and withdrawal. After this assembly of emotion with Move 2, Emily moves forward to shape an encounter for Ella to share this newly formulated fear of disappointing Sophie and linking it with her action tendencies of getting frustrated with Sophie and withdrawing from her instead of sharing that fear directly. Ella tells Sophie, "I get frustrated and pull away from you when inside I'm terrified that I've disappointed you again."

There is a good possibility that while Emily uses Move 4 to process this encounter, Sophie may react with disbelief, reluctance, or a direct attack. Emily is learning to keep her own balance in these moments. She knows the value of Ella's discovery of the links between her inner emotional processing and her behavioral moves toward Sophie. She will revisit these links many times with Ella going forward. If Sophie has difficulty trusting this new disclosure from Ella, Emily will use an immediate intervention of catching the bullet before repeating Move 2 with Sophie to assemble and distill her experience in their recurring pattern.

When Sophie reacts to Ella's disclosure with, "That is all rubbish! She has no fear. She doesn't care about my feelings!" Emily gently and firmly interrupts and follows the *catching bullet* format (outlined in Chapter 4), beginning with tracking the present moment process. "Sophie, when Ella told you how she fears your disapproval but instead of sharing that fear, typically gets frustrated and pulls away from you to avoid hearing your disappointment in her, you reacted in disbelief." Next, she adds a conjecture to reframe the intention:

> It must be so hard to believe that all this time, when Ella has gotten frustrated with you and walked out of the room, she was running away from hearing you were disappointed in her! You had no idea she is afraid of hearing that you are not happy with her!

Emily is checking whether this conjecture fits for Sophie. If Sophie agrees, Emily may invite an encounter for Sophie to respond with authenticity to Ella. "Can you let Ella know this is so new that it feels impossible to trust just now?" In spite of reactivity and bullets, Sophie and Ella are in the process of recognizing and stabilizing their protective, imprisoning pattern.

Flowing with Tango Moves 2, 3, and 4 toward Stabilization in EFIT. Moves 2, 3, and 4 with Sahra illustrate how Move 2, assembly and deepening, is extended furthered by blending with Moves 3 and 4, shaping and processing encounters.

Through Stage 1 stabilization, Sahra identifies a familiar pattern across relationships. She recognizes:

> The more alone I am and receive others' dismissive and critical responses, the more I take on others' suffering and try to help them. The more I fail to get others' appreciation and approval, the harder I try to make them happy. Inside I am filled with fear of being unwanted, unlovable, and abandoned even by God – fearing I will be punished.

Sahra survives the many challenges of her life in a similar pattern. Her childhood sexual abuse, abandonment by her father, her mother's emotional absence and criticism, racist experiences of exclusion and dismissal, especially in graduate school and in her residency, and several broken, abusive romantic relationships are all responded to with a similar pattern of dismissing her own needs and emotions and trying harder to help others.

She is beginning to stabilize her emotional chaos and pattern of spinning from one dangerous relationship to another. She is able to engage with core emotions of bottomless grief. Her present-day grief is most closely tied to the losses of her mother – not only from her mother's actual death – but equally as poignant and alive today, is the loss of the mother she knew, when she sank into a deep depression after *Aabo,* Sahra's father, left the family. She also touches the shame and fears she carries about hell and judgment from her mother.

Sahra notices a familiar pattern come to life – longing for her mother's approval, feeling her life depends on getting her mother to see her worth, and sinking into shame and fear each time she fails to get a warm, affirming response. "One trigger for this pattern I've lived all my life and still seem to be repeating across relationships is seeing, in my memory, my mother's vacuous face, looking lonely and depressed." Sahra owns the meanings she makes, as, "I have to save her. I can't be relaxed or happy if she is depressed." She also owns her action tendencies:

> It's like I say, "Let me suffer with you. I will embrace it all. I will give, give, give to you without limits, swallowing your insults and invasions." I keep playing games to help her because she will not receive direct help, nor will she ask clearly for help.

Sahra speaks as if her mother were still alive. She is, in fact, very much alive in Sahra's internal world. Echoes of her mother's cryptic, blaming message implying she should do more to make her happy, weigh heavily on Sahra who feels caught in a repeating pattern of dismissing her own needs and taking on the weight of others' distress. She recognizes how she relives this pattern across relationships and in her internal world with herself as well.

Messages of judgment and disapproval from her mother continue to play in Sahra's head, even though her mother is no longer living. "It is mission impossible to do enough for others!" declares Sahra, clearly caught in a pattern of seeking approval and love, failing to get it, and continuing to expend more and more energy to prove her worth and goodness.

Weaving between Moves 2 and 3, Emily shapes various imaginal encounters for Sahra to speak with her mother, with her estranged father, with her recent romantic partner, with her supervisor at work, and some encounters for Sahra to dialogue between two aspects of self. She processes the impact of these encounters with Move 4.

She also processes the spontaneous encounters that occur between herself and Sahra. At one point, Sahra mentions how enraged she feels with the racist treatment she experienced at work that day, "My supervisor dismissed my expertise because of the color of my skin!" Almost immediately, she drops into shameful meaning-making. Looking straight into Emily's eyes, she says with a defeated look, "I must be a bad person deserving of burning in hell!" Emily begins with a tracking reflection to acknowledge that this shameful meaning showed up after Sahra noted how enraged she is. "True" whispers Sahra.

Refocusing, Emily says in a soothing voice:

Can we go back a moment, and can you tell me how it is for you? That, for a brief moment, before that dreadful fear of hell showed up, you looked in my face and said, "I am enraged that my supervisor dismissed my expertise because of the color of my skin!"

Emily's voice is stronger and more forceful. "How is it to share that rage with me and have me fully attending and feeling enraged as well, just before the old familiar shaming message took over and muffled your rage?" Encounters with the therapist emerge spontaneously at times. Processing the encounter between therapist and client is one of the most effective ways to make the most of these moments. Sahra, flushing slightly, reflects on how challenging it is to stay in touch with her core anger. She notes that putting those shameful words out loud is already helping to shrink their power and leaves her feeling determined to return to her experience of rage!

Integrating Stage 1 Change (Stabilization) with Tango Move 5

By the end of Stage 1, the problem is reframed as the pattern – the repetitive moves and meanings, the ongoing bodily felt stressors, all fueled by underlying attachment fears, vulnerabilities and longings. The essence of stabilization is linking the elements of emotion into a coherent whole, where no one is the bad guy, but clients are painfully stuck in their best attempts to protect their relationship (EFCT) and manage difficult emotions (EFIT). To integrate and validate the first change event of stabilization, the EFT therapist uses Move 5 to *go meta – to the game not the ball* and links the pattern to the core underlying emotions that fuel the experience.

First, we'll drop into Emily's validating work with Wayne and Jessica and then with Sahra as they integrate the stabilization change event of Stage 1.

Tango Move 5 in EFCT to Validate and Integrate Wayne and Jessica's Stabilization. Using Move 5 with Wayne and Jessica, Emily links the elements of their repetitive pattern together, to form a positive reframe of their relationship distress. What a long way they have come in these 15 sessions. Their focus has shifted from fights over children, housework, and in-laws, toward the fears and concerns that throw them off balance. Emily recalls their rigid pattern, where the more Jessica pursued for contact and response, the more Wayne stiffened up and turned away. She remembers how Jessica, in exasperation, had begun to withdraw as well. Wayne is less numb and not so quickly frustrated. His shaking foot and his cramping neck have calmed considerably. Jessica's rapid flipping between anger and tears has slowed down measurably, although both anger and tears do still erupt.

Box 8.2   Markers of Stabilization in EFCT

- Each partner has an experiential sense of the alarm bell that rings for them in the relationship and how they typically react to this threat.
- Beginning to see how their behaviors pull their partner into the cycle and how their reactive position triggers their partner's core fear.
- Discovering, naming, and expressing the vulnerable emotions and longings underlying positions of pursuit and withdrawal.
- Partners accept their unique pattern as a reframe for their relationship problem.
- Partners co-create with the therapist their own meaningful story of how the pattern defines their relationship and how they create this pattern. A sense of efficacy emerges: "If we created this, maybe we can make it better."
- Partners are aware of and sometimes able to stop their automatic reactivity.
- Less reactivity means there is more safety in the relationship.
- A less hostile, more engaged, hopeful relationship is emerging where the repetitive pattern, which does recur, is less rigid and hurtful.
- Interactions are more fluid, but the basic organization of interactions has not changed.
- A new kind of dialogue is emerging. Instead of rapid reactivity, partners are beginning to be emotionally engaged with each other. Conflicts are calmer; partners feel closer.
- Each partner's experience of self and other is less constricted.

Pursuers Are:

- Relieved to see their partner is not indifferent or uncaring but is hiding to protect themself from the enormity of their partner's actions.
- Accessing longings for connection; still very angry and mistrusting, but less hostile, and beginning to talk about their sadness and desperateness.

Withdrawers Are:

- Relieved to see that their partner is not being hostile because of random aggressiveness, but because they are making a desperate response to the withdrawer's position of hiding.
- Speaking about their paralysis instead of just going numb.

Markers emerge which indicate that they have stabilized (see Box 8.2). Earlier in therapy, Wayne could not hear Jessica's fears without immediately being triggered into defensiveness and offering indirect counter-attacks framed as "suggestions for ways to take better care of yourself." He is now able to lean forward with interest and to speak congruently and say things Jessica might not like to hear, such as, "I am struggling—it is very difficult to listen to you right now, I feel so badly that I just want to run. It feels a lot safer to just get out of the way when I hear how I have let you down."

Jessica, in turn, is awestruck with his honesty. "I don't want him to feel badly, but it is *so good* that he is letting me in to what is going on for him! I am actually getting to see Wayne!"

They recognize what throws them off balance and pulls them into their cycle. For example, in de-escalation, Jessica says, "I get it! My loneliness moves me to ramp up, and that primes your fear of losing me, which moves you to back far, far away. That fuels my loneliness and fear that you'll never really be with me, which moves me to get angrier and more accusatory and then silent, and on and on it goes."

Wayne joins in, "Of course, the more frantic you get, the further away I go. I'm freaked out at the degree to which I have unsettled you. There's no chance for me anymore. I feel like that at work where I am the only black man getting passed up for promotions even though I am the most qualified guy for the job, and I just need to get away. But now I get how dreadful my disappearance is for you, and why you yell even louder to call me back. It never works though. I do more and more of what you are telling me not to do," he says with a chuckle.

They have shared these fears and owned their action tendencies with each other. Jessica is beginning to taste the rejection and exclusion Wayne lives with every day of his life as a black man. The cycle happens less often; sometimes, they can stop it midway and reconnect afterward, though it can take a while. Emily remembers her joy in the moment Wayne and Jessica said, "Nothing has really changed, and yet everything is different." This is cycle stabilization.

Tango Move 5 in EFIT to Validate and Integrate Sahra's Stabilization. Emotional balance, safety, and a sense of agency are achieved in Stage 1 as clients recognize and accept that their patterns for engaging with self, others and the existential realities of life are what shape their suffering (Johnson, 2019). Like all EFIT clients in stabilization, Sahra internalizes that she is not to blame for her problems, and at the same time, she feels a new sense of agency to discover how her repetitive strategies for coping are keeping her in a repetitive cycle of distress (see Box 8.3). Several encounters with her imaginal mother, who is now deceased, with her estranged father whom Sahra does not want to see in real life and several other significant others, in addition to her encounters with Emily, the therapist, and some intrapsychic encounters are all helping Sahra to stabilize and feel much more accepting and aware of the pattern as the problem. She feels emotional balance and a new sense of hope and agency.

How EFT Therapists Engage While Guiding Clients through Stabilization

The main answers to the question about *how* EFT therapists deepen awareness of clients' self-protective patterns and evoke the experience and expansion of the core fears driving those patterns, revolve around providing a genuine, empathic, unconditionally accepting presence, while tracking present patterns and being familiar with the EXP scale (Klein et al., 1969,1986) as a predictor of client outcome (Kailanko et al., 2022; Pascual-Leone & Yeryomenko, 2017). When therapists develop a manner of engaging with clients that facilitates clients' increasing moment-to-moment

---

Box 8.3   Markers of Stabilization in EFIT

In EFIT, Stabilized Clients:

- Are more balanced emotionally – less reactive or numb.
- Are more aware and accepting of their own active process of emotion (as cascades of trigger-perception-feeling-meaning-action).
- Are more discovery oriented and open about inner experience and interpersonal encounters.
- Are more able to focus and outline key repetitive patterns.
- Are aware that their real problem is their pattern for coping and not self or other.
- Tell a more coherent narrative.
- Have a new sense of hope, efficacy, and direction.

emotional awareness and depth, they offer transformative therapy. *Emotional depth* means the capacity to reflect upon emotional experience as it emerges and expands. In addition to the EFT interventions already discussed, particularly the RISSSSSC manner that contributes to deepening clients' emotional experience (using Repetitions, Images, Simple, Soft, Slow pace, Specificity, Somatic cues, Client's words), there are several guidelines that can help therapists offer an *accessible, responsive, engaged* presence. The following guidelines can help a therapist to offer the safety of an exquisitely attuned, culturally humble, empathically curious therapeutic presence that clients need to complete the first change event of stabilization.

Ground Self as a Therapist

It is important for an EFT therapist to be emotionally balanced and attuned internally in order to process distressed clients' emotional experiences. Trusting the unconditional acceptance of the EFT model can help an EFT therapist to find a calm, centered place within. Knowing you are not alone but have the option of consulting with a colleague or EFT learning buddy for encouragement after a difficult session can also be calming.

A colleague or supervisor's voice saying, "It's all right. You are being present. That is what's most important" can help to balance you emotionally. EFT therapists can recognize "I can feel my heart pounding, sensing an 'Uh oh' danger moment" and then imagine a soothing presence, and a calming voice saying, "It's all right. Just notice you are feeling nervous. Be present. That is your best gift. Your anxiety is probably also the clients' experience." Knowing the power of mirror neurons to feel what another is feeling, an EFT therapist can trust that some experienced anxiety may be resonant with one or both partner's experience.

Resonate with a Felt Sense of the Client's Experience

Resonate in your own body with a felt sense of the client's emotional experience. When a client reports butterflies in their chest or a knot in their stomach, for example, feel that sensation in your own body. Walk around in the client's experience to taste it, sense it, feel it. Grasp the existential enormity of clients' different experiences. For example, one partner fears their partner does not care; another fears that they are not respected by their partner. Attune to the core fear of an individual client who has been so badly injured in relationships that they repeatedly step back whenever they dip a toe into emotional waters.

Be very humble in your resonance. Curb your tendency to be certain of your conjectures. Regardless of how good a therapist you are and how many times you have been told you effectively find words for clients' experience that precisely captures what they feel but couldn't put into words, remember to be tentative in your responses, continually inviting clients to let you know if they feel you understand and encouraging them to share the precise nuances of their experience. For example, a client of color alludes to ongoing experiences of exclusion. After validating how difficult that must be, a culturally humble therapist who has not experienced racial exclusion realizes their reflection may have felt minimizing and invites the client to say more about this.

Reflect From the Heart by Facing Your Own Existential Fears and Helplessness

Use empathic imagination to sense what each person's experience in their repetitive pattern must feel like and how it makes sense that each one reacts in the ways they do. Repeat, not only the label for an emotion while remaining distant from the experience, but physically lean in and reflect in a slow pace, matching clients' emotional tone while also having a felt sense of the client's distilled emotional experience. Vocal tone and pacing can be evocative and soothing. Resonate with each client like a responsive mother resonates with an upset child, noting signs of somatic movement in the client. With differences of intersectionality, be courageous to acknowledge that your own experience may be quite different and invite the client to say more. Reflect, taste, explore, evoke, heighten, and validate emotional experience so that a client can fully experience the present moment and a partner can hear the other's experience.

Immerse Yourself in the Unfolding Process of Each Client's Emotional Experience

The active elements of emotion remain significant after core emotion has been distilled. Repeating elements helps to keep the emotional experience alive. Return, again and again, to the importance of the cue that sets the emotional cascade in motion. That is, recall *when* this emotion process begins. Repeat the trigger for the emotion process. An EFT therapist never stops making explicit the action tendency element of emotion, how it is linked to the cue, and evoking the concrete, vivid, specific, granular story of the client's bodily felt core emotion. The meaning-making part of emotion is very important. Depth of experiencing includes "the degree to which clients engage and explore their feelings moment-by-moment as part of the process of personal meaning making" (Pascual-Leone & Yeryomnko, 2017, p. 654). In fact, as Kailanko et al. (2022) remind us, depth of emotional experiencing is less about intensity of emotional experience and more about *active reflection on meaningful emotional material*. That is, depth of emotion is the integration of the cue, bodily felt sense, meaning, action impulses, and distilled core emotion. The somatic part of emotion is very important as well. Thus, tracking where there is a visible shift, such as clenching in the body, movement in the face, or a change in voice tone, noting specifically what was observed, and inviting a client to expand on what they were experiencing as the bodily cue took place, has been shown to deepen experience in the moment (Kailanko et al., 2022). In EFCT, while working with one partner, a therapist also tracks bodily reactions of the observing partner.

Hold a Curious Awareness of Each of the Elements of Emotion

Use tracking reflections, patiently and repetitively, with a couple or individual client. Repeat the cue and link it to the action tendency with Move 2 until you can evoke more of the underlying experience. An EFT therapist is relentlessly curious and empathic, expanding on the emotional handles in each client's story.

Conclusion

Attuning with the EFT Tango Moves, therapists lead clients to step through the first change event of stabilization. In EFCT, following the stabilization change event, partners have a clear picture and an inner felt sense that the real problem in the relationship is neither one of them, but is, in fact, this automatic survival dance they are pulled into when their bond of love is threatened. With this awareness, partners disempower the cyclic pattern from unraveling their attachment bond and damaging their connection.

One might see the first change event in EFCT as calming troubled waters. There is some truth to that, as the couple does become calmer. Their fights are less hostile, and times of shutting-down are less rigid and shorter. Moments of calm and laughter emerge. The more blaming spouse seems less blaming and somewhat softer at times, and the more withdrawn partner seems less defensive and somewhat more present. Stabilization or de-escalation is more than calmer waters, however, as there is an active ownership of how each one pulls the other and how each one gets pulled into the old pattern. There is a sense of efficacy and hope of changing the pattern.

The attachment bond has yet to be restructured into a safe, secure bond of interactive reaching and responding. The basic system has not changed, and the old familiar pattern will resurface with very troubled waters if deeper, systemic, emotional changes are not made. The steps toward lasting change, where new emotional music creates a new dance, have yet to happen. Stage 1 leads to stopping the automatic recurring pattern, thereby creating a secure base from which to begin creating the Stage 2 change events (see Box 8.2). In Stage 2, the newly discovered and acknowledged emotions underlying the pursuit and withdrawal will be expanded, reprocessed, and used to shape new risks of reaching and responding that reshape the attachment bond into a positive one of mutual caring and comfort.

Likewise, in EFIT, with stabilization clients have an increased awareness of how they are shaping their worlds, recognizing their typical patterns of automatic physiological fight, flight or freeze reactions to perceived threats, the meanings they make about self and others in the moments of threat or distress, and their habitual action tendencies and emotional reactions (see Box 8.3). This awareness and sense of being an active player in shaping their experience is empowering and gives them a sense of agency and choice, though they have not yet reshaped their worlds. They are more able to focus and outline key, repetitive patterns in which they get caught. In stabilizing, by owning how they shape their worlds, clients are more balanced emotionally, less reactive or numb, and more aware and accepting of emotional experience. They are more discovery oriented and open about inner experience and interpersonal encounters. This capacity to tell a more coherent narrative is filled with a growing sense of hope, agency, and direction.

Get Ready... The Clients Are Coming!

Be sure to check Chapter 8 Support Material (routledge.com/9781032151335) for chapter summary and guidance to review each client case, imagining you are Emily, preparing for your therapy day by identifying your clients' basic patterns and core emotions.

Part III

Restructuring Attachment in Stage 2

Introduction to Part III

Restructuring Attachment in Stage 2

Defining love as an attuned and emotionally responsive presence is relevant to the change process in EFCT and EFIT. Stage 2 of EFCT creates a seismic shift where clients "open up emotionally and become more attuned and emotionally responsive to each other's vulnerabilities and needs. And we all know that this is what love is all about in the end. It's all about emotional presence" (Johnson, 2016c).

The role of emotion in creating lasting change and restructuring attachment bonds and views of self and other is featured in Part III. Two factors identified as key to creating change in EFT come to the fore in Stage 2: Deepening emotional engagement and shaping affiliative encounters with attachment figures (Brubacher & Wiebe, 2019; Greenman & Johnson, 2013; Johnson, 2019). Emotion is the agent of change as EFT therapists help couples to reshape their despair and disconnection into loving, lasting bonds filled with laughter, caring, and comfort. Likewise, emotion is the agent of change in EFIT as individuals are helped to reshape depression, anxiety, and post-trauma reactions into flexibility and resilience, and, using emotion as a guide, are helped to shape a positive sense of self in affiliative engagement with others. In Stage 1, EFT therapists focus on the role of emotion in organizing and stabilizing patterns of interaction, whereas in Stage 2, they use the power of emotion to fuel the two change events of engagement and softening. These corrective emotional experiences transform a romantic relationship into a safe haven and a secure base, and restructure individuals' distress into an expanded view of self and constructive engagement with others.

"To change a powerful interactional cycle, and to have that change last, therapists need 'dynamite' (Nichols, 1987). To harness the power of emotional responses may be the most effective route to that change" (Johnson, 1998, p. 2). In Stage 2, the therapist helps clients to first, deepen engagement with their core underlying fears and needs, and second, to increase mutual sharing, reaching, and responsivity between partners in EFCT and with imaginal significant others in EFIT. The therapist facilitates new engagement with underlying emotion, initiating corrective emotional experiences by disclosing emotions and needs in a new way to a relevant other. As these new reaches and responses change the emotional music, new views of self and other emerge. The therapist summarizes and validates the new reaches and responses, and heightens how clients are creating a new, positive dance of safer and more secure interactions.

To call this a seismic shift is not an overstatement. The overarching goal of EFT, to reshape distress into attachment security with others and within self, is achieved in Stage 2. Support from attachment neuroscience shows that secure attachment bonds not only have a significant emotion regulation function (Coan & Sbarra, 2015); they actually change how the brain responds to threat (Johnson et al., 2013). Relationships that were once dominated by unacknowledged, unexpressed fears of rejection and abandonment, and rigidly held views of self as unlovable and of other as dangerous or unreliable, shift into safe harbors. In this shift toward safety and security IWMs are

DOI: 10.4324/9781003242673-13

changed: *Self* is experienced as worthy, competent, and lovable, and *Other* (the partner in EFCT and at least some others in EFIT) is experienced as safe, accessible, responsive, and emotionally engaged.

Corrective Emotional Experiences

Key elements of shaping corrective emotional experiences are that emotion needs to be alive in the client and it needs to be attended to in an emotionally engaged way by the therapist. Both therapist and client need to have an alive, bodily felt sense of the present moment emotional experience. The therapeutic relationship needs to feel safe enough that the client can engage with the therapist as, together, they assemble and order the client's *emotional soup* into coherent words. Accessing and clarifying formerly underlying, unfamiliar, implicit core emotion become possible in the safety of the attuned relationship. Having "the social proximity of a close other, a trusted therapist or an attachment figure, can influence the perception of threat in the brain and reduce anxiety, thereby changing the essential nature of key emotional experiences *as they occur*" (italics added; Johnson, 2009b, p. 279). This is the essence of a corrective emotional experience. Change happens *in the moment* of experiencing and coherently expressing core emotion in an in-session encounter. The corrective emotional experience activates new meanings, new action tendencies (motivation to interact in new ways), and a new bodily felt sense of self and other that can reprogram the brain. "Neural circuits are shaped and reshaped as they are challenged," writes Johnson (2009b, p. 279), referencing neuroscientist J. Coan.

Engagement and Softening

The two EFT Stage 2 change events are *engagement*, presented in Chapter 9, and *softening*, presented in Chapter 10. Both change events have been identified as key elements in restructuring relationship-specific secure connections which equip couples and individuals with resilience against stress, reducing risk of depression, PTSD, and physical health concerns (Dalgleish et al., 2015; Greenman & Johnson, 2022; Wiebe & Johnson, 2016).

There is a predictable order in which these change events occur. In EFCT, the more withdrawn partner engages with their own emotional experience and then takes the assertive risk with their partner to become a fully engaged player on the relationship field. That engagement is needed for it to be viable for the more anxious, critical partner to *soften*. *Softening* is the process of risking to reach from a position of vulnerability to ask for attachment fears to be soothed and attachment needs to be met. Similarly, in EFIT, a client needs a new depth of emotional engagement and clarity with their emotional experience, before they can assertively and coherently reach for and receive interpersonal validation, soothing, and an expanded view of self.

The therapist's five-move macro intervention, the EFT Tango, organically takes clients through the Stage 2 restructuring change events of engagement and softening. "The basic process of change involves three steps" (Johnson, 2019, p. 145), also known as Steps 5–7 of client change (see Box 9.1).

Significant Differences

The EFT clinician sees and hears common differences in clients with over-regulating strategies (also called withdrawers in EFCT) and those with hyperactivating strategies (also called pursuers in EFCT). Those who default to suppressing, de-activating strategies typically discover and express emotional pain, grief, and exhaustion. They dread rejection and long for acceptance, protection from attack, and assurance that they are wanted and needed. Those who tend toward hyperactivating strategies typically express rejecting anger (Myung et al., 2022), fearing abandonment, and longing to feel important, loved, and assured of the other's engaged presence. Avoidant withdrawers and anxious pursuers engage somewhat differently in the emotional change processes. More withdrawn partners engage little by little through the course of therapy, whereas more pursuing partners make significant shifts much later in therapy (Burgess Moser et al., 2015). While avoidance is found to decrease over the course of therapy, relationship-specific attachment anxiety does not shift significantly until the actual softening change event. Even after a former withdrawer engages and remains engaged, a more pursuing partner could continue to seem anxious, critical, and mistrusting until after the softening change event.

Knowing that there are nuanced differences between how EFT influences change with more anxious individuals and with more avoidant individuals can help an EFT therapist to be patient with the process and to trust the model. For example, research is continually discovering nuanced variations in how attachment strategies orient clients to respond differently to interventions of heightening with repetition to evoke and deepen somatic experiencing. While repetition may more deeply engage a suppressed withdrawer, it may in fact heighten an anxious pursuer beyond their window of tolerance (Kailanko et al., 2021a). Most importantly, the therapist needs to be attuned to all verbal and non-verbal cues and contain or heighten as needed.

The pinnacle encounters for clients in Stage 2 change also look significantly different between engaging withdrawn clients and softening anxious pursuing clients. EFCT therapists expect withdrawers and pursuers to act differently when they risk reaching to ask their partner for what they need to meet their attachment needs. The engagement change event is associated with a more withdrawn partner stepping forward and stating needs and wants in an assertive manner (Johnson, 2020), whereas the softening change event is associated with a more pursuing partner reaching with vulnerability and softness to the now engaged partner to ask for reassurance.

Myung et al. (2022) were surprised to find the absence of assertive reaches in their study of the final withdrawer engagement encounters. Given the incremental nature of the engagement change event, they suggest it is likely that the more assertive expressions may have preceded the segments analyzed in the Lee et al.'s (2017) studies. While soft and vulnerable expressions are part of both the engagement and softening change events, assertiveness is an important part of engagement. As an incremental process in Stage 2, engagement includes risking to assert what they need to remain engaged in the relationship. These needs are usually centered on needing acceptance without demands to be a different person, needing an opportunity to be heard, to participate in, and to influence the relationship, and sometimes, also needing permission to make mistakes without their partner erupting or walking off in anger or despair.

The relevance of these differences between clients using different attachment strategies applies to EFIT as well. Throughout all of therapy, an EFT therapist attunes to the client's emotional process with a contextually relevant attachment frame. This attachment frame helps a therapist to recognize one client's suppression or seeming nonchalance as a valid, survival strategy, while also recognizing how that suppression is also blocking them from processing their distress. A contextually relevant frame helps an EFT therapist to appreciate another client's rush of panic or disgust followed by shutting down as another valid strategy, also with problematic consequences of rigid depression and anxiety. EFT therapists attune to each client's emotional cascade (perceived threat, bodily response, meaning making, action tendency of suppression or hyperactivation) and to their implicit attachment fears in this process.

In EFIT Stage 2, a therapist facilitates coherent, assertive engagement with suppressed experience. The assertiveness in the engagement change event can be a statement of needs with a clear decision to step away from a particular unsafe relationship or it may be engagement with a part of self that has been habitually dismissed, such as a trauma-survivor-self or a person in grief whose anger and pain have been effectively blocked from awareness. (Numerous video examples of EFIT clients coping with trauma and grief can be found at steppingintoeft.com.) A disregarded, despised, or fragile younger self, whom a client has been trying to ignore, may also emerge in the engagement change event with surprisingly clear messages of needs and wants.

Softening change events in EFIT occur between self and an imaginal other, where clients experience new safety and acceptance toward and/or from an imaginal safe other. Softenings also occur toward previously disregarded or unacceptable parts of self when clients embrace a newly emerging part of self with welcome and appreciation. Integrating two parts of self or two attachment strategies that were previously working against one another into a secure resourceful bond is another way that the final change event of softening in EFIT shapes change. (See case example in Brubacher, 2017.) EFIT softenings can include a softening toward and welcoming of a part of self that was once experienced as self-critical, now becoming a supportive ally with excellent foresight and encouragement, or a compassionate, welcoming affirmation of the worth and strength of a vulnerable, younger self who had previously felt disregarded and unworthy. Engagement and softening change events are shaped interpersonally (with imaginal others and with the therapist) and intra-psychically (between parts of self), all restructuring internal working models of self and other.

In Chapters 9 and 10, we continue to explore what EFT therapists see and hear, what therapists and clients do, and *how* they do it.

9 Working with Emotion to Shape the Engagement Change Event

> Emotion is then the music in the dance of adult intimacy. When we change the music — we change the dance. (Johnson, 2020, p. 62)

The change event of engagement is remarkable for partners and individuals alike. After risking stepping forward into relationship with self and other, there is no full disappearance, regardless of the response(s) of the other. Fresh emotional music is playing. New emotion moves the client into new actions and meanings, and a new interactive dance ensues. The first Stage 2 change event is called *re-engagement* or *engagement*. Johnson (2020) uses both terms. As mentioned in Chapter 1, I prefer *engagement* since *re-engagement* implies that a client has previously been engaged with their own emotional experience and engaged in relationship, and over time has drawn back. While it is surely true that some individuals, over time, have become less and less emotionally engaged, other withdrawn partners and deactivating individual clients have a lifetime survival pattern of downplaying their own and others' emotions and needs. It is truly a transformative change event to discover acceptance when they risk engaging, first with self (clients taking Step 5), and then fully in relationship, asking for needs and wants to be met (clients taking Step 7).

The terms *withdrawer, avoidance,* and *suppressing* are used in EFT with respect for how the strategy of deactivating can be adaptive. Deactivation can be a necessary survival strategy for survivors of sexual, emotional, racial, ethnic, and cultural trauma. In the attachment-base of EFT, coping strategies are seen for their strengths and only as problematic when clients are stuck in automatic repetition of strategies that threaten their emotional health or important relationships.

The Beginning of Stage 2 Change

In the *Engagement Change Event* for couples, the previously withdrawn partner shares attachment fears and needs, and from an emotionally engaged and assertive position, asks for what they need to remain engaged and to have a safe and secure connection with their partner. This request is made from what Johnson (2020) calls a position of entitlement; it is a new balanced, assertive position, an emerging sense of actually being worthy of care. Wayne calls taking this new position, *really weird.* "I have never asked for something for myself before," he adds. The goal in EFCT is to have the more withdrawn partner engage with and disclose their attachment fears and longings (in the more intrapsychic Step 5), and from that place of newly engaged awareness, to step assertively into the relationship and closer to their partner, asking for what they need to feel safe to remain present and engaged (reaching with a Step 7 request).

Similarly, in EFIT, Stage 2 change events begin with a client engaging deeply with their assembled core emotion to formulate a message of need. These change events culminate in a coherent, assertive expression of need to a significant imaginal other (IO), to the therapist, or between parts of self. Attachment theory holds that everyone needs another's response, to mirror their worth, in order to integrate a sense of value and competence into one's working model of self.

DOI: 10.4324/9781003242673-14

Withdrawer Takes the Lead in Stage 2 EFCT

As a bottom-up model, developed from what couples have shown is the path to lasting change (Johnson, 2020), the engagement change event precedes the softening change event. Neither partner would feel safe if a critical pursuer were to expand and express vulnerable emotions and needs to a partner who is withdrawn and emotionally unavailable. A pursuer's vulnerable expressions of pain or soft tears are likely to trigger a more withdrawn partner to feel overwhelmed and to become unresponsive in the face of their partner's distress.

EFCT therapists flow creatively with the EFT Tango as they help clients move into Stage 2, helping partners (taking Steps 5 and 6) to engage with intrapsychic emotional experience, share core fears, and process the encounters where these fears are shared. The ordering of who is invited first to assemble and deepen their emotional experience in Stage 2 is not rigid, though it is more often the withdrawn partner who is invited first. The process of partners' Steps 5 and 6 change can be "intertwined and reciprocally determining" (Johnson, 2020, p. 166). A reduction in hostility of a more critical partner may encourage a more withdrawn partner to risk stepping forward; a decrease in distancing from the more withdrawn partner may encourage a more critical partner to risk some softening. Where the order is important is in clients' Step 7 reaches. The engagement change event of a withdrawn partner stepping *into* the relationship with assertiveness and openness and asking for needs and wants to be met, must precede the softening change event of a pursuer's vulnerable request for reassurance to have their attachment needs met.

Metaphorically, EFT therapists invite the more withdrawn partner onto the dance floor first, helping them to engage with their own experience and to risk stepping into the relationship in a more assertive and engaged manner. The person "who once cringed and placated now begins to become assertive" (Johnson, 2020, p. 149). After the engagement change event, in EFCT, there are two partners on the dance floor, ready to create a new relationship dance of secure reaching and responding.

In the case of a withdraw–withdraw pattern, such as Phil and Julie where both partners use avoidance and self-reliance to cope with attachment threats and fears, neither partner will feel safe to venture out first. An EFT therapist will typically first engage the more accessible (least withdrawn) of two withdrawing partners. With continual support, empathy, and validation from the therapist, the more accessible of the two withdrawers will be able to take the lead into alien, frightening emotional territory and make it safe for their partner to follow.

Literature on culturally sensitive EFT reminds us that good EFT is, first and foremost, flexible and responsive to clients' process *in their social context*. The depth of emotional experiencing that EFT therapists seek to evoke in Stage 2 is about much more than vulnerability. In learning to be an EFT practitioner, Emily initially thought that EFT is all about *getting clients to experience and express vulnerability*. In fact, Nightingale et al. (2019) refer to this as "traditional EFT" (p. 239) and offers in its place a culturally sensitive approach that attunes to how racial oppression organizes Black women's and Black men's emotional responses. This accentuates the need to prioritize clients' context. Culturally sensitive EFT is EFT at its best. Emily sees now that vulnerability is not the way to *begin* the change process, nor does it fully capture the end goal for all clients. "Rather," she muses, "The end goal is all about shaping accessibility, responsivity, and engagement (ARE) with core emotional experience, which potentiates sending and receiving clear messages." This is true for EFCT and EFIT.

EFIT Clients' Stage 2 Change Also Begins with Engagement

As described in the introduction to this section, there is an analogous process in EFIT of *engagement* preceding a *softening*. Engagement with core fears, vulnerabilities, and longings that drive what Johnson (2021) calls *the pattern of emotional protection, the constraining prison, and the problem-perpetuating process* are distilled, deepened, and disclosed before facilitating a softening with another or between parts of self. "Clients' engagement with themselves and key aspects of their narratives, revisited at deep levels of experiencing, give way to powerful corrective emotional experiences" (Johnson & Campbell, 2022, p. 142). The individual client is supported to linger longer in deepened core emotion that has been too frightening, unfamiliar, or unacceptable to face. In the engagement change event, this emotion is fully faced and reprocessed, beginning to shift working models of self and other.

Entering Stage 2, Max has stabilized his pattern of avoidance, discovered interpersonal sources of support in the therapist and in his sister, and awakened his own motivation to journey into feared territory. Stabilization has readied Max to begin the process of facing his most dreaded traumatic memories that are filled with shame, guilt, remorse, and terror. Stage 1 engaged encounters with the friend as Max remembered him before the fatal accident, elicited a sense of love from the man for whose death he is responsible. Validating encounters between his current-day self and his young-adult self, who felt shattered from his experiences in jail, strengthened Max's courage to explore dreaded emotional experience. This stabilization indicates readiness for more intense Stage 2 exploration to shift his negative view of self into one of worth and competence, and to form positive and caring relationships with others even as he grieves the loss of his long-term partner.

What EFT Therapists See and Hear as Clients Step into the Engagement Change Event

An EFT therapist sees and attunes to indications of readiness to move into the Stage 2 engagement process. Although Stage 2 flows organically from the stabilization achieved in Stage 1, it is significantly different from Stage 1. An EFT therapist sees and hears some of the following markers that indicate client readiness to begin Stage 2.

Signs of Safety and Balance

Markers of stabilization (see Chapters 8 and 13) and a growing tone of safety between partners signal a couple's readiness to begin Stage 2. Similarly, an individual client's readiness for Stage 2 is marked by emotional balance and a capacity to focus on difficult experience. They have a clearer narrative, are more able to outline key patterns, and have a sense of direction and hope toward achieving their goals.

Emily observes a different tone in the room with several of her couples – the withdrawers are staying more involved for longer periods of time before stepping back into familiar places of safety. Typical withdrawer moves of distancing and defending are happening less frequently and less rapidly. In place of a routine shrug of apparent nonchalance, an intellectual analysis, or a rapid-fire counterattack of self-defense and shutting down, the more withdrawn partners are remaining in conversation longer. At the same time, stabilized pursuing partners can tolerate more uncertainty before suddenly becoming reactive (Box 8.2).

Emily also notices hope and stability in her individual clients. Max, for example, who has used avoidance to manage the impact of his traumas for decades, demonstrates markers of stabilization (Box 8.3). He still feels like he has these *monster-in-a-box* feelings but now he can see himself more clearly. He is ready to listen to the *monster feelings* of resentment and pain that he has tried to ignore. He sees that he is on a hopeful path toward change even as he identifies fears and traumatic memories that he is frightened to explore.

Emotional Handles of Withdrawer's Core Fears

An EFT therapist is on the lookout for emotional handles to explore the hidden misery or despair of a withdrawn partner or individual caught in deactivating patterns. "Behind the mask of indifference is bottomless misery and behind callousness, despair," wrote Bowlby (1944, p. 39). EFT therapists watch and listen, moment-to-moment, for subtle signs that a client who typically deactivates core emotion is touching the core emotion that was identified in Stage 1 (Step 3); that is, the fear that moves them to automatically withdraw, go numb, or become defensive. Emotional handles to open a withdrawn or avoidant client's world can be images ("the look like just before the bee stings;" "nothing to hold on to"), bodily movements (tightening jaw; facial cringe), reported bodily sensations ("a knot in my gut;" "a cube of hate in my chest;" "pain rushing down my arm"), or a sudden exit or interruption.

Images. Wayne identifies that he gets half-way up the mountain of trying to get it right for Jessica, and then gets a sudden sinking feeling in his gut that he will never get it right, so he braces for defeat, nonchalantly offers to run an errand, and refuses to engage. "Sinking feeling in his gut" and "bracing for defeat" are emotional handles for Emily to take hold of to help Wayne assemble more of his core emotion.

With Sophie and Ella, Emily hears an emotional handle to begin assembling Ella's core fear of being annihilated. "Sophie's demands tug on my trouser leg, as if she will never let go until I am dragged into the dust and annihilated!" "Dragged into the dust and annihilated," repeats Emily, using Move 2, to assemble and then deepen Ella's core fear and misery in that poignant image.

One poignant emotional handle for Max's underlying fear is his dread of one day remembering the scene of the accident and seeing his dead friend's mangled body on the ground. Entering Stage 2, he has more emotional balance; he feels hope and courage to face the dreaded image of the scene of the accident and the frightening turmoil this image evokes.

An emotional handle to open into Sahra's core emotion is her phrase of "reaching for a response, then backing away in defeat and cold isolation."

Bodily Movements, Nonverbal Signals, or Reported Bodily Sensations. In a withdraw/withdraw couple, emotional handles are frequently very subtle, such as Julie's sigh and Phil's poker face. Emily recognizes these as common signs of core emotion in withdraw/withdraw patterns. With these emotional handles, she can reach in and deepen the fear on the leading edge. "As Phil's face went still, I noticed, Julie, you had that familiar sigh that you link to your tendency to go silent when you sense that Phil has disappeared. Is that what is coming up for you?" Reported bodily sensations such as "heart sinking" or "clutching tightness on the back of my neck" are also emotional handles signaling unexplored depths.

Avoidance as a strategy for engagement is difficult to detect at times. Emily is learning that for Wayne, as a black man in a world of persistent racial discrimination, survival outside the home has literally depended on holding back and tamping down all emotion. Jessica and Wayne have identified how this survival strategy also plays out between them in their self-protective pattern. Attuning to his nonverbal signs, Emily notices Wayne sit back with tension on his face. Tentatively, she reflects what she notices and checks whether it is linked to Jessica's comment that she is disappointed that he slept on the sofa again. Wayne, initially surprised at her comment, feels safe enough entering Stage 2 to say, "Yes, it is! I automatically step back hearing, 'Oh oh, I've done damage. She is upset. Now I've done it!'"

Max says, he doesn't feel the fear of remembering Léo's body as much as he used to, and then speaks of their old saying, "Live fast, die young, leave a beautiful corpse." A chill runs through Emily's spine as Max hints at the trigger of his fear – Léo's corpse – and she conjectures at the frightening topic, "That must be painful to remember he didn't have a beautiful corpse." "Oh yeah!" utters Max. Although he has a slight smile and muted laughter, his voice seems to be cracking and he looks down. Emily feels herself tearing up and asks Max what is happening as he smiles, looks down, and his voice breaks. "I'm fighting tears," Max says, pulling out a handkerchief to blow his nose. Together they explore the emotional handle of Max's bodily signals, linking his cracking voice, holding back tears, and looking down to his chilling fear of seeing Léo's body and feeling the emotional turmoil he has avoided for decades.

Sudden Exits – An Expected Part of the Process

Another observable sign that an avoidant client's core emotion might be on the leading edge is an abrupt exit from emotional exploration. Sudden exits suggest some core emotion may have arisen. Interruptions from a partner suggest the observing partner may have detected vulnerability and stepped in to block it. Withdrawers' exits from emotional exploration are frequently very subtle, such as dismissing the significance of what they just expressed, intellectualizing, suddenly changing the subject, or stopping themselves midsentence. An EFT therapist expects sudden exits from emotional experiencing. It is very common for avoidant clients to deepen emotional experiences in fits and starts, exiting from deeper levels of emotional experiencing and needing help to re-engage (Lee et al., 2017; Rheem, 2012). Emily finds it helpful to recall that backing away from high levels of experiencing is an avoidant client's familiar pattern of emotional protection. "Of course, that is how you have survived – by touching the emotional heat and backing away for safety." She is undeterred, knowing this process of deepening, exiting, deepening, disclosing through engaged encounters, and processing the encounter, is the engagement change event in its incremental process (Lee et al., 2017). Emily sees exits as a meaningful moment to track with Move 1, reflecting present process. Then she flows into Move 2 assembly, replaying the emotional handles to engage the client more deeply. Next, she shapes an encounter with Move 3. She is confident that this flow of Moves 1, 2, and 3 is a reliable way to re-engage avoidant clients when they exit. (See Chapter 13 for more on exits and interruptions.)

The tone in Phil's voice heightens ever so subtly and his pace increases as he recounts Julie asking him to buy the groceries *before* getting the car washed. Emily repeats the bodily signals of emotional arousal that she notices, "Your voice got a little louder and faster, Phil, as you said that." Phil pauses. "I hadn't noticed – but yeah!" He chuckles, gradually recognizing, "It was a little difficult to have her tell me when to do what, but it was fleeting." "If that fleeting moment of difficulty had words…?" wonders Emily aloud, to which Phil replies, "If it had words (pause), no (more silence) nothing." Phil completely exits from the conversation, looking up as though he had just entered the room. Gently and persistently, Emily returns to this *fleeting difficult moment* again and again. Gradually this emotional handle of "a fleeting difficult moment" opens into some "mild annoyance." Phil finds the courage to allow Emily to help him assemble his reluctance to speak up to Julie when he is annoyed with her telling him how to do things. Eventually Emily helps him to distill and engage with his core fear of upsetting Julie and losing her to "a bout of frozen depression."

Images, bodily signs, or sudden exits are all emotional handles, indicating that a high level of emotional experiencing is on the leading edge of awareness. An EFT therapist recognizes these handles as golden opportunities to seize in order to help clients expand present-moment emotional awareness, beginning with Move 1 reflection and tracking, followed by Move 2 assembly and deepening.

New Dynamic Emerging

In addition to these many emotional handles opening doorways to expand avoidant client's core underlying fears, an EFT therapist sees and hears the emergence of a new dynamic through the

Stage 2 engagement change event. The most salient observable aspects are a previously avoidant client's growing openness to explore their inner experience and a newly discovered longing for closeness and connection. Typically, an avoidant withdrawer has felt averse to close connection. Closeness to others and to one's own experience has not been safe or desirable. Habitual deactivating strategies create patterns of self-protective distance from others and from one's own emotional experience. "I have never really turned inward to notice me and to see how it feels to be left alone, in danger, with nothing to hold on to," Wayne admits, engaging in deeper intrapsychic exploration in his Step 5. His avoidant strategies have helped him cope with the ongoing racial stressors and daily danger cues he faces as a Black man in the outside world, but as he and Jessica have de-escalated, he recognizes how his self-sufficiency isn't always serving him well in their relationship. Deeper emotional exploration in his Step 5 culminates in his disclosing to Jessica that he is lonely and very concerned about her disapproval.

In Stage 2, there is an emerging awareness on the part of a habitually withdrawn client that they have longings and needs for connection and support. Finally, in Step 7 when a more withdrawn client makes the courageous, assertive reach to ask for their attachment needs to be met, the dynamic shifts substantially.

Asking for something for himself feels very foreign for Wayne. After asking Jessica, "Can you tone down the yelling and stay with me? No more turtling?" Wayne acknowledges how odd that feels to ask for something for himself. He looks like he has surprised himself with saying these words to Jessica. Her heart melts in response to his courage and his expressed need for her to tone down her voice, even as she cringes with embarrassment for memories of how harsh she can get in her desperation to get a response from him.

In her Step 7 request, Ella asserts to Sophie:

I want to feel safe committing to you, knowing you won't give up on me! I need to know you want me even though I let you down sometimes. If I risk depending on you, can you assure me you will not give up and walk away? That you will stay?

Max says:

I have never looked at me in this way! For decades I have tried to fight off frightening flashbacks – and now to see myself and feel my grandmother's loving presence also looking at me, all alone and terrified, is amazing! I have always been too ashamed to let her see me… and now we are here, together! It's like we are in the same zone! She is not judging me. She always knew my dad was too harsh. She is the warmth of compassion. She is weeping when she sees me go to jail!

In his Step 7 encounters, Max reaches to grandma and to Léo.

What EFT Therapists and Clients Do to Shape the Engagement Change Event

Entering Stage 2 has an element of increased risk. EFT therapists respect that moving into depths of emotional waters is very risky for clients who have survived by using deactivating strategies. Thus, they are prepared to support clients with tenacity and respect for the incremental process of bringing their core, underlying emotions to life. They recognize that clients are unlikely to take a sudden plunge into deep waters or continue swimming comfortably in new emotional depths. EFT therapists are ready to enter the emotional waters gradually with their clients and to creatively bring them back to manageable levels of heightened emotional intensity, after they step out for reprieve.

Table 9.1 delineates themes of what clients and therapists do to create the engagement change event. In addition to the themes, it includes the microelements of change (aka client steps), the therapist moves and micro-skills that are used to facilitate these steps, and the typical levels of client emotional experiencing during this process. *Workouts for Stepping into EFT* and Chapters 2–4 of this book detail the therapist moves and micro-skills in each move.

As therapists are deepening emotional experience in Stage 2, it is especially important to pause and be mindful of intersectionalities of race, culture, gender, sexual orientation, socio-economic status, neuro-diversity, and so on, and to listen deeply to *how* clients wish to tell their stories. Empathic conjectures need to be used very judiciously. Empathic reflections and process tracking need to be balanced with evocative responses. Rapid assumptions of understanding, conveyed with reflections, validations, or conjectures, can convey reluctance to truly listen and can feel like white dominance or an imposition of a position of power (F. Villodas, personal communication, October 2022).

Table 9.1 Themes of the Engagement Change Event

Themes	Client Step	Therapist Interventions: Moves and Micro-skills	EXP Levels*
1. Assemble and distill core affect	Client Step 5	Move 2 Assembly Evocative responses and questions, empathic conjecture, reflecting core emotion.	Levels 2–3
2. Distill and deepen core affect	Client Step 5	Move 2 Deepening evocative reflections, heighten,	Levels 3–4
3. Disclose core affect	Client Step 5	Move 3 SHAPE encounter **S**harpen, **A**nticipate, **H**eighten, Direct to **P**resent message, **E**ngage	Level 4
4. Series of encounters	Client Step 5	Moves 3 and 4 SHAPE and process series of encounters	Level 5
5. Process encounter with recipient of disclosure	Client Step 6 (respond to partner's disclosure)	Move 4 Evocative responses and questions, heighten,	Level 4
6. Promote acceptance / authentic response	Client Step 6	Move 3 to SHAPE response from recipient **S**harpen, **A**nticipate, **H**eighten, Direct to **P**resent message, **E**ngage.	Level 4
7. Shape encounter to assert needs and make request	Client Step 7 (reach and request)	Move 3 to shape specific reach to state needs embedded in core fear and to request these needs to be met.	Levels 5–6
8. Shape encounter for partner to respond and other to receive	Client Step 7 (respond and receive the response)	Moves 3, 4 and 5	Levels 4–6

Adapted from Lee et al. (2017)
* For details on EXP (levels of depth of emotional experiencing) see Chapter 2 and Box 12.1.

What Clients Do in the Engagement Change Event

A key facet of attachment science is that change takes place *in relationship*. Stage 2 change events are changes *within* and *between*. A deeper engagement with self and one's own emotional experiencing (within) needs to happen before clients are able to send new, more clear interpersonal signals (between).

The fundamental elements of what clients do in the engagement change event are deepening their emotional experiencing and risking participating in vulnerable and assertive disclosures and responses. Assertiveness for a more withdrawing person is indeed vulnerable! For deactivating clients, speaking assertively can feel as vulnerable as soft, tender reaching does for hyperactivating clients. The entry into Stage 2 is marked by the emergence of newly formulated emotional experience and moments of emotionally engaged encounters, initiating a "watershed in the therapy process" (Johnson, 2020, p. 149). Stage 1 shapes the stable, secure base that provides enough emotional balance for deeper levels of exploration in Stage 2, where, with the therapist's help, clients disclose messages that evolve from their deeper intrapsychic exploration. The newly formulated messages begin to shape powerful new *broaden-and-build cycles of connection* in EFCT and EFIT.

In couple therapy, the withdrawn partner engages more deeply with their core attachment fears, disclosing them incrementally to their partner. Thus, the withdrawer's Step 5 can be more of a series of gradual steps than one distinct step (Lee et al., 2017; Rheem, 2012). When the therapist uses Move 4 to process an engaged encounter, the partner, in Step 6, either welcomes this new view of their partner or struggles to accept it. Either reaction can be expected. Some receiving partners, like Julie, respond to a disclosure with deep appreciation. Julie's heart melts when Phil is able to describe his fear of upsetting her and losing her beneath her blanket of depression. Other partners receiving an encounter are shocked to hear their withdrawn partner disclose underlying emotions. Jessica is stunned to hear the enormity of Wayne's dread of losing her. Others are disbelieving and become triggered, as Sophie does when Ella begins to disclose her fatigue at trying to please her. Sophie is skeptical when Ella shares her fears of rejection and annihilation –fearing that she will totally lose herself trying to get it right for Sophie and still fail.

The more pursuing partner is likely to continue to remain guarded and very anxious (Burgess Moser et al., 2015), even as the previously withdrawn partner begins to have a voice. A new cycle is emerging, however. The previously withdrawn partner discovers and reveals hidden parts of self (such as enormous fears of hurting or getting hurt) and steps more fully than ever into the relationship with newly asserted needs for acceptance or support.

As doubtful and guarded as the pursuing partner may be, with the therapist's help they are supported to respond with a congruent response to their newly engaging partner's disclosure of core emotion and fear (a pursuer's Step 6). Authenticity is more important and more believable than feigned warmth and acceptance. Sophie says to Ella, "I don't quite believe this is really you. I hear you and I'll try to be accepting – but this is all too much for me to take in just now." The more withdrawn partner's engagement, which evolves gradually in bits and pieces, is a change event and it will not disappear completely, even when the pursuing partner becomes triggered by it. Partners are co-creating an up-to-the-minute dance to new strains of emotional music.

Partners' non-accepting reactions to a withdrawn partner's increasing engagement can be normalized when seen through a culturally sensitive lens. For example, Nightingale et al. (2019) illustrate how racial oppression organizes emotional responses and tends to "elevate attending to Black men's needs while Black women continue to suffer" (p. 240). This understanding helps the therapist, in the case they present, to validate the pursuer's protest of the therapist's support of the withdrawn partner's engagement:

> Black women are always at the end of the line. We are always expected to put everyone else's needs first. I'm sick of that… Micro-aggressions left and right. I have an unemployed husband,

who may be trying, but still, it's all on me. Nobody cares. If I complain, folks say, "Girl, get it together. Ain't nobody got time for your pity parties?" But I can't stop. I don't know how. (p. 139)

It makes total sense that the therapist's support of the more withdrawn male partner became overwhelming for the female pursuer, and it was necessary to validate her reactions and her authentic response to him. The therapist validated the pursuer's reaction with culturally attuned empathy and the pursuer's critical reaction evolved into the following vulnerable disclosure:

Weak is what I think White women do. You know, they fall apart over every little thing. I don't want to be that. I'm proud of being a Black woman. I don't have time to be weak. I don't want Mark to think I'm weak. (Nightingale et al., 2019, pp. 139–140)

Her expressed, vulnerable fear of her husband, Mark, seeing her as weak pulled him to respond with warmth and support. This also illustrates a common EFT theme – that withdrawer engagement evokes pursuers' fears and leads organically into the softening change event discussed in Chapter 10.

Following this new interaction (withdrawer's Step 5 disclosure and pursuer's Step 6 response) and while emotion is fully alive, the more withdrawn partner, with the therapist's help, listens to what their attachment fear tells them they need from their partner. In their Step 7 request, the withdrawn partner steps forward and assertively states what they need to remain an active participant in the relationship, as described previously in the "new dynamic emerging," where Wayne requests of Jessica that she tone down her voice and stop turtling.

Similarly, in EFIT, clients step into new territory with the movement into Stage 2. With emotional balance, safety, and a sense of agency achieved in Stage 1, clients are ready to engage with what has been hidden. Max notices with his sudden "awakening" at the ending of his long-term relationship, that he has been carrying this weighty *monster-in-a-box* for a long, long time! He is ready to engage with his stories of resentment and pain that he has been trying to ignore for his whole life. EFIT clients in Stage 2 gradually come to internalize that they are not to blame for their problems. At the same time, they are empowered to discover how their typical strategies for coping are precisely what is trapping them in a repetitive cycle of distress.

Sahra's assertive engagement, first with her own emotional process and then in encounters with several others who have injured her (friend, mother, father, ex-partner, abusive babysitter), shifts her view of self from self-doubting, collapsing, needing to apologize immediately or deserving punishment when others do not respond with understanding, warmth, or safety, to someone who can safely speak congruently without needing the other to change. Sahra, to her imaginal mother says, "Yes, I have resented you. But I also wanted to help you. I've felt so guilty for leaving you in Ukraine, yet I've done all I could to bring you to America." In a series of encounters, her imaginal mother, in Sahra's perception, moves from defensiveness to confusion to genuine curiosity. The first six themes of engagement (see Table 9.1) are shaped in a series of encounters with her imaginal mother, where Sahra discloses her core fears. Theme 7, asserting her needs to her imaginal mother, is an empowering and important moment of change for Sahra. She tells her imaginal mother that she needs to be seen as a good daughter, as a competent professional, and that she needs the kind of compassion from her *now* that she remembers from when she was six years old. Engaging with this clear, assertive message to her imaginal mother, she experiences a sense of hope that her mother may actually be proud of her, though in this encounter her imaginal mother is not yet able to communicate that. Nonetheless, Sahra's engagement is a substantial corrective emotional experience that grounds her in a sense of knowing herself and having legitimate needs for her mother's love. Her engagement, first with her inner emotional experience and then in dialogue with an image of her mother, is shifting her view of self as someone whose voice matters.

This engagement strengthens her sense of self across relationships. Her shifting view of self and other extends into changes she makes with others in her inner world, including her father, her ex-partner, and her abusive, childhood babysitter. Her view of other will continue to expand as she discriminates reliable others from those she cannot trust.

What Therapists Do to Facilitate the Stage 2 Engagement Change Event

Change is happening. As Emily sees and hears markers of readiness to begin Stage 2 she wonders, "Can I take the plunge into greater emotional depths? Do I know how to help withdrawn Wayne continue to deepen and expand his emotional experience? Do I know how to be racially humble and validate that not showing fear and vulnerability is part of his survival strategy, reinforced by the fact that 'racial priming makes vulnerability more dangerous … [and that] it is never safe for a Black man to be vulnerable' (Guillory, 2022, pp. 201, 161–162)? I need to be patient with myself and prioritize attending to each partner and not impose expectations of white pacing or vulnerability. I will contain and validate Jessica, as she hears more clearly how she is affecting Wayne, even if she dissolves in a puddle of tears or silent exasperation and I will keep my focus on helping Wayne to engage with his core attachment emotions and their embedded assertive messages that have not felt safe for him to express."

Knowing that there are identifiable therapist moves (of the EFT Tango) and interventions that facilitate withdrawer engagement helps Emily relax. Throughout therapy, she returns to Move 1 to reflect present process but she senses that the interventions to rely on most heavily for engagement change events are summarized in the flow between Moves 2, 3, and 4. Encounters evolve out of Move 2 assembly and deepening, using evocative questions and responses to engage a withdrawn partner in their own experience, along with reflecting and heightening newly emerging emotional experience, and making empathic conjectures by closely attuning to the leading edge of attachment-significant experience.

In Stage 2, therapists use Move 2 assembly and deepening, at a slower pace, persistently, and beginning with intrapsychic present-moment exploration. This leads directly into shaping new encounters between partners in couple therapy and with IOs and between parts of self in EFIT with Move 3. The final reach/request of the engagement change event evolves out of this deeper emotional experience and expression. Many encounters are shaped to create Stage 2 engagement. An EFT therapist can maximize the process of engaging the withdrawer "by accessing, exploring, and heightening emotions and by creating more enactments between partners in an attempt for the more avoidant partner to let in new relational experiences" (Dalgleish et al., 2015, p. 272). Through these deeply engaged encounters, interpersonal needs are discovered and then disclosed. Using moves of the EFT Tango, therapists help clients to risk *reaching to request, respond, and receive.* They flow in attunement with clients, using Move 2 assembly and deepening, Move 3 to shape a "request encounter" to have attachment needs met, followed by another Move 3 to shape a response to the courageous request. Finally, Moves 4 and 5 are used to process the impact of the reach and response and to integrate this transformative exchange.

In EFCT, Move 2 is directed toward one partner at a time, while also monitoring reactions of the observing partner. The goal of assembly and deepening is toward shaping new interactions between partners. Thus, as the therapist focuses on assembling, deepening, and expanding the emotional experience of the withdrawer (the experiencing partner), they stay in contact with the pursuer (the observing partner). An EFT therapist always attends, as much as possible, to both partners' present-moment experience. A couple therapist can explicitly include the observing partner through making eye contact while interacting with the experiencing partner and by including mention of their significance while heightening the other's experience. For example, while speaking to

Ella, Emily includes the observing partner, Sophie, by referring explicitly to her as she says to Ella, "You are terrified of never measuring up in *Sophie's* eyes."

In EFIT, during encounters, the client's perceptions of the IO's reactions are evoked and welcomed. When Sahra speaks to an image of her mother, Emily asks, "How do you picture your mother as she hears this message from you?" The therapist attends to both the client's inner experience and their felt sense of the IO's response or non-response. When an encounter is between two parts of self, the therapist attends to the client's present-moment internal experience of each of two parts of self in dialogue. After exploring how Emily guides her couples through the first Stage 2 change event of engagement, we will examine how she uses the same interventions to guide her EFIT clients to engage in experience that they are avoiding, and from there, to formulate coherent, empowering statements of need.

EFT Tango Moves to Facilitate the Engagement Change Event in EFCT. Emily is building confidence in doing Stage 2 work by attuning and guiding clients through their change process with the EFT Tango. She is coming to trust that she can follow emotion and shape emotionally engaged interpersonal dialogues that shape lasting change. She is encouraged by Thompson and Samoilow who wrote, "In session, client process is our guide and the [EFT] tango allows us to improvise and follow the affect in the room, rather than being disappointed because the couple isn't doing what we had planned for them" (p. 4). I do not need to impatiently "take clients through the steps of change," muses Emily with a sigh of relief:

> Rather, as a process consultant, I need to trust the empirically-validated interventions of EFT to guide me in attuning and facilitating change. Client steps of change will evolve as clients are ready and the map of their steps of change can orient and ground me on this journey.

With the comfort of the five moves for attuning to her clients, and the map of client change in the background, Emily relaxes to reflect on how her couples organically move through the steps of change in Stage 2.

EFT Tango Moves to Help Deactivating Partners Distill, Deepen, and Disclose Core Fears (Clients take Step 5). First, with Move 2, the therapist helps the withdrawer to expand and deepen core emotions, fears, longings, and aspects of self that were outside of full awareness, and then, with Move 3, helps them to disclose this newly engaged emotional experience to their partner. As described previously, the survival strategy of avoidance is to dismiss and ignore one's own and others' needs for closeness and connection. There is an adaptive quality to this strategy of distancing from others' disapproval and from internal awareness. "Withdrawal and immobilization can be functional responses to impossible or dangerous situations in which the experience of vulnerability might be overwhelming (Porges, 2011), such as finding oneself dependent on an unpredictable attachment figure" (Kailanko et al., 2021a). Partners are typically more tuned into signs of possible disappointment from their partner than they are to the knot in their own stomach or to the rumblings below the surface that they work hard to ignore. Suppression, of course, interferes with a capacity for closeness (Gross, 2014).

Common core emotions and emotional meanings of withdrawn partners include pain and hurt (especially of feeling unworthy or inadequate), helplessness (to ever be enough), despair, shame, exhaustion (at trying relentlessly and unsuccessfully to please the partner or to keep the partner happy), and grief (at not feeling fully accepted or appreciated). There are subtle differences in how withdrawers engage with disowned internal experience. "I see one look of disapproval, and I shrink away—I can't bear to face letting my partner down again," acknowledged one withdrawn client. "I stop myself before I even move, so convinced I'll never measure up that I don't even try," said another.

Gradually, after exploring triggers, action tendencies, bodily arousal, and meanings made, withdrawers access an awareness of fear. Frequently, the fear is some variation of fearing rejection at disappointing their partner mixed with exhaustion from striving endlessly to keep the peace and to gain approval. Another common variation of a withdrawer's fear is that of being suffocated, silenced, annihilated, or remade into who their partner wants them to be. Embedded in the fear of being suffocated or remade is the implication, "If who I am is unacceptable in my partner's eyes, and if I comply with their demands, I will totally lose myself."

Emily, with Move 2, explores Ella's experience beneath her self-protective surface of nonchalant withdrawal. Ella acknowledges:

> I do worry every day. I worry that I am going to lose Sophie. Her constant demands are slowly killing me. I feel like the frog who boils to death in a pot of water it doesn't even recognize is slowly getting hotter and hotter.

Lingering with and expressing attachment emotions and fears in a more fully engaged manner than before, is the newness of Step 5 for the withdrawer. While engaging moment-to-moment with the elements of core emotion, the descriptions, the images, the associated meanings, and the bodily felt sensations expand and become clearer. This depth and enormity of fear or pain has not been expressed before, and it can be risky indeed for a withdrawn partner to linger in these new depths and then to share them with their partner.

Before shaping a Stage 2 encounter, an EFT therapist ensures that the client experiences the emotion to be alive in the present moment. With Move 2 assembly and deepening, Emily helps Wayne to expand what he calls the dread he first recognized in Stage 1. (Emily conceptualizes it as "fear" but uses Wayne's word "dread," to more closely match his felt experience.) He discovers that his dread paralyzes him, slumping him at the bottom of the mountain he wants to climb to please his lady. Sighing, Wayne says:

> I feel so useless and inept. I end up feeling all I do is get it wrong and miss the mark with her—as if nothing I do will make any difference. Futile really. I am almost certain I am going to lose her at some point. Not one day goes by that I don't live in dread of losing her.

Shaping an encounter with Move 3, Emily invites Wayne:

> Can you turn to Jessica and tell her how overwhelmed you get—how it sems futile to try to please her and that you feel doomed to see her pull away from you in disgust and how this dread stops you dead?

Wayne ventures:

> Yes… I do get overwhelmed. The message that I disappoint you stops me dead. I am convinced I can't meet your expectations and will be falsely accused of something. But I stop—I do hold back and totally freeze. It is somehow safer to be accused of doing nothing than to be accused of doing the wrong thing. I do need you. I need to feel safe. I want to feel close.

Emily heightens Wayne's dread of being falsely accused and of losing Jessica. She also highlights his emerging new position. Wayne asserts, "I am tired of walking on eggshells—I want to let you see who I really am."

EFT Tango Moves to Process the Encounter with Recipient and Promote an Accepting Response (Clients take Step 6). Emily uses Move 4 to process this newly engaged disclosure from Wayne. After asking Wayne how it is to be sharing this, Emily asks Jessica how it is to hear this.

Jessica is stunned. She claims she has not seen this part of Wayne before, definitely not the part of needing her and wanting to feel close! She says she never really grasped that she has any impact on him. She has been perceiving that she does not matter – that he does not need her. Emily is surprised that Jessica is so bewildered, since she thinks they have discussed this before. Then she recognizes what must be happening: Wayne is engaging more deeply than ever, acknowledging needing to feel safe, needing Jessica, and wanting to be close. These are definitely new things for him to be sharing and he may be triggering disbelief or mistrust in Jessica.

EFT therapists help the observing partner to see, hear, and feel the impact of the emerging withdrawer's disclosure, to receive this new view of the partner, and to respond with an authentic encounter. Observing partners sometimes welcome the disclosure with open arms and other times are skeptical and reactive. Seeing a new view of one's partner can be disorientating. With Move 4, therapists support the observing partner to receive and integrate the new disclosure, using evocative questions such as, "What is it like to get this new view of your partner?" Move 4 questions are directed specifically at what was just shared, often repeating particular elements of the disclosure, as shown in italics in the following dialogue. To Jessica, Emily evokes:

> What happens for you as Wayne shares that *not one day goes by that he doesn't live in dread of losing you?* What is it like for you to have him turn and share with you that *he does need you – does need to feel safe and wants to feel close to you?* What happens for you as you hear this?

The EFT therapist reflects and repeats the disclosures of "new" emotional experience to maintain focus on the *new view* of the experiencing partner, while also validating the observing partner's present experience. A therapist validates confusion or surprise ("You hear the words but are too surprised/confused to trust it") or receptivity ("What a relief for you to hear that you are so important he freezes in dread of not being enough *for you!*").

Emily sometimes feels discouraged when a receiving partner expresses uncertainty, disbelief, or even anger at this significantly new view of their partner. She quickly recalls, however, that these reactions are understandable, given many painful years of seeing the partner in a totally different light. Acceptance of a "new partner" is not easy. It can shake the assumptions of the entire relationship. Jessica says, with some perplexity, "He's like a stranger to me! I don't know this part of him!"

In the face of partner reactivity and inability to receive the withdrawer's disclosure, an EFT therapist's mantra is twofold: "Empathy for non-acceptance is key"; and "Keep the *new view* in sight." Here, Move 1 reflection of present process is vital. Empathic responding validates that it is still too risky to accept a new attachment picture, such as, "I do matter; he is not uncaring, he is afraid of losing me." That new view simply doesn't fit with the meanings they have endured for many painful years. Keeping the new view in sight – by repeating the withdrawer's disclosure – is important because the new view contains the antidote attachment seed that has power to transform the relational bond. For example, Emily supports Jessica in her confusion as she encounters this "new" spouse, while also repeating the new view of Wayne (in italics), "It is so confusing to see *Wayne as living in dread of losing you, needing you and wanting to feel safe and close with you,* when you've seen him as totally self-sufficient for so long."

The therapist empathizes with the more pursuing partner's non-acceptance in a soft, slow, simple, tentative tone, checking if they are accurately reflecting the receiving partner's experience:

> This is way too hard for you to accept—that he dreads losing you? You don't see him like this. Too hard to take in that what has looked like nonchalance and self-sufficiency is actually his

deep dread of getting it wrong with you and losing you? Just too difficult to trust that *your approval matters that much to him*, yes? That he longs to *feel safe and close* to you? (Italics show the attachment significance.)

An EFT therapist learns with experience that genuine empathy does indeed move the couple forward. Move 4 is not used to change where clients are but to reflect accurate understanding of their present process.

A withdrawer's (Step 5) disclosure that can be very difficult for a receiving partner to hear is a fear of being consumed or suffocated by the pursing partner. "What?!" shivers Sophie (the pursuer), in response to Ella's disclosure of her fear of "being sucked dry." "Ella is saying that I am too much, isn't she? She thinks I want to destroy her? I feel terrible to hear this—I knew I was too much! No one ever thinks that my wishes are reasonable!" Once again, the therapist's empathy for Sophie's non-acceptance of the withdrawer Ella's disclosure of attachment fear is key. Emily validates:

> Of course, it is very difficult to hear Ella admitting her fear that she loves you so much that she would let you suck her dry, that she would give up everything about herself just to please you and to be enough for you!

Emily can see Sophie calming just a little, as she validates how troubling this is for her. She emphasizes that indeed this is Ella's fear. It is not that Sophie wants to destroy her, but that Ella loves Sophie so much she is afraid she would give up everything just to make their relationship work.

With Move 3, an EFT therapist shapes a genuine response from the observing partner toward the engaging, previously withdrawn partner. They hope to shape an affiliate (warm, accepting, engaged) response from the observing partner, however, if acceptance is not their reaction, an authentic response owning reluctance to trust the disclosure at this time is shaped. A therapist asks a receiving partner who accepts this new presentation of their partner, "Can you turn and tell your partner how much it means to you?" Having the observing partner express acceptance is very reassuring for the experiencing partner. Alternatively, a therapist asks a receiving partner who mistrusts this new disclosure to respond authentically, "Can you turn and tell your partner you hear the words, but it is just too difficult to trust this yet?" The word "yet" plants a seed of hope that the trust will evolve.

When the receiving partner discounts the withdrawer's new disclosures, the EFT therapist contains aggression or dismissal by validating the difficulty of trusting the new disclosure. The therapist empathizes with the lack of readiness to trust at this time, linking the difficulty and disbelief to the couple's repetitive cycle and to this partner's own attachment fears and needs. They validate and explore blocks to acceptance, such as confusion, disorientation, fear, or anger.

The therapist also processes the observing partner's non-acceptance with the disclosing partner (in this example, the more withdrawing partner), helping them to understand their spouse's non-acceptance, "It is still not safe for your partner to trust that this new you is for real." By validating that, in this moment, the partner is not yet able to hear and accept this newly disclosed aspect of the engaging withdrawer, an EFT therapist plants seeds of hope that the new disclosure will be become believable and acceptable as they rebuild the trust that the negative cycle has damaged.

After non-acceptance has been validated and disclosed to the partner, some acceptance and trust frequently emerge. Whether or not the pursuing partner has fully accepted the formerly withdrawn partner's new disclosure, there is usually a readiness within the withdrawn partner to continue the journey toward engagement and to step more fully into the relationship (as they will do in their Step 7).

EFT Tango Moves to Shape Encounters to Assert Needs, Make a Request, and Respond (Clients take Step 7). To help the withdrawer access what they need from the partner to feel safe to live fully in the relationship, the therapist needs to help the partner fully experience the core emotion that was previously expanded and distilled (in Step 5). The therapist may use some Move 2 deepening to bring the core emotion alive again in order to help the withdrawn client to access clearly what they need from their partner, and to find the courage and motivation to risk asking their partner to meet their needs and longings.

Core emotion, alive and fully felt, is the most reliable information about core needs (Frijda, 1986). Withdrawers typically explore pain and grief (Myung et al., 2022) and we know that emotional pain is a complexity of anger, sadness and fear of loss and devaluation (Vangelisti, 2009). Unexpressed needs can be accessed from core emotion, for example: Fear and pain of rejection can give a partner direct access to a need for reassurance and comfort; fear of being consumed can evoke a need for reassurance that it is safe to show up and to express oneself without being judged or remade; and, fatigue and grief from placating can evoke a need to be seen and heard and a longing for safe engagement and connection.

The therapist invites the client to linger in their bodily felt fear of rejection or annihilation or whatever granular, nuanced word best captures their fear in the moment. Lingering, to heighten the client's fear, the therapist invites them to listen to what this core fear tells them they need from their partner. After they find words for their need, the therapist, using Move 3, directs them to take the risk to ask their partner for what they need. It may be a request to "tone down the judgement" or "temper your temper" or to "assure me you can accept me with all my failings and won't give up on me." The therapist guides the client to make this emotionally engaged request which then pulls for a connecting response. The partner is supported to respond right away to this courageous request.

This is a remarkable new interaction of *request and response*. Using Moves 4 and 5, the therapist processes the impact of this dialogue, heightening and summarizing what has taken place. It is noteworthy in that withdrawing partners rarely send clear messages of needs and wants. Taking the risk of stepping fully into the relationship by stating needs and wants shifts the basic pattern of avoidance and placating when under stress, to one of stepping closer to their partner with assertiveness and engagement. This step marks the Step 7 withdrawer engagement change event. This change event might not appear like a monumental shift because avoidant partners engage gradually in the relationship from the early sessions of therapy (Burgess Moser et al., 2015). It is, however, a very important shift to facilitate and to witness, since without taking the risk to step forth and express their needs, the withdrawer remains in a position of hiding and the basic dance will not change. This change event initiates an interpersonal dynamic of effective dependency – reaching, responding, and receiving – that will be completed with the second round of Stage 2 and the softening change event.

It is important to distinguish a partner's fully bringing themselves with needs and wants, into the relationship and risking speaking from a position of entitlement and need, from that of trying harder to please their partner and doing more of what is demanded of them. A withdrawer's incremental engagement in therapy can be deceptive for beginning EFT therapists, who can misperceive that a withdrawer has re-engaged in the relationship just because they are spending more time in the relationship, are sharing more, or are more compassionate and caring. With closer attunement, a therapist might discover that the relationship is going much better because the more pursuing partner is thrilled with the withdrawer's changes; however, the more withdrawn partner might continue to remain largely unaware of his or her emotions and needs, and rarely, if ever, reach out to ask clearly for support or to be heard. When avoidance remains the dominant coping strategy, the withdrawer has not yet claimed full residency in the center of the house but continues to live on the edges to maintain peace or to protect themself and the relationship. They need the therapist's support to engage fully – to take risks to access attachment needs and to step openly and assertively into the relationship, to clearly state needs for support and influence.

Lingering in difficult emotions is likely to be one of the most challenging things for a therapist new to EFT. This is understandable since it is also very difficult for partners to remain there. In Julie and Phil's withdraw–withdraw cycle, Julie trepidatiously takes the lead into Stage 2 saying, "It is so scary to stay in that fear, I can barely stay there long enough to find the words." Emily helps Julie to stay and expand that very fearful place, and in her Step 7, Julie continues ever so carefully, "You pushed me for what you wanted. I lost my voice. It happened over time. I am hurting. I need you to hear, but I am so afraid you will push more or disappear again." Emily reflects and heightens.

When Julie's attachment needs begin to emerge, Emily asks Julie to risk turning to Phil. Julie discloses:

> Inside I shut down—afraid to stand up to you. Afraid you will disappear again, and I need you to be close to me. I am desperate for you to hear me and stay with me—not too close—but don't leave me. Can you assure me you really want me for me? That you really are interested in who I am? Can you ease up on your intellectualizing and really hear me?

This is a huge moment, filled with emerging confidence and immense risk for Julie.

Phil's response is complex. He is deeply moved by Julie's courage and assures her, without hesitation, that he doesn't want to leave her, that he definitely wants her and is interested in her. He is also sufficiently emotionally engaged that he knows he cannot glibly promise to stop intellectualizing and pulling away. He is honest about his intentions, as well as the likelihood he will resume old habits. Nonetheless, this is a substantive change event. Julie's courage to make this request of Phil and Phil's honest responses are precisely what Julie needs in the moment. It is a big step toward a more secure bond between them, paving the way for Phil's engagement change event.

Wayne shares his newly discovered longings to be close to Jessica. He discloses, to Jessica, his core dread of hurting her, getting hurt, and losing her; failing to be what she wants him to be; and his dread of disappointing her. Then, with Emily shaping a Move 3 encounter, he moves into his Step 7 reach, asserting, "What I need is your reassurance that you still love me, even when I let you down. That you want me despite my imperfections. I need you to stay with me – don't turtle away when I upset you!" Emily knows this moment of Wayne's reach to Jessica is an absolute treasure. After Wayne risks reaching and requesting Jessica's reassurance, Emily heightens the moment and supports Jessica's response. This time, Jessica joyfully receives Wayne's message of "dreading" to lose her; dread which she says sounds "terrifying." Wayne shrugs and demurely exclaims, "It is terrifying!" She embraces his request for reassurance of her love, "That is all I want to do, is reassure you of my love. I just don't know how to do it well when I am afraid that you're disappearing."

Emily recalls hearing a supervisor say, "Expanded emotion opens a door into a new world." At the time, it sounded too magical for reality; however, she is thrilled each time she experiences that, indeed, expanding emotional experiences and disclosing them in interpersonal dialogue does indeed open doors into new worlds of self and relational discovery.

Some pursuers, like Jessica, are thrilled to see their partner taking this assertive risk to reach for support and they readily respond with full reassurance. Others, such as those caught in more attack–attack patterns, like Sophie and Ella, respond differently. During Ella's engagement, Sophie remains guarded and disorientated, and unable to respond with full assurance. It is not uncommon for pursuers to be disorientated and initially unable to embrace the withdrawer's assertive engagement. The good news is that an EFT therapist can trust the change process. The change event of the withdrawer having claimed a newly engaged position in the relationship will have a lasting impact, whether the pursuer is welcoming or distrustful.

In summary, by shaping an encounter with a specific request, therapists help withdrawers to step forward to state what they need in the relationship to feel more valued, wanted, hopeful, and safe to be themselves with their partner. They help clients to take a stand from a position of increased efficacy, accessibility, and emotional responsiveness, rather than the previous distant, inaccessible, and reactive position. They help them to disclose a newly discovered desire for closeness and connection, and to ask for what they need to stay engaged. This is the essence of withdrawn clients moving from their Step 5 disclosure of core fear to Step 7 engagement. Statements such as, "I feel small and inept with you and live in fear of you really seeing this and leaving me, so I go numb, defend and withdraw," evolve and crystallize in Step 7 into a clear request, "I am exhausted from feeling small in this relationship. I want to be close. I need to know that you want me and appreciate me. Can you hold back your criticism, stop threatening to leave me and show me you want me?"

For a withdrawer, it is extremely risky to step in the direction of closeness. The EFT therapist needs to be attuned to this risk and to be directive in shaping and inviting this reach toward connection. A withdrawer's vulnerability and sense of risk might appear more assertive than weepy, though there could also be tears. Tears or no tears, stepping close to express attachment needs is, nevertheless, a huge risk with a significant impact.

EFT Tango Moves to Facilitate the Engagement Change Event in EFIT. Although the steps of Stage 2 change are detectable in EFIT (Johnson, 2019, 2021), the movement between EFIT steps and stages is much more fluid than in EFCT (Johnson & Campbell, 2022). There is ample room in EFIT for a therapist to flow with the EFT Tango, putting the client's change process in the foreground and moving artfully between stages.

Consider an engagement change event in EFIT that is created in a similar manner to engagement in EFCT: A client, whose default strategy is to deactivate, first of all engages with an expanded awareness of their own emotional world in their socio-cultural context. This involves bringing newly emerging internal experience fully alive and coherently formulating this emotional experience in words. In the self-protective pattern, deactivating clients typically tune out internal experience and primarily tune into possible signs of disapproval or attack. With the therapist's help, the client explores bodily felt core attachment fears and discloses this expanded view of self to an imaginal significant other, to the therapist, or between parts of self. Similar to EFCT, in EFIT a new pattern of effective dependency is *initiated* with engagement.

In Emily's stabilization work with Max, they identify his pattern of minimizing the losses and trauma he has survived. He clearly recognizes his pattern of downplaying the situations he has had to endure and pushing emotions into the background. He owns how this has been his strategy to manage some of his biggest terrors and losses. In spite of trying to ignore them, they have stalked him for decades. In particular, he identifies his childhood sexual abuse and his terror of having a conscious memory of the scene of the accident where his friend was killed. The other part of his recurring pattern is to *subjugate himself*, doing what others ask of him and silently resenting how much of himself he gives up. He identifies many losses and grief that rarely, if ever, does he allow himself to touch. Entering Stage 2, Emily guides Max to develop a growing capacity to feel the grief of his many losses, including the loss he is living with from his long-term relationship ending.

Distill, Deepen, and Disclose Core Affect. Encounters created by the therapist using Moves 2 and 3 help a client to take Step 5. First, the therapist helps the EFIT client to engage more with emotions – fears and longings – that were previously assembled. Using Move 2, lingering longer and more deeply in the assembled core emotion, a therapist helps the client to expand fears, pain, grief, core assertive anger, and aspects of self that were outside of full awareness. Then with Move 3, the therapist shapes an encounter to support the client to disclose this newly engaged emotional experience to an imaginal other (IO), to a part of self or to the therapist.

After a difficult week of loneliness and grief regarding the ending of his relationship, the strongest emotions for Max are guilt and shame over his friend Léo's death. Fear of remembering Léo's body at the scene of the accident continues to linger. Emily helps him assemble his emotion. The trigger is the silence in his home – a daily reminder that his partner is no longer with him. Anxiety and tension fill his chest (bodily arousal). He describes his difficulty sleeping as he acknowledges his fidgeting in session (body; action tendency). In this heightened state, the tension in his chest reverberates with thoughts and fears of the future by himself (meaning making). The guilt and shame surrounding Léo's death become full center, followed by the bodily felt horror of the consequential time he spent in jail. "I have a mantra," he says, "And I feel calmer when I use it: You can't change what happened in the past" (action tendency of brushing overwhelming emotion aside).

When Emily checks about his fear of remembering the scene of the accident, Max is quick to say, "It is always there! I know how badly he was hurt, and I don't ever want to see that." Emily assembles and deepens Max's core emotion of remorse, experienced as a tightness in his chest and respectfully invites him to picture Léo the last time he spoke with him, alive. She wants to build enough safety for Max to eventually address the body he fears facing. Emily uses Move 3 to shape an encounter for Max to tell Léo how sad and sorry he feels that he died that night. After Max speaks to this imaginal Léo, Emily processes the experience with him. Much to his surprise, Max experiences Léo looking accepting and not at all angry. He hears the imaginal Léo say, "It wasn't your fault. I got in that car too. I wanted to go street-racing too."

As Emily flows between shaping and processing encounters between Max and Léo, Max sighs, "It takes a little bit of the weight off, that's for sure. And it's going to help me release some of my shame and guilt, that's for sure. It will help with that process." Max dips into experiencing pure sadness and grief over the loss. It is a refreshing sadness that is no longer constricted by guilt and shame.

Process Encounter with Discloser and Recipient. Processing engaged encounters with Move 4 and potentially shaping additional encounters help a client to take Step 6 of client change (see Box 9.1). With Move 4 processing, the therapist helps the client to process the impact of the encounter: First, eliciting how it was to share this deepened disclosure, and second, by inviting the client to reflect on how the IO is receiving this message. If it is safe to hear from the IO they will be invited to speak from the IO, in their voice.

As previously described, in EFT, the goal is to promote an accepting response from the recipient. Acceptance, however, is never forced. If the recipient of the disclosure is unable to be accepting at this point, the therapist will shape an authentic response, such as an expression of reluctance or disorientation. If the client perceives the imaginal recipient of their disclosure or an internal part of self to be dismissive or hostile, the therapist holds the client in this difficult place with validation and support, and then uses Move 3 to help shape an additional assertive message.

When Sahra first addresses her imaginal mother to acknowledge how frustrated she is with her for not protecting her when she was young, and more recently, for not cooperating with Sahra's attempts to protect her, her mother bristles and becomes defensive, "You never appreciate how much I do for you!" Non-acceptance or defensiveness from an imaginal parent can motivate a client to send an even stronger message in response, asserting legitimate hurt and loss, and taking a new, more assertive position with the internalized parent (Johnson & Campbell, 2022). Therapists are

---

Box 9.1 Stage 2 Microelements of Client Change

EFCT: Therapists are finding it easier to learn EFT by keeping the therapist moves and micro-skills in the forefront and client steps of change in the background. Nevertheless, clients' specific steps that empirically validated research shows lead to lasting change (Johnson, 2019, 2020) remain the same, and it is helpful to know the terrain of client change.

First, each partner, in turn, distills and deepens their core attachment fears that were discovered in Stage 1, and risks disclosing them clearly and in an emotionally engaged manner to their partner. (Step 5: Distill, deepen, and disclose core fears and emotion.)

Second, the partner receiving the disclosure is guided to respond with acceptance, or if acceptance is not available, with authenticity. (Step 6: Process and respond to partner's disclosure.)

Third, the disclosing partner risks requesting what they need to meet their attachment needs and the receiving partner is guided to respond with reassuring comfort and care. (Step 7: Request, respond, and receive new-found security.) The *reaching and responding* are corrective emotional experiences that shift views of self and other, ameliorating individual emotional distress and forming secure interpersonal bonds (Ganz et al., 2022; Johnson, 2019).

EFIT: Therapists guide clients to take three similar steps in Stage 2.

First, the therapist helps clients to explore more deeply, across relationships, core emotions, themes and patterns that were discovered and assembled in Stage 1. Deepened emotion is disclosed in encounters with inner experience, with IOs, and with the therapist.

Second, a series of deeply engaged emotional encounters with images of significant others, between parts of self, and with the therapist, reveal expanded aspects of self and other. Except for cases where a client does not want to hear back from an IO, such as situations of abuse and danger, they are also guided to explore their perceived responses from IOs. "Whether the encounter is positive or negative, new emotional music invites the client to try a new kind of dance with this other person, often at a different level of connection" (Johnson & Campbell, 2022, p. 83).

Third, powerful corrective emotional experiences are created wherein clients are supported to send clear messages of needs to IOs and between parts of self or to the therapist. The therapist guides clients to receive and integrate imaginal and real responses wherein view of self and view of other are transformed. "In this experience, vulnerability is embraced and owned in a way that leaves the client feeling more whole and more balanced, and ironically, more powerful" (Johnson, 2019, p. 91).

---

frequently reluctant to shape encounters with hurtful others because they fear the IO may respond harshly, however, the hurtful response is, in fact, what the client is already living with internally. Engaging in realistic encounters in the safety of the therapeutic relationship can help a client to take a firmer stance and to clarify, for example, as Sahra does:

What you did was indeed worse than what you are hearing. Let me tell you again! I will not accept your dismissing my pain. When you laughed at my career goals, it crushed me to the core. I have never felt as confident and as clever as I did before that day.

After Max tells imaginal Léo that he is sorry for his death, Emily has a brief moment of fear about processing the encounter but then she trusts that it is safe to flow with Move 4. She invites Max to describe how he experiences Léo as he expresses his remorse to him. Emily guides him to formulate an imagined response from Léo, by asking, "What do you, as Léo, want to say to Max, who is filled with regret and remorse and guilt for your death?"

Later, Emily shapes an encounter for Max to tell the imaginal Léo that his time in jail was hard on him. He is reluctant to do so, saying, "That seems like a very big ask!" She slices it thinner and invites him to let Léo know that it feels wrong to tell him that jail was hard on him. Flowing with Move 4, Emily processes this "thinner slice" with Max.

Emily: How is it to tell him, "It doesn't seem right to tell you that jail was hard on me"? He's the one that died and you're the one that suffered. How is it to be letting Léo hear this from you?

The response Max is about to make may seem surprising but it reveals the power of fully engaging with clients' present-moment experience, without trying to help them change it.

Max: It makes me feel like that's a possibility. Being able to articulate that makes me feel like there's a possibility to change the feelings that I have around it, which is good. Gives me hope.

Emily: Risking telling him, "I don't feel I have a right to say this but your death and my going to jail has been hard on *me*." Taking that risk, having that courage, feels hopeful? And when you closed your eyes and you took the risk to tell him what felt not right, what did you notice in your image of him? How did his face look? What did he look like when you told him that it's been hard on you? (Move 4, checking the perspective of the recipient of the encounter.)

Max: He looked forgiving. (Pause) And, really, I think he would be, like… We all lived pretty fast, you know? Live fast, die young. Leave a beautiful corpse. We were all pretty wild, right? So, because of that, I don't think he would hold the kind of grudges that somebody else might, because…

Emily: So, just savor this. Notice how it is to see that Léo looks forgiving. Léo looks like he understands. Yes? (Tracking, reflecting, evocative question for more Move 4 processing.)

Max: It… it… it's good. It makes me feel like maybe I can turn the corner around this.

Emily: What do you feel like telling him? What do you feel like telling the Léo that looks forgiving and understanding and that gives you some hope?

If the recipient of a disclosure is the therapist, the therapist will offer a transparent response about their experience of receiving this disclosure. If the encounter was made between parts of self, the client will be invited to respond from the receiving part or, depending on the situation, to process more deeply their experience of this intimate contact between two parts of self.

Shape Encounters to Assert Needs, Make a Request, and Elicit a Response (if Appropriate). Using Moves 2 and 3, encounters are shaped to help a client make a reach or a request in the engagement change event that restructures internal working models of self and other. Core emotion tells us what we need. As core emotion is distilled, deepened, and disclosed, the needs embedded in that core emotion can usually be discovered. Encounters are then processed with Move 4.

Max: (Speaking as imaginal Léo.) I would tell him that I love him.

Emily: Yeah? That's a powerful message. You want to tell Max that you love him. It's amazing you can tell him that! He's carried so much guilt and blame and shame for your death, and now, you're his buddy, saying, "We did this life together. Live fast, die young, leave a beautiful corpse?" Do I remember that right?

Max: Yeah. Yeah, that's the saying.

Emily sees this moment of Max sensing Léo's love, to be an amazingly serendipitous, safe opportunity to help him to face one more layer of his terror. The interpersonal safety of speaking to an image of a friend he expected would be angry and is now loving, is striking.

Emily: Can you tell him, "I don't think your corpse was very beautiful. It has haunted me for ages."

Max: (20 second silence, with his eyes closed.) It's an interesting… It's interesting. I imagined feelings. I imagined feeling guilt and sorrow and love and remorse… all sort of mixed together.

Emily: (Move 4.) What's coming up?

Max: I just… I have a… I have a little bit of peace. Which is not something that I ever had.

Max does not express a request explicitly in words to Léo, however, it has the impact of a Step 7 reach where he tells his deceased friend about his remorse, his responsibility, his sadness, and his need to be seen as one who is grieving and loving him.

Emily: Right. Imagining the mix of guilt and sorrow, love and remorse to your image of Léo is giving you some peace that you haven't felt before!

Max: The idea that I can forgive myself is powerful! It's what I've been trying to work towards throughout this whole process. The idea that I can address these things and for it not to be all this overwhelming negative emotion… I can feel a little bit more neutral.

Max participates in more Stage 2 engagement encounters with Emily and between parts of himself. Little by little, he engages with feelings that he has boxed away at a safe distance. The boxed away feelings are coming closer to his awareness, and he now says he feels like he is carrying a heavy weight, like a *monster-in-a-box* in his head. The young-adult self asserts to his current-day self, "It is too heavy to carry inside. I need you to listen and help me carry this dreadful weight!" Max wants to face all this heaviness that he carries. He engages with his fears of seeing Léo's dead body; with his shame and guilt for street-racing and being responsible for Léo's death; with the ongoing, threatening impacts of his time spent in jail. His engagement includes exploring resentments for how much he has subjugated himself, put aside many parts of himself, and bypassed many of his longings to be kind to others.

To guide Sahra through engagement with her imaginal mother, Emily assembles her grief and anger that her mother let her down by refusing to move to America with her when she got into medical school. With Emily's help, Sahra assembles her *emotion story*:

I can't understand that she wouldn't let me help her. During her entire struggle with the cancer that finally took her life (trigger), I perceived she was blaming me. I heard and still do hear that I am not enough as a daughter. She has never liked me for who I am (meanings)! Admittedly I tried to convince her, to change her (action tendency)! Something broke between us when I came to America! Well, it broke when I was young, but her refusing to join me, refusing to support my career, refusing to let me help her, pushed us further apart. I fought to convince her to come here where I could care for her – where I could get her the best medical care!

Emily helps Sahra to share her core emotions in a series of encounters with her imaginal mother.

Her imaginal mother's reactions begin with initial defensiveness. Emily has learned not to be rattled by this or to panic that the encounter is *going badly*. Sahra's imaginal mother protests, "I gave up my career for you – when your father left. You didn't need to leave me now. You know I couldn't leave Ukraine. I can't leave this town… one day your father may come back looking for us." Not thrown off-balance by her mother's typical defensiveness, Sahra engages more clearly with her own experience and speaks directly to her imaginal mother, who gradually becomes confused and then curious to hear what Sahra has to say.

From her core anguish (anger with her mother; grief at her isolation and their disconnection; fear of abandonment and rejection), she accesses what she longs for from her mother and is able to shape a direct request to her, "Please see my goodness. I need your kindness and compassion. Please see how hard I have tried to help you! Let me know you see me and care about me."

To Emily, Sahra says, "Regardless of her response, I already feel such relief to find those words. I just need her kindness and compassion. I deserve that!" She wipes tears of joy and celebration. "I couldn't have done this without you," she says to Emily, smiling. The session is coming to an end and Sahra says, "I want to have more conversations with her – conversations like this that we never had in real life!" Engaging with a coherent voice for her own experience leads to a softer and ironically more confident, powerful view of self. The process to reach repair with her mother will be completed in a softening change event, an attachment injury resolution process, included in the online support material for Chapter 16 (routledge.com/9781032151335).

HOW EFT Therapists Guide Clients through the Engagement Change Event

Much of *how* a therapist works in Stage 2 to shape corrective emotional experiences is similar for both the engagement change event described in this chapter and the softening change event described in Chapter 10. There are, however, some identifiable differences in working with clients using deactivating, commonly thought of as withdrawers in EFCT, and clients using hyperactivating, typically described as pursuers in EFCT (Kailanko et al., 2021a; Lee et al., 2017), as mentioned earlier. Stage 2 work involves helping clients to expand and step into deeper levels of their own emotional experience than they experienced in Stage 1. Heightening clients' emotional experiencing to Levels 4 and above on the Experiencing Scale (EXP; Klein et al., 1969, 1986) is considered necessary for Stage 2 in-session change (Kailanko et al., 2022). EFT therapists, working with emotion as a *perception-feeling-meaning-action process* know that the deeper levels of experiencing that need to be attained for Stage 2 change include not only feeling affect, but also more deeply reflecting on meanings, insights, and behavioral responses as they are occurring. It is from deeper levels of emotional experiencing that new meanings, new views of self and other, and new motivation for interacting emerge. From these shifts, new *broaden-and-build cycles of effective dependency* are formed. In addition to using the EAR of empathic attunement (Box 1.3) to continually monitor and check that your clients feel you are accurately attuned, *how* EFT therapists guide clients through the greater depths of the transformative Stage 2 change events could be summarized by identifying the following key elements:

1. **Therapist presence.** The quality of a therapist's presence can predict higher levels of client experiencing needed for Stage 2. Therapeutic presence is impacted by the therapist's vocal quality and their emotional balance. (Details given in online support material.)
2. **Somatically focused interventions.** Tracking, evoking, and commenting explicitly on somatic signs of emotional experiencing in the present moment can increase client depth of experiencing, in particular, for those using deactivating, down-regulating strategies, featured in this chapter.

3. **RISSSSSC Manner.** EFT therapists guide clients to *risk* exploring greater emotional depths in the following manner: Repeat, use Images, use a Simple, Slow, Soft voice, be Specific, reflect Somatic signals (such as changes in voice or bodily shifts) and use Client's words.

4. **Situating clients on the EFT map of change**. Knowing where clients are on the EFT map of Stage 2 change (Box 9.1) helps an EFT therapist to determine *how* best to intervene to keep emotion alive during Stage 2.

Check Chapter 9 Support Material (routledge.com/9781032151335) for an expanded description of the above elements of how EFT therapists guide clients through the engagement change event.

Conclusion

This chapter focuses on engagement, the first of the two Stage 2 change events. Withdrawers or those who survive by using deactivating strategies have an overly determined sense of independence and self-reliance. In some social contexts, particularly for those marginalized due to race, ethnicity or culture, down-regulating strategies are needed for survival. The deactivating strategy functions to avoid any emotional state that would interfere with the main goal of keeping the attachment system deactivated, and evading emotions that are associated with a sense of threat and vulnerability (such as fear, anxiety, anger, sadness, shame, and guilt). Clearly, in withdrawer engagement (Step 7 of EFCT), the therapist invites the withdrawer to risk doing the very thing that goes against their survival strategy: Risking stepping *into* relationship toward an intimate partner with vulnerability and assertiveness, taking a stand to voice their wants and needs. Similarly, inviting an EFIT client to request their needs and wants is a huge risk and a potentially life-altering move.

In EFCT, the withdrawer's new engagement with self and with their attachment fears and needs, followed by assertive stepping into relationship and reaching for connection is a corrective emotional experience. This new position is a lasting shift. Although, the old pattern is likely to resurface, and in a couple relationship, the pursuer is most likely to remain critical and mistrusting, the former withdrawer remains much more engaged with self and in the relationship. There are now two players on the field. The first change event of Stage 2 that initiates a new positive cycle of reaching and responding has occurred.

In EFIT, the main goal is similar, in that shaping relational safety and connection fosters a positive working model of self and some others, and the confidence to discriminate who can be trusted. In the engagement change event clients become more open to their own experience and freer to explore emotions previously experienced as unapproachable, unfamiliar, and/or unacceptable. Clients need help to process unimaginably intense emotions and impulses to action in order to shape more effective strategies for engagement (Bowlby, 1988). During engagement, an EFIT client has corrective emotional experiences that begin building emotional flexibility and resilience, and secure connection across relationships.

Get Ready... The Clients Are Coming!

Check Chapter 9 Support Material (routledge.com/9781032151335) for a summary of the key ingredients of facilitating the engagement change event. There you are also guided to review the five client cases and to identify key features of each client's engagement and to prepare for a next session with them.

10 Working with Emotion to Shape the Softening Change Event

[L]ove is not only an end for therapy; it is also the means by which every end is reached... Psychotherapy changes people because one mammal can restructure the limbic brain of another. (Lewis et al., 2000, pp. 169, 177)

The seismic shift of a softening – the second Stage 2 change event in EFT – is the focus of this chapter. In couple therapy, a softening event is when the more anxious, pursuing partner softens and takes a new position in the relationship. By definition, a previously hostile, critical partner accesses and deepens attachment emotions, and "from a position of vulnerability and within a high level of emotional experiencing" (Bradley & Furrow, 2004, p. 234), risks to reach to their partner who is now engaged and responsive, asking for contact comfort and for their attachment needs to be met. This is an interpersonal corrective emotional experience that includes the pursuer's vulnerable reach to their partner, the now-engaged withdrawer's reassuring response, and the pursuer's full reception of this response. The Rs of Reaching to Request, Respond, and Receive, form this ultimate bonding event, a seismic shift that reshapes the entire relationship into a secure bond of reaching and responding with comfort and care.

In EFIT, a softening is also an interpersonal corrective emotional experience wherein an individual client risks distilling, deepening, and disclosing their core attachment fears, discovered earlier, with an increasing depth of emotional experiencing. The softening change event begins in EFIT, as in EFCT, with the disclosure of a distilled and deepened core fear that continues to define views of self and other. The fear could be fear of isolation, rejection, abandonment, or injury. Disclosure of this deepened core fear at a level 5 or 6 on the Experiencing Scale (EXP; Klein et al., 1969, 1986; see Chapter 2 and Box 12.1) lays the foundation for discovering the need embedded in this fear. In the increasingly alive emotional depths of Klein et al.'s Levels 5–7, new edges and felt shifts of emotional experiencing emerge. Fresh ways of knowing and of listening to the needs embedded in core emotion arise. A series of dialogues (or engaged encounters) culminates in a pivotal, vulnerable reach or statement of need. Through emotionally engaged encounters, EFIT clients move into the accessibility, openness, responsiveness, and full engagement that characterize secure attachment within self and with others.

A softening in EFIT redefines a client's sense of self as worthy, loveable, competent, and resilient. It also redefines the view of other, distinguishing reliable others from unreliable and unsafe others. The Stage 2 softening in EFIT may involve detaching from unreliable and hurtful others, while at the same time shifting the working model of other to include some others as trustworthy. Confidence that some others are reliable and safe emerges. This shift in view of other is significant, in that it heightens a client's confidence to discriminate between others who are trustworthy and those who are not. Stage 2 change events can redesign a world that has been painted as dangerous by despicable, cruel acts of others, with expanding islands of safety. Experiencing safe interpersonal connection as an antidote to interpersonal injury is a core tenant of EFT.

EFIT Stage 2 softenings can occur across various relationships. Examples include (1) a perceived softening *from* an imaginal other who was previously experienced as hostile or

DOI: 10.4324/9781003242673-15

dismissive, showing love, empathy, and remorse for how hurtful they have been. This redefines a client's view of self and other, even if the client chooses to detach from that relationship in real life; (2) a softening and bonding between two internal parts that were previously discon- nected, critical, or dismissive of each other; (3) an experienced softening *toward* an imaginal other; (4) a softening with a spiritual figure.

The significance of a softening is the profound shift it creates in a client's felt sense of security with others and within self. There is an expanded sense of self as competent, lovable, and worthy, a fully alive self with meaningful, open connections with others and confidence to choose between reliable and untrustworthy others.

EFCT therapists witness some moments of softening through Stage 1; however, these softer moments continue to fade and to be replaced with critical demands or frustration. Eruptions of the repetitive pattern frequently reappear in couples, despite the withdrawing partner being engaged. Until the actual softening change event occurs, anxious pursuers default to anxious attachment strategies, sending unclear messages of fears and needs. Unmet longings for contact comfort fuel rigid, self-protective, pursuing behaviors. The EFCT softening change event, however, transforms a relationship into a safety zone, setting the relationship on a trajectory of bonding as "an eternal process of renewal" (Johnson, 2013, p. 215).

A softening is found to be crucial to success in EFT (Johnson & Greenberg, 1988) and is known as the watershed event in the EFCT process of shaping secure bonds (Bradley & Furrow, 2004; Dalgleish et al., 2015; Johnson & Greenberg, 1988). Couples that complete the softening event "are more likely to display higher levels of emotional experiencing and expression and greater attuned responsiveness, and to move out of relationship distress at the end of EFT than couples who do not achieve this change event" (Burgess Moser et al., 2015, p. 233). Researchers examined session-by-session changes in a sample of 32 couples, finding significant decreases in relationship-specific attachment avoidance, and in the couples who completed a blamer soften- ing, also a significant decrease in relationship-specific attachment anxiety (Burgess Moser et al., 2015). In other words, avoidance reduces throughout therapy, but the blamer-softening change event is necessary to reduce attachment anxiety. This change event is considered to be the most difficult change event and is also recognized as the most common impasse that EFT thera- pists encounter (Johnson & Talitman, 1997). A common impasse to a softening is a relationship trauma or *attachment injury*, discussed at length in Chapter 16.

EFIT clients can easily slip back into old patterns of emotion regulation, despite moments of change during Stage 1; however, Stage 2 shifts have more lasting impact. In the deeper engage- ment of Stage 2, softening events are created, "where small shifts come together to form sig- nificant new dramas that take people to the heart of their vulnerabilities and existential choices... moving into and through core pain and fear into a new sense of balance and agency" (Johnson & Campbell, 2022, p. 171). EFIT change events, parallel to the EFCT softening, open the door for in- dividual clients to move into *broaden-and-build cycles* of full engagement with life, with their own experience, and with others. This security is marked by a positive shift in view of self and other, with more flexible, interpersonally effective ways to engage with the existential dilemmas of life.

As in previous chapters, having defined the change event, we will explore the aspects of a sof- tening by examining what EFT therapists see and hear, what therapists and clients do, and *how* (the manner by which) therapists guide clients through a softening.

What EFT Therapists See and Hear as Clients Move through a Softening

Therapists see and hear signs that indicate when clients are ready to begin a Stage 2 softening. There are also notable elements that they see and hear throughout the process that culminates in the softening event.

Engagement of Previously Withdrawn Partners or Individuals

Markers of readiness to begin Stage 2 softening with couples are signals that the more withdrawn partner is engaged. Engaged withdrawers exude a different quality of presence than when they defaulted to avoidance and defensiveness. It is obvious that they are in a new position to attend and respond to their partner. They appear more involved, assert themselves more freely, and are less quickly triggered into reaction and defense. This means there is now a viable secure attachment figure toward whom the more pursuing partner can risk reaching (Bradley & Furrow, 2007).

While the distinction between the engagement and softening change events is less significant in EFIT, EFT therapists do see similar markers of clear engagement with emotional experience. Individuals who are engaged with their emotional experiencing have an increasing ability to articulate experience with confidence. They have a voice to assert fears and needs that were previously entangled in emotional chaos or hidden from their own awareness.

An Anxious Partner or Individual Client Withdrawing

It can be disorientating for a therapist new to EFT to see a more pursuing partner withdrawing or an anxious individual downplaying fears and needs. There are, however, several ways that an attachment perspective makes sense of anxious individuals' withdrawing or deactivating behaviors.

First, anxious strategies frequently include a pattern of withdrawal in exasperation or futility when partners do not get the response they are seeking. This self-protective strategy of withdrawal can appear despite a more withdrawn partner being engaged. Until the softening change event has occurred, a pursuing partner remains anxious about the reliability of receiving their partner's response. It is also not uncommon to see a trauma survivor who may have engaged deeply in previous sessions, suddenly revert to the safety of blocking all emotion and sensation. EFT therapists have a *felt-sense understanding* of how pulling away and shutting out the very person one wants close can seem like the safest move for a highly anxious client.

Likewise, in EFIT, therapists can resonate with clients' numbing and suppressing as the only apparently safe alternative when they are on the verge of risking to experience and express deeper and more vulnerable emotions. Emily understands that when Sahra abruptly loses touch with her emotional experience, saying, "I just lost connection," or, "I just got out of it," that she is exceeding her window of tolerance. She is overwhelmed. At these points, Emily typically validates Sahra's overwhelm, offering soothing and containment, frequently checking if she is aware of *when* she loses connection. The "*when question*" can help an individual identify the triggering moment and thus gain coherence and regain emotional balance.

EFT therapists recognize that attachment fears and needs for safety are running the show in intimate relationships and in individual clients' worlds. EFT therapists can feel in their own bodies how daunting it is for partners to imagine risking expressing vulnerable emotions or reaching to others who have hurt them or let them down. Pursuers may respond with a range of undifferentiated emotions, including harsh criticism toward their partner mixed with withdrawing in shame and self-loathing. Knowing that clients who have a history of traumatic attachments, typically use a mix of avoidant and anxious responses helps therapists normalize withdrawal behaviors in anxious pursuers.

Second, pursuing partners in couple therapy are frequently guarded and cautious. It is risky to trust that the newly engaged partner will stay present. *View of other* remains tenuous. ("Will you continue to show up?") View of self is also shaky. ("Am I loveable or worthy?") It is difficult to trust that one is deserving of their partner's newly engaged presence. Fears related to views of self and other can trigger withdrawal in anxious pursuers. Recognizing that withdrawal in a pursuer is an understandable reaction increases an EFT therapist's capacity to be empathically present. Without this understanding, an EFT therapist could become frustrated or disoriented when a pursuer withdraws.

In EFIT, the same attachment fears arise. Fears are related to view of other ("Can I count on them?"), view of self ("Am I worthy of love?" "Am I wanted?" "Do I belong?"), and fears of reaching ("Can I risk reaching to anyone?") EFT therapists understand how extremely vulnerable it is for clients to access and process these fears. For individuals with a trauma history, fearful avoidant strategies ("Come here, go away") have protected them from unsafe others. This mix of avoidant and anxious responses is likely to come to the fore during this extremely vulnerable exploration in Stage 2. It is not uncommon to see an EFIT client, having engaged in their experience, to uncharacteristically retreat and minimize their experience. "I just went numb," says Sahra as she begins to approach her unresolved terror of a recent traumatic experience with her daughter's father. Emily recalls the dance between Sahra's deepening of emotion and sudden numbing as she reprocessed a traumatic incident. She recalls that her calm patience, slow pacing, soft voice, and trust in the regulatory function of this deepening/numbing dance made it gradually safer and safer for Sahra to return to exploring core fears and anguish around the trauma. When an individual suddenly seems to retreat from exploration and progress, it may be a sign that this anxious client has exceeded their window of tolerance for intense emotion and needs the therapist's help to contain, safely regain focus, and re-engage them emotionally.

Emotion Online and Distilled

A therapist looks and listens for verbal and non-verbal indications that a client is engaged in a present-moment felt flow of inner experiencing, that is, that the client's emotion is *online*. If emotion is online, it is more than a concept or a word. It is available to the entire system of affect, bodily sensed arousal, cognition, and action impulses. It is *fully felt* at a Level 4 and above on the Experiencing Scale (EXP; Klein et al., 1986; see Chapter 2 and Box 12.1).

An indication that the core attachment fear is online is when a client describes the physical sense related to the emotion (heart pounds, stomach aches, lump in the throat) or shows visible signs of experiencing a bodily felt sense of the emotion (sighs, tears, swallowing). A marker that the core attachment fear is distilled is when a client can link the felt emotion to other elements, such as the trigger, the attachment meanings, the felt experience, and the action tendency, and can find simple words to describe the fear. Sophie not only says she is terrified of meaning nothing to Ella (core fear and meaning), she also feels the fear in the back of her throat (bodily arousal) that says, "Be careful—act strong. If Ella sees how much I need her, she will turn away." A therapist looks and listens carefully for these signs, since emotion needs to be online and distilled to choreograph a successful Stage 2 softening.

Emily begins to shape an encounter for Sahra to address her imaginal abusive ex-partner. They have distilled the message Sahra wants to share and as Emily helps her anticipate the encounter, Sahra confirms she is feeling safe enough to do so, however, there are long, silent pauses. Emily monitors very closely to see if Sahra is still within her window of tolerance. "My heart is racing – I want to talk to him – I just need time to work up my courage." From time to time, she looks at Emily as though drawing strength from her presence. At one point Emily worries that Sahra may be numbing out, so she evokes a grounding element of emotion – the action tendency, "What do you feel like doing?" "I feel like running," Sahra admits with a slight giggle, which tells Emily that Sahra is still engaged with her inner process. Emily validates the courage it takes to anticipate speaking to an imaginal, abusive other when what she really feels like doing is running away. "I just need more time," says Sahra again, and then she begins, "You hurt me..."

At the Core, Attachment Longings and Needs Are Not So Different after All

Throughout much of therapy, there seem to be significant differences in the attachment longings and needs of avoidant, withdrawing clients and those of anxious, pursuing clients. As the softening change event is experienced, anxious fears of "Can I count on you?" and avoidant fears of, "Am I worthy of love and appreciation?" blend together. Each client touches a core need to trust that a *significant other* is solidly there for them in a safe, validating, responsive manner.

In spite of significant and persisting differences between withdrawers' and pursuers' strategies for coping, Emily is amazed to experience, time and time again, that when partners get to the end of Stage 2, similar attachment needs and longings emerge. No longer are anxious pursuers and avoidant withdrawers so different. Engaged withdrawers access longings for connection, a focus typically heard from anxious pursuers. Softened pursuers access longings for acceptance, typically the purview of more withdrawn partners. Emily is thrilled to witness that while pursuers and withdrawers express their distress in different words, images, and actions early in therapy, after they distill core fears of rejection, annihilation or abandonment and access their deepest needs, they discover similar needs – to know the other is fully there for them, in an emotionally accessible, engaged, and responsive manner (Johnson, 2008). At the end of Stage 2, both partners are more comfortable expressing fears and needs, and reaching for comfort (Greenman & Johnson, 2013).

The longings and needs of pursuers and withdrawers coalesce through Stage 2 change events. Both partners discover how their safe connection can strengthen a sense of self as worthy of love and acceptance, and a sense of other as reliably present. We see this convergence at the close of the softening change event in the first EFT training video. Dr. Johnson says to Prue, the softening pursuer:

> Maybe [you'll need] a little time just to get the feel that he is not dangerous and that he is not going to disapprove of you – in a sense that he's not going to disapprove of you as much as you sometimes disapprove of you. It's funny how you [Mark] were talking in the beginning of how much you needed Prue's acceptance, approval, affirmation… and now it's like Prue, you are talking about that – you are saying how much you need his acceptance (transcript taken from video; Johnson, 1993).

What EFT Therapists and Clients *Do* to Co-Create a Softening

Recognizing that it is common for most beginning EFT therapists to struggle with how and when to intervene in this most crucial of EFT change events, EFT therapists and researchers Bradley and Furrow (2004) set out to examine successful softenings. From examining videos of successful softening events, they developed a mini-theory of this change event to guide therapists through it. A further process-research study of the softening change event, showed that therapist presence, as shown in vocal quality, is a predictor of deepened client emotional experiencing, and deepened emotional experiencing is at the heart of this change event (Furrow et al., 2012).

Although the EFIT literature does not distinguish between *engagement* and *softening* change events in Stage 2 restructuring, Emily is delighted to discover repeatedly that as she flows with the EFT Tango through Stage 2 in EFIT, engagement organically precedes a softening. The corrective emotional experience of softening restructures the individual's view of self and other and launches them into secure *broaden-and-build cycles* of new engagement with others and with their own emotional experience. Reaching for interpersonal support and growing confidence in self becomes the new *broaden-and-build cycle*. Snapshots of softenings in EFIT follow the examples of EFCT softening events, first with Wayne and Jessica and then with Ella and Sophie, presented according to the softening themes that Bradley and Furrow (2004, 2007, 2010) identified.

A Snapshot of Wayne and Jessica's EFCT Softening Change Event

A softening in EFCT is like a second round of Stage 2. In Stage 2 withdrawer engagement, Wayne, the more withdrawn of the two, was the experiencing partner, while Jessica, the more pursuing partner, was the observer and responder. In this second round, Jessica engages in emotional exploration of her attachment fears and needs. Emily shapes encounters for her to disclose core attachment fears and to risk reaching and asking Wayne, who is now engaged, to meet her deepest attachment needs.

Jessica had been very moved by Wayne's words in his engagement, "Stay with me – don't leave; don't turtle away from me." At the same time as she welcomed his request and responded enthusiastically, she became frightened, "I hope I won't leave," but her core fears were ignited, as typically happens for pursuers in engagement change events. Even though it is precisely what the more pursuing partner was longing for, their partner's new assertive engaged presence can also intensify fears for the pursuer: Fears of view of other ("Will you stay present? Is this for real?") and fears of view of self ("Am I worth staying engaged for?" "Am I too needy, too demanding, that my partner will see me as pathetic or simply too much?")

Jessica can sense that Wayne is more present and that he is remaining engaged. She begins to feel that she is important to Wayne, but this newness remains tentative for her. She fears he won't remain accessible and that she won't be able to find him when she needs him (view of other). In contrast to her view-of-other fears, she does repeatedly experience that he is remaining engaged; however, this stirs even deeper fears – fears of not being lovable to him (view of self). Her fears have yet to be distilled, deepened, and disclosed. Then Emily will support her to access from within distilled core fear, what it is that she needs from Wayne to soothe the fear and will support her to risk reaching to him with a clear request.

Using Move 2 assembly and deepening and Move 3 shaping an open, vulnerable encounter, Emily guides Jessica to deepen, distill, and disclose directly to Wayne, her fears of abandonment and longings for connection in an emotionally expanded and increasingly vulnerable way. Jessica courageously discloses to Wayne her terror of abandonment and feeling undeserving of his love, taking her Step 5. Processing the impact of this encounter with Jessica and then with Wayne, Emily flows between Tango Move 4, processing how it is for Wayne to hear this vulnerable and courageous disclosure, and Move 3, shaping more encounters. She supports Wayne to process this view of Jessica as terrified of losing him, yet too terrified to ask for his reassurance. He describes how it pulls for a new depth of compassion and care for her. Emily supports him to take in this newly vulnerable experience of Jessica and to respond to her from that place of compassion that is awakened by Jessica's softened position. As Wayne shares his authentic, engaged response to Jessica, he takes his Step 6 on the EFT map of client change.

Next, Emily facilitates the pivotal moment of softening that is often likened to jumping off a cliff. She heightens Jessica's fear of reaching to Wayne, while at the same time envisioning a picture of safety (seeding attachment), "You could never, ever reach to Wayne and ask him to assure you he loves you, just as you are – that you are his precious one and he is here for you? Never, ever take the risk to ask him and imagine he would reach back with all the comfort and assurance you long for." "No, no," Jessica hesitates, "Too scary to ask… when he sees how needy I really am, (view of self) he just might shrug his shoulders and walk off in disgust" (view of other). Emily feels in her own gut how terrified Jessica must feel. She also sees Wayne patiently leaning in, waiting for Jessica and she says softly to her:

> Wayne is right here, leaning towards you with a tender, patient smile. He says he is all in – that he wants to hear from you and that he has a whole new respect and compassion for how alone

you are feeling just now. Can you give him a chance? Can you take the leap? He is right there. He will catch you.

Emily invites Jessica to take the emotional risk of putting her life in Wayne's hands. Jessica, with heart pounding and fingers twisting the tissue in her hands, prepares to take the leap. Guided by Emily, she turns her newly expanded emotional experience into a reach – a request to Wayne (Bradley & Furrow, 2004; Johnson, 2020). She takes the risk from her most vulnerable, shaking heart and trembling hands, to ask him to meet her need, "Can you see how much I need you? Can you assure me you love me like this and you won't turn away from me anymore?" (This is her Step 7.) Wayne's immediate, tender response is full of reassurance and love, and all three are moved to tears. After a long pause for each of them to absorb the enormity of this bonding moment, Emily confirms that Jessica is receiving the assurance from Wayne. She then flows with Move 5 to validate their attachment needs and to heighten and integrate the courageous reaching, responding and receiving – the most important and powerful moment of bonding and transformation.

Themes in Sophie and Ella's EFCT Softening Change Event

Describing in more detail what EFT therapists and partners do in the softening change event, the following case example of Ella and Sophie illustrates the themes of Sophie's softening, according to expanded themes of the original blamer softening mini-theory (Bradley & Furrow, 2004, 2007, 2010; Table 10.1).

Ella, the former withdrawer is re-engaged and has a voice for the parts of self previously left out of the relationship (Johnson, 1993). When Sophie becomes impatient with her for spending so much time on her computer, or chatting on the phone with her son, Ella expresses her attachment needs and longings with assertive engagement, "I want to be close to you! I don't want to turn away from you, but it hurts to hear your disapproval. You're exhausting me with your demands; I need to know I'm enough for you." She talks about wanting to be close, too, and longing to feel wanted and valued. She thrills with delight at responses of appreciation from Sophie.

The cycle reappears, however, and Sophie begins the next session with some typical complaints:

> It happened again this week! Just when I needed her and hoped we'd have some time together, she left me all alone and spent all evening working at her computer until her son called and then she talked with him for an hour!

Emily notices Sophie's typical complaint and whining, while also tuning into the attachment channel – *being left alone, without Ella.* To attune as best she can to Sophie's experience, Emily feels within her own body, something of the sensation of being left alone and set apart from the most important person in one's life, the one you have been missing all day, who becomes emotionally absent and seemingly more interested in her work and her family than in you. Emily draws on her own lived experience of the feeling of being left alone. As discussed previously, the therapist's use of their own somatic experience is shown to help deepen client experiencing (Kailanko et al., 2022).

Emily attunes to how lonely and upset Sophie must feel at not being able to connect with Ella. She invites Sophie to be aware of what she is feeling as she complains about Ella, "Just notice how are you feeling right now, as you talk about being all alone without Ella." Sophie asserts, "I am angry!"

Then, as Emily validates her anger at feeling left out, Sophie's eyes soften. Emily conjectures in a soft, slow voice, "From that sad look in your eyes, I wonder if, under your anger, there isn't some

Table 10.1 Themes of the Softening Change Event

Themes	Client Step	Therapist Moves and Micro-Skills	EXP Levels
In themes 1–4, guide clients through the Ds: Distill, Deepen, and Disclose core attachment fears.			
Theme 1: Accessing core fears	Client Step 5	**Move 2 Assembly and Deepening** – with RISSSSSC manner. **Move 3 Shape Encounter** – to disclose the distilled, deepened fear.	Levels 2–3
Theme 2: Shoring up the engaged withdrawer	Client Step 5	**Move 1 Reflecting Present Process** – tracking, reflecting, conjecturing, and heightening partner's engaged presence.	Levels 3–4
Theme 3: Experientially imagining the reach	Client Step 5	**Move 2 Assembly and Deepening** – seeding attachment with evocative responding to paint a new picture of reaching and receiving comfort.	Level 4
Theme 4: Processing fears of reaching	Client Steps 5 and 6	**Move 2 Assembly and Deepening** – heightening, empathic conjectures, evocative responding, reflecting underlying emotions, and reframing in context of attachment needs, in a RISSSSSC manner. Expand and deepen 3 fears: fear related to view of other; fear related to view of self; fear related to reaching. **Moves 3 and 4** – to shape and process encounters with both partners.	Level 5
In themes 5–8, guide clients through the Rs of: Reach/Request, Respond and Receive.			
Theme 5: Actual reach	Client Step 7	**Move 3** – to shape this unique encounter, inviting a vulnerable reach with a specific *request*.	Levels 5–7
Theme 6: Engaged withdrawer reaches back with support	Client Step 7	**Moves 3 and 4** – Invite immediate response, evocative responses and questions, heightening.	Level 4
Theme 7: Process the reach with engaged withdrawer and softened pursuer	Client Step 7	**Moves 4 and 5** – to heighten the reach and response, evocative questions and reflections. Promote an affiliative response.	Level 4
Theme 8: Validate newly experienced emotions and attachment needs	Client Step 7	**Move 5** – to validate newly experienced emotions and attachment needs.	Levels 3–4

Source: Adapted from Bradley and Furrow (2010).

deep sadness at feeling alone?" She assembles the elements of emotion, linking them together to evoke more of the core underlying fear:

> You hear Ella happily talking online with her son for an hour, after an evening of working on her computer (replaying the cue) and you say, "She's left me all alone again. I'm just not important to her!" (reflecting the automatic attachment meaning Sophie makes) and you flip into anger and complaint (reflecting her reactive, surface emotion and action tendency) when

underneath you feel all alone – so afraid you are unimportant to her (in a tentative, soft tone, conjecturing at the emotional meanings and core underlying fear that Sophie has previously formulated). Is that it?

Emily checks for confirmation from Sophie as to whether the attachment conjecture fits with her present-moment experience. Sophie's eyes widen as she nods at Emily. The doorway into the first theme of the softening change event has opened. EFT Tango moves and micro-skills are noted below with each theme.

Theme 1: Accessing Core Fears. Use Move 2 Assembly and Deepening, with RISSSSSC and Move 3 Shaping an Encounter to disclose the distilled, deepened fear.

Emily: (Evocative responding.) You feel angry right now as you say, "There she is – her mother and sister and son are her real family, and I really don't belong. Try as I may, I just don't belong!" (Evoking an attachment longing.)

Sophie: That's it. I'm not in her inner circle. I am not her real family! I don't belong! (Therapist's evocative responding helps Sophie express a clear, congruent message of her worst attachment fear.)

Emily: What happens when you touch this deep dreadful place – where you long to belong in Ella's world? You try to belong and then you have this sense of, "If I make one mistake, everything will slide away – she'll be gone and I'll be all alone again with nothing to hold on to." You began sharing that with Ella, and then went suddenly silent. What's happening inside? (Heightening images and somatic cues.)

Sophie: It's as if I have a rock here. (Pointing to her chest.)

Emily: A rock in your chest. (Pause, gazing at Sophie, attuning to the enormity of the moment.) Your eyes fill with tears and the rock says…? (Reflection, tracking somatic cues, repeating image, evocative question.)

Sophie: Always waiting – waiting for – for somebody to walk away from me.

Emily: That's what you live with, this fear, this heavy rock in your heart that signals dread, dread that you are going to lose; especially dreading that you are going to lose Ella? (Reflecting, tracking, RISSSSSC manner: Repeating images in simple, soft, slow voice, somatic cues, specific attachment fear, client's words, conjecturing that the fear is specific to Ella, not just "somebody will walk away.")

Sophie: Yes!

Emily: This is an old, old feeling. You've described having this sheer terror ever since seeing your mother's casket lowered into the ground – feeling totally alone after your mother died. (She was seven years old when her mother committed suicide, and her father had been in and out of hospital most of her life.) And this old sheer terror of being alone is reinforced over and over again in your cycle with Ella, isn't it? (Evocative responding by replaying a cue of the dread of abandonment.) She is here now, but over and over in your negative cycle she has disappeared from your sight! And the fear and dread are totally alive just now. (Validating, heightening.)

Sophie: (Nodding.) And inside I hear, "She's gone. Gone for ever!"

Emily: So you know this feeling of always expecting to lose. You live with this feeling a lot – so afraid you are going to lose – that you feel this rock in your heart. You have lost so much and, in this moment, you feel the fear of losing Ella. So, can you tell Ella about this rock in your heart that says, "I'm always on this edge of danger – that there will be no one to reach for – that you will just walk away from me?"

Sophie:	No, no, can't show her. I can't let her see my sadness or my loneliness. She won't want to hear it. No one wants to hear about death, about loss. She only wants to see happiness.
Emily:	"Don't show this terror to Ella! Only show her the happy me!" When you're this sad and lonely, you don't want to show that, so you really try not to show it, yes? So afraid you've already lost her? Never show it to her? Never! (Heightening, conjecture.)
Sophie:	Mm-hmm. (Nodding her head vigorously.)
Emily:	You never want her to see the heavy rock in your heart, the panic that you've lost her this time for good?
Sophie:	No!
Emily:	And the panic spills out like that "fire hose of disapproval" you were talking about. (Evoking the fire hose image that is code for the intensity of Sophie's underlying fear that pours out as criticism.) Can you turn and tell Ella that the fear of being alone is too big to share with her? (Slicing it thinner.) It's just safer to hold it all back and try to look happy. That you are terrified she will not be able to hear your fear?

Theme 2: Shoring up the Engaged Withdrawer. Use Move 1 Reflecting Present Process – tracking, reflecting, conjecturing, and heightening Ella's engagement and Move 2 Assembly and Deepening, with evocative responding, and empathic conjectures about the attachment experience.

To shore up the withdrawer and set the stage for a safe encounter, the therapist comments that Ella is leaning in, listening intently. To make the picture of Ella's engagement and desire to respond vivid and alive for Sophie, Emily conjectures at the implied longing in Ella's bodily expression.

Emily:	You are leaning right in there, Ella, almost as if you are saying, "I want to hear from you. I do want to know about this rock of fear in your heart. I am very interested in your fears," yes?
Ella:	Absolutely! I don't run from sad. I don't run from fear! I run from disapproval. (In the negative cycle she has been running/withdrawing from Sophie's complaints and disapproval.)
Emily:	You wouldn't run from this sad, lonely place at all? (Ella: No!) You would run right towards her? (Ella: Yes!) You'd run right in. (Ella: For sure!) She would pull you right in? (Conjecture and heightening attachment image.)
Ella:	Absolutely, I'm not going anywhere! I want to know everything about you! I don't need you to be perfect. I just want to know what's underneath the "fire hose" force that I have been running from. I'm not running any more – I want to know you!

Theme 3: Experientially Imagining the Reach. Use Move 2 Assembly and Deepening, seeding attachment with evocative responding to paint a new picture of reaching and receiving comfort.

Creating a picture of safe connection also heightens the experienced fear in the present moment. The therapist wants to both seed attachment security and to heighten the fear and bring it alive.

Emily:	(To Sophie.) You can't imagine saying, "I am terrified Ella, come and be with me – I need to feel you with me. I need to know you care?" You could not say, "Ella, I am so afraid everything will fall away. I am so afraid of that *white marble wall with nothing to hold on to.*" (Repeating the image Sophie has used to describe her loneliness in this relationship, and

through her entire life.) "Can you come and show me you will never leave me?" You could never, ever say that?

Theme 4: Processing Fears of Reaching. Use Move 2 Assembly and Deepening, with evocative responding, reflecting underlying emotions, heightening, empathic conjectures, and reframing in context of attachment needs, all in a RISSSSSC manner; also use Moves 3 and 4 Shaping and Processing Encounters with both partners.

The fears that EFT therapists expand and process here are fears embedded in negative working models of other and of self. Fears related to view of other are fears that the other will not respond or will respond in a hurtful way. ("How can I trust that you will really be there for me? That you will really love me when no one has ever been there for me?") Fears related to view of self are fears of being unlovable and undeserving of a safe response. ("How could you really love me when I am so critical, weak, needy, or pathetic?") Fears and working models of self and other become vividly alive, frequently triggering similar emotions and memories from within this relationship and earlier relationships.

Expanding and Deepening Fear Related to View of Other.

Sophie: People always walk away from me – seems no one wants to talk about loneliness. I am alone, against a cold white marble wall, with nothing to hold on to.

Emily: Always waiting – holding your breath, waiting for everyone to walk away. Cold white marble – so very alone – cold and afraid that no one cares, not even Ella. (Heightening.) "So afraid I'll never feel I really belong to Ella's inner circle, never sure she will *be with me*," is that it? (Proxy, first-person, empathic conjecture in the attachment context of fear of view of other.) What is happening in your body in this cold, hard fear of being alone, of never quite belonging to Ella's world? (Reflecting core fear, evocative question, to access the bodily arousal of the core fear.)

Sophie: I feel a lump of fear in the back of my throat, like the moment you bury someone and you know they're out of your life forever.

Emily: You're always on the edge of danger – fearing there'll be no one to turn to, to stay with you. So, when Ella is busy, and especially when she talks happily with her son, you get this same lump in your throat and it says, "She's gone – not interested, not caring about me," yes? (Deepened and distilled in the cycle.)

In a soft, slow, tender voice, Emily shapes an encounter (Move 3) for Sophie to tell Ella about her enormous fear that is there all the time, a fear that Ella will walk away. (Unreliable view of other.) After Sophie discloses this fear to Ella, Emily processes the encounter (Tango Move 4) with Sophie and then Ella, inviting each, in turn, to notice how they feel sharing and receiving this vulnerable fear. Receiving assurance from Ella that she is fully present now, Sophie's fear shifts, as is typical for pursuing partners at this point in therapy, toward a fear related to view of self and terror that she is unlovable and unworthy.

Expanding and Deepening Fear Related to View of Self.

Sophie: Maybe she will be there – but it's me, as if I have a sign on my head that says, "Walk away!" I am too much, not important – I am pathetic. My sadness, my loneliness are *far* too much! It's not pretty; it's disgusting.

Using Move 2 assembly and deepening, Emily helps Sophie to expand and clarify this emerging fear: "Your deep fear is that if Ella sees how very much you need her, she will not want to be close to you? That she will not like that needy part of you?" (Simple reflection of fear related to view of self.)

Sophie: Right! To me the loudest invitation to get people to leave is to say, "I am sad," or, "I'm hurting." That's kind of the sign you hold up when you want people to leave. She'll back away. She won't like to hear about this.

Emily: Your deep fear is that if Ella hears how lonely you feel –how very afraid you feel about being left alone, how very, very much you need her comfort and her presence –that she will not want to be close to you, that she will not see you as lovable, yes? (Soft, tentative voice, checking to see these words are matching precisely with Sophie's internal experience.)

Expanding and Deepening the Fear of Reaching.

Sophie: I can't show her my sadness. I can't tell her I am lonely. I just can't ask!

Emily: You fear, "I'll reach and she won't be there. She'll be too busy. I'll show her this dreadful rock in my heart, and she'll take one look and go, 'Yuck!'?" (Heightening fear of reaching.)

Sophie: I can't reach – she will turn away too. Everyone else has, and she will too!

Emily: (Again checking in with Ella, the engaged withdrawer, as she prepares to shape an encounter with Sophie with Move 3.) How are you doing as you are leaning in, listening so intently to Sophie? (Reflecting somatic cues.)

Ella: I need to hear about this lonely, frightened place – I would be there. I don't ever hear that she *wants me.* I just can't take her anger and disappointment with me, but I do want us to be close!

Sophie: No, no – I don't believe it!

Again, in soft, slow, simple words, Emily invites Sophie to tell Ella directly about her immense fear, this time her fearful view of self, that in Ella's eyes she is too much, unlovable; in fact, how very scary it is to even imagine reaching to her from her lonely "unlovable" place. (Shaping a clear message related to fearful view of self and fear of reaching.)

Theme 5: The Actual Reach. Use Move 3 – to shape this unique encounter, inviting a specific *reach to request to have attachment need met.*

The actual invitation for the experiencing partner, in this case Sophie, to ask Ella to meet her attachment need while the fear is fully alive, is very directive. In this specific engaged encounter the therapist invites the client to take Step 7, the softening change event of Stage 2. Emily confirms that Sophie's attachment fear is alive, vivid, bodily felt in the moment, and that Ella is accessible and engaged. She understands the importance of the fear being *at a boil* (Bradley & Furrow, 2004) – what Klein et al. (1986; EXP) identify as Levels 5–7. "The therapist makes a simple request to reach, yet the heightened affect of the client makes this one of the most intense moments in the EFT process" (Bradley & Furrow, 2007, p. 31).

It is important that the pursuer experience an intense sense of risk while making the reach because that heightened fear opens them to receive the corrective emotional experience of their partner's engaged response. An engaged response, to a vulnerable partner's reach, is the antidote to fear that restructures the relationship and both partners' internal worlds. The bigger the risk

Sophie takes, the stronger the antidote to her fear that Ella's engaged response will provide and the stronger the bonding will be.

When Sophie's fear of reaching to Ella is *at a boil*, Emily invites her to take the leap, "Can you tell Ella what you need from her to help with this lump of panicky aloneness and sadness in your heart? What do you need from her right now?" (Evocative question, directed at earlier identified bodily sensation of fear.)

Sophie: I just need her to see me.
Emily: (Persisting with directing Sophie to reach with a request.) Can you ask her? Right now, she is here. (Heightening awareness of partner's accessibility.) Can you ask her? She is leaning right in, saying, "Ask me. Give me a chance to show you I *am* here." Can you ask her?
Sophie: (Haltingly, with a soft voice, barely above a whisper.) Can you see how much I long to matter to you as much as Craig (her son) and Min (her sister), and as much as all your work commitments? When I am a big, needy inconvenience for you, can you make time for me? Can you assure me I am important?
Emily: How could she help to assure you, you are important? (Focused on specific reach.)
Sophie: She could move in and hold me and tell me.
Emily: Can you ask her? (Prompting the reach.)
Sophie: (Quivering.) Can you?
Ella: Of course! (She moves close to Sophie.) You are my precious one!

From within a fully alive, bodily felt fear, Sophie reaches and experiences Ella's soothing response. For Sophie, it is an unprotected leap off a cliff, counting on Ella to catch her and meet her attachment need for an engaged response to her deepest fear.

Theme 6: Engaged Withdrawer Reaches Back with Support. Use Move 3, Shaping an Encounter to prompt a response if one is not offered spontaneously and Move 4 Processing, with evocative responses, questions, and heightening.

Emily gives space for Ella to respond to Sophie. Ella puts her arms around Sophie and holds her while she sobs, uttering soothing tones, assuring her this is the part of her she especially loves and cares for.

With Move 4, the therapist heightens the engaged withdrawer's response to the now softened pursuer's reach. Emily heightens the very loving response Ella offers to Sophie, highlighting the message Ella is sending of how precious Sophie is to her.

Theme 7: Process the Reach with Engaged Withdrawer and Softened Pursuer. Use Move 4 Processing, with evocative questions and reflections, with both partners.

For the corrective emotional experience to be created between partners, there needs to be a felt sense of risk and an antidote response. The therapist reflects how the sense of risk and the engaged response from the other partner is transforming the fear. Following the reach and the response, the therapist evokes each one's experience, and reflects and heightens how this is strengthening the trust and bond between them.

Checking to see how Sophie is receiving Ella's response, Emily supports both partners to share the impact this reaching and responding is having on them.

Sophie: I thought she would say yes, but it was still so risky to ask.
Emily: What is happening in your chest now? (Evocative question, with a somatic focus.)

Sophie: It's light!

Ella: (Reflecting, as withdrawers frequently do at this point.) This helps me, too. I need to know you need me. You seem angry and shut me out so much. I can do feelings. I can hear your fears and loneliness. I am not afraid that this part of you will ever be too much for me!

Using a mix of Moves 4 and 5, Emily heightens the reach and response, building on the image of light and the warmth of holding each other close, which is so much more comforting and reassuring than the cold, lonely, white-marble existence that they have endured in isolation for so long.

Theme 8: Validate Newly Experienced Emotions and Attachment Needs. Use Move 5 Integration and Validation. Emily validates the new experience they have created together – how new it was for Ella to see and hear from this shaky, vulnerable side of Sophie. She reflects how much this new reach/request from Sophie pulled Ella close. She heightens Ella's desire to be there for Sophie, feeling stronger and more deeply loved, after hearing Sophie's vulnerable expressions of needing her. She validates that both are becoming increasingly capable of sharing their deepest attachment fears and reaching to the other for comfort and support.

Conclusion on Themes of EFCT Softenings. While the above themes are not rigid steps to be followed sequentially, they offer a meta-perspective of what clients and therapists do to co-create softenings. They offer guidance for facilitating the two key elements that predict success in Stage 2 of EFT: Deepening emotional experience and shaping intimate dialogues about attachment fears and needs. Softenings can occur as one event in therapy or as several smaller softenings over time, and sometimes a softening can occur between sessions. Regardless, the EFT therapist is always there to evoke, shape, heighten, process, and consolidate the change event. The "therapist's ability to deepen and distill the attachment-related fears, informed by views of self and other... is critical in facilitating a softening reach" (Furrow et al., 2012, p. 40).

Snapshots of EFIT Softenings

Softenings also occur in EFIT. As Emily reflects on her experience with several EFIT clients, she is struck by the power of this relational model. Following the momentum of emotion and shaping interpersonal encounters literally brings order, coherence, and agency to EFIT clients' chaotic worlds, redefining and softening working models of self and other.

Softening from Another and between Parts of Self. Sahra, in an imaginal encounter with her estranged father, very vulnerably discloses the depth of pain that his departure caused her and that left her questioning her own goodness, "Mother gave us this hope that you might come back one day. I lived my entire childhood wondering if I could be a better daughter, would you come back? Would mother be happy again?" She begins to weep. "My hopes were always clouded by my doubts of you. I could never count on you (view of other) and my heart was murky with an invasive fear that somehow I was not good enough (view of self)." As Emily processes this brave encounter, asking Sahra, what happens inside her body as she looks at this image of her father hearing his weeping daughter share this heart-breaking story, Sahra stops. "Wait a minute!" (Her voice gets louder.) "Let me tell him something more! How could you do that to us? You were wrong – mother deserved better! We deserved better!" In her imagined responses from him, she initially hears defensiveness, but she persists. As she tells him how much they struggled to recover from his abrupt departure, her assertive claims are mixed with weeping. "Your departure changed mom forever! You absolutely shattered our world! Her voice softens as she weeps, faltering between her words, "I miss him so, so much, but I am also annoyed with him for leaving!" This time as Emily processes with Move 4, Sahra begins to see her imaginal father's shame and remorse for having abandoned her! With a brightening face, Sahra says, "He may not get it, but it feels so good to share this with him and imagine him actually stopping to listen to me!"

Her focus shifts from her imaginal father to her vulnerable, tender six-year-old self. "She is so tiny and so beautiful! Looks like her dad – has his skin color, just a little lighter, and his curly hair. She did not deserve this and all the trauma that followed!"

Emily invites Sahra to engage more with her beautiful little child-self. She validates her weeping for the little girl that her father abandoned and shapes an encounter for Sahra to comfort her. Looking at an image of her six-year-old self, Sahra says, "She looks frightened and she doesn't even know how much strife is coming! But I just want to hold her and shield her and promise her of her goodness – and let her know I will always believe in her."

Directly to her imaginal six-year-old self, Sahra says, "I will hold on to your goodness little one – I will not let anyone take that away from you! I'm here to listen to you, Tiny – to all your fears and feelings!"

In dialogues with her imaginal father that extend over several sessions, Sahra feels empowered standing up to him. She tells him how deeply he hurt her and how she carries the hurt to this day! To an imaginal father she says, "I am tired of feeling I am to blame. I long to know I am a loveable and worthy daughter in your eyes. I want to hear you admit you were in the wrong!" Emily invites her to check back with her image of her father, knowing it is a risk, but also knowing she can support Sahra in whatever imagined reply her father gives – knowing they are only making explicit Sahra's inner world. In a soft, firm tone, Emily says, "Do you want to ask him – can you ask him, 'Can you see I was an innocent, beautiful six-year-old and I didn't deserve this life-shattering event you wreaked upon us. I needed a loving father to depend on. I needed the father who looks like me to stay with me'?"

Sahra says, "Yes I want to take the chance…" and she addresses him. The risk in this vulnerable yet assertive request marks a powerful shift for Sahra. It is the transformative *risk to reach and ask for needs to be met*, that makes this Stage 2 change event so powerful in shifting views of self and other, and restructuring self and system.

Her imaginal father appears to slink away in shame, but not before he acknowledges, "You did deserve a loving father. You were beautiful. I broke your heart. I broke your world! I am in awe of who you have become today!" As Emily helps her process that imagined response, and the picture of what Sahra describes as "a pathetic old man slinking away," an old memory resurfaces, "I remember he used to tell me he thought I was very clever. Very determined! I like to hold onto that. It warms my heart." He changed – he is pathetic now – but I will hold onto that image of me, looking clever and determined in the eyes of my father as I remember him at six-years old. He knows he lost a good daughter!"

The dialogues with an imaginal father shift Sahra's sense of self from, "What's wrong with me that my own father would abandon me?" to emerging depths of holding him totally responsible for his departure! Sahra continues not to trust that her father would be reliable and is unready to attempt to contact him in real life. Nevertheless, this softening and strengthening change event shifts her overall view of other and her sense of effective dependency. About her father Sahra says:

> He is not dependable; I don't forgive him for how he hurt us and my mother, but now I feel more worthy and able to discriminate between those I can trust and those I can't trust. I don't blame him anymore. I just feel neutral about him. Before I couldn't trust anyone because I feared there was something about me that made people leave me. Now I am clearer that what he did was not my fault!

More EFIT Softenings with Sahra are available in Chapter 10 Support Material: A softening with a spiritual figure and a softening between two parts of self (routledge.com/9781032151335).

Snapshots of Max's Softening Encounters with an Imaginal Other. Max's softening is unique in that he is wrestling with fears and guilt related to his responsibility for his friend Léo's death in a street-racing crash where Max was the driver. Max's pivotal Stage 2 softening unfolds over several sessions, expanding his sense of self and softening his views of self and other. Encounters of walking directly into the scene of the accident and speaking directly to Léo's imaginal body create a corrective emotional experience for Max. He experiences a powerful, bodily felt shift in view of self from that of a harmful human being to one of being loved and affirmed for his worth, fully accepted and acceptable, and connected to others.

The transcript below is of Emily and Max reprocessing his terror of consciously seeing Léo's mangled body at the scene of the accident. This series of imaginal encounters, with Léo, began in Stage 1.

Max has come far in lifting the weight of shame related to the death of his friend, Léo. He has engaged in encounters with an imaginal Léo as he remembers him, alive. In those encounters, Max asserted his responsibility for driving recklessly while street-racing. He told Léo of his remorse, and to his surprise, Léo was not angry. Max felt acceptance and love flowing between them and felt they recovered a sense of connection. Emily is uncertain if she has completed the work of helping Max to reprocess what he has identified as his greatest guilt and fear that has haunted him for decades: Consciously recalling what Léo's body looked like at the scene of the accident. Up until now, she has titrated the risk of exploring this fear by shaping encounters with his friend as he remembers him while he was still alive. In this session, she checks with him if that fear is still alive.

Max: It's always there at the back of my head. I know he suffered a massive amount of trauma. Talking to my friend who had to identify the body, he never really was okay after that. I think that's part of the reason that I have this fear.

Emily: (Move 1, reflecting, validating the enormity of this fear.) So deep to always have in the back of your mind this fear that one day you might have a conscious memory of Léo's body at the scene of the accident! (Being transparent with Max about the process, she continues with some trepidation.) I have been feeling like we walked close to the edge when I invited you to speak with an image of Léo as he looked when he was still alive. I didn't say that to stay away from your biggest fear. I just felt that was a starting point. But I would feel I was doing you a disservice if we didn't revisit this core fear still in the back of your head.

Max: Yes.

Emily: Does that make sense?

Max: I understand completely, yep.

Emily: You're saying that having visited him in your imagination and saying to him in your imagination, "I don't think you had a beautiful corpse," has taken away some of the edge of that fear? (Validating stabilization. Max looks down.)

Max: I would say yes.

Emily: Uh huh. And yet, just hearing me say, "I don't think you had a beautiful corpse," you looked down. It is a painful thing to hear, isn't it? (Reflecting bodily signal of alive fear, part of Move 2.)

Max: It is. (Pause.) I've always wanted to be a person that didn't cause a lot of damage in this world – to be a gardener of people. You know, like lived a good life, didn't harm himself and didn't harm other people. And I've done a bad job of that. (Longing.)

He validates his own grief and says he needs to feel sad – that his grief is much better than the terror he has worked hard to ignore.

Emily: So much sadness in, "Look, I always wanted to be a good person who didn't let others down. I wanted to be a kind gardener and I have lived feeling like a harmful person for so long!" You're saying, "I need to feel sad about that. I need to feel the grief, that I was the driver of the car where Léo was killed." (Validating his sadness and grief, to keep him engaged.)

Max: Yep. Engaging with that sadness means that I can engage with the memories and the trauma and the history, and make different choices; whereas before, I was just blocked.

Emily: Right.

Max: Which is a change.

Emily: You kept away from the sadness. And in a way, today you're saying, "I – it felt too terrifying to go there. I was afraid I would just see Léo's mangled body."

Max: Yeah. I didn't think I could accept the sadness because I didn't feel like I was improving or correcting anything. So, it was an overwhelming reminder that I was this harmful person. (He shudders.) Whereas now I'm changing. I'm *actioning* this guilt. I am expressing it honestly – not like before. I used to pretend maybe I wasn't driving the car when he died. Totally deceitful! This sadness is manageable. It's not overwhelming.

Emily wants to keep Max as fully engaged as he can tolerate, treading the fine line between challenge and overwhelm. She is also feeling fearful of inviting Max to look at what has terrified him for decades, and yet, feels she needs to create the safety for him to do so.

Emily: And can that kind gardener take your own hand? Can that kind gardener walk back into that scene of the injury and say, "You've already seen this. You can see it again. You know what it is to feel Léo's love. That man that died has forgiven you, and it's not going to kill you to look at the scene and see how bad it is." (Drawing on his internal resource of his kind gardener who wants to nurture others to help them grow.)

Max: Yeah, I can do that. I am more fully aware of myself. (Wiping tears, sniffling.) And what I am capable of. (Signs his emotional flexibility and resilience are growing.)

Emily: More aware of you. And you wipe the tears! (Heightening his signs of emotion.) This is really sad to walk into that scene and see Léo's body on the ground. Almost like you're saying, "I am getting to be the kind gardener I've always wanted to be, and I've come back to see you."

Max: Yeah. His body is just a grey shape. (Pause.) It's not super graphic. My brain doesn't make it graphic. It's just a body, it's just a shape. (Whispering to his image of Leo's body): I can make better choices, and I will make better choices. I am sorry!

Emily: How are you doing? As you stand in that scene. What is happening in your body?

Max: I'm okay, I don't have that tightness that I normally get. I'm a little sad but I don't have that tightness. (Confirms shift in bodily felt sense.) There's still sadness. There are still regrets, but there's also a sense of a belief in myself that I haven't had in a long time.

Emily: (Smiling; deeply touched.) Yeah?

Max: I've always "believed in myself." (Making air quotes.) And I've always been quick to articulate that I believe in myself, but deep down, I've had something akin to an imposter syndrome about myself. (Shifting sense of self.)

Emily: Right. Yeah. Because deep down, you had a picture of yourself as a harmful person. That's a big shift from a sense of yourself as harmful to being a kind gardener – someone you can trust and like. You always felt like there was something imposter-like about believing in your goodness, believing in you. And now, you are saying, "This is me. I'm beginning to notice I do have that kind-gardener heart. I can return to the scene of the accident and tell Léo how sorry I am and still feel his love."

Max: Yeah, I just lost it, lost touch with myself for a long time. (Long pause.) This is new for me – I can feel sad without feeling tight!

Emily senses an opportunity to invite Max to make that special, transformative "ask" – the risk to reach and request what he needs. This special encounter seems to be such an important aspect to complete this seismic change event, so she herself takes a risk and asks Max to make a request.

Emily: There you are in this dreaded scene, and you are ok. Léo's body is not overwhelming you. Can you ask this grey shape of Léo's body for what you need at this moment? What could you ask of him to soothe that fear you have carried for so long?

Max closes his eyes and in his typical way, sends Léo his "ask" silently, as tears roll down his face. Twenty seconds pass and he looks up at Emily with a big smile.

Max: I felt my question to him and I felt his assurance back. (Long pause, then looks right at Emily in another engaged encounter.) I think part of the reason I struggled with this a lot is that one of the ways that I dealt with this was I told everybody that I hadn't wanted to race – but that my friends pushed me to do it and I gave in. I said I gave in to pressure from my friends – passing the blame – when it really was something I wanted to do. I feel like I was disingenuous. I lied. I carried that around a lot.

After Max's an engaged encounter with Emily where he shares his guilt for lying about the street-racing that killed Léo, with Move 4, Emily processes this final encounter.

Emily: Now you can revisit that. "The worst of it is that I felt bad that I lied." Putting that out loud to me, what is that like?

Max: It feels like progress, that is what it feels like.

Emily: Ah, this is the lingering "yuck" that you felt. You felt guilty about wanting to be this kind gardener when you still had that lie in the closet?

Max: Yes! Yeah, it was a way of deflecting my own blame for myself, and a way of deflecting conversations so I didn't have to revisit this thing over and over again.

Emily notes the significance of his transformative shift from avoidance to openness, reinforcing the view that avoidance is the kryptonite of emotional disorders. EFT research illustrates the need to target and monitor avoidance (Wiebe & Johnson, 2016).

Emily:	(Move 5, summary and integration.) In a way, avoiding the whole truth was a self-protective move to help you survive, yes? (Reframe). And it had its cost because you've been fighting all these years with guilt – guilt over your lie, guilt over Léo's death, and fear of a conscious memory resurfacing. Now with your courageous moves of interacting with Léo's imaginal body, sharing your remorse and responsibility, and receiving his love and acceptance; and sharing with me your lingering guilt about your deceptiveness, you are connecting with this growing sense of being the kind gardener of people with a very strong commitment to help others. You've been open and honest with me and with an image of Léo and you have graciously received each of our responses to you. You have moved close to this shape of Léo on the ground and discovered that your own sadness and regret doesn't destroy you. You can now feel that you are a good person. A good person with much regret, remorse, and love.
Max:	Yes. (Deep sigh!) I feel like I've accomplished a lot.

The support material for Chapter 10 (routledge.com/9781032151335) summarizes themes of what therapists and clients do to co-create a softening change across both modalities of EFCT and EFIT.

How EFT Therapists Guide Clients to Co-create Softenings

They key ingredient to co-creating softenings lies in deepening emotional experience, within clients' window of tolerance. Softenings are deliberately shaped, with emotionally vulnerable reaches of requests for attachment needs to be met, followed by engaged responses. "The EFT therapist must intentionally work to deepen and reprocess attachment affect to connect these felt experiences to underlying attachment needs" (Furrow et al., 2012, p. 47). Furrow et al. found the levels of heightened emotional experience separated successful from unsuccessful softening attempts.

Micro-Skills for Softenings

The EFT therapist has a reliable set of micro-interventions for guiding clients through a softening, and as previously noted, the implicit *manner of the therapist's presence* is of most importance. "In the softening change events… [M]oves 2, 3 and 4 of the Tango are intensified and often repeated a number of times to shape specific new levels of deeper experiencing and discovery" (Johnson & Campbell, 2022, p. 90).

Move 2, assembling and deepening emotion, comprises the following micro-skills: Reflecting and validating emerging, previously hidden core emotions; evocative questions and responses to access attachment fears related to models of self and other, fears of reaching, and attachment needs; heightening (especially fears of view of self and other and fears of reaching); empathic conjectures about current attachment fears and longings; and, reframing in the context of attachment fears and needs.

In Move 3, shaping softening encounters, it is important to build emotional intensity and depth of engagement while setting up the encounter and to maintain it during the actual disclosure. The acronym SHAPE is useful to delineate the complex process of choreographing encounters: SHARPEN the message to share; HEIGHTEN with repetition; ANTICIPATE the moment of contact, visualizing the other and maintaining sufficient safety while heightening the sense of risk; direct client to PRESENT the message; ENGAGE if client exits or needs to be refocused. Micro-skills used in Move 3 include, conjecturing, seeding attachment, and heightening to shape encounters. Encounters are shaped for three main purposes – to share the core fear, to reach to the other with a specific request, and for the partner or significant other to respond, unless an EFIT client specifies they do NOT want to hear back from an unsafe other. A specific encounter is shaped for the client to make the Step 7 reach to request what they need. This unique reach is typically followed, not by Move 4 processing, but rather, an immediate invitation for a response from the partner or relevant other.

Move 4 evocative questions function to heighten and process the experience of the request and the response. After many or several repetitions of Moves 2, 3, and 4, integration can be done with Move 5, validating attachment needs and, in EFCT, heightening the new secure bond and summarizing how partners created it together, and in EFIT heightening the shifts in views of self and other, and the new sense of agency and hope.

As Emily focuses on how to co-create softenings with her clients, whether individuals or couples, she ponders Johnson's (2019) message that softenings are co-created through deepened emotional experiencing disclosed in interpersonal dialogue. She knows her growing edge is seeking guidance about *how* to facilitate the depth of experiencing needed for shaping the kinds of emotionally engaged dialogues that shape change

Therapist Manner for Deepening

The manner by which a therapist deepens emotion through the softening change event is closely related to the Stage 2 engagement change event described in Chapter 9, but there are some differences in how to deepen emotional experience with withdrawing, more avoidant clients and with pursuing, more anxious clients. A difference, noted by Kailanko et al. (2021a) about repeating somatic experience in EFCT is also relevant for EFIT. Heightening with the RISSSSSC manner includes reference to somatic signals, however, Kailanko et al. found that while repeating somatically focused interventions leads to deeper experiencing and expression for withdrawing clients, anxious, pursuing clients tended to decline in depth of experiencing with somatic repetition. It appears that repetition of somatic experience can become too much for anxious clients and they thus reduce their experiencing to a more manageable level to remain within their *window of tolerance*. Emily remembers to stay closely attuned to her own emotional experiencing and that of her anxious clients during softening events to balance containing with heightening.

Guidelines for shaping softenings are to balance heightening with safe containment; to monitor therapeutic presence through voice quality and with a somatic focus; and to build emotional depth and intensity before and during encounters. More details about deepening to shape softenings are available in Chapter 10 Support Material (routledge.com/9781032151335).

Summarizing the Map of Stage 2 Change

The seismic shift of Stage 2 change is fueled by the power of emotion. By deepening emotional experiencing and shaping affiliative, interpersonal encounters, therapists help clients to create lasting change. Before briefly recapping the Stage 2 change process, it is important to explore how this seismic shift in EFT can look dissimilar across different cultural contexts, in light of varied expectations regarding emotional experience and expression.

Contextual Impacts on Emotion

Giving precedence to how REC (race, ethnicity, and culture) organize emotional responses and impact survival strategies for responding to threat (relationally and culturally), EFT therapists need to flexibly honor unexpected twists and turns on clients' Stage 2 pathways toward change. The EFT therapist does not follow a map from an objective distance but rather with flexible attunement to the subjective ways that each client experiences and expresses the universal, yet individually nuanced, contextually informed fears and needs for secure human connection.

One size does not fit all. While initially developed from observing white, heterosexual, middle-class couples, the EFT model with its client-centered focus, must implicitly give precedence to REC influences. Muslims, Latinos, Asians, Indigenous, African American, LGBTQ+, immigrants, neurodiverse individuals and socio-economically diverse identities will all have differently nuanced ways of experiencing and expressing emotions and needs. REC factors need to be acknowledged, particularly when working to facilitate emotional depth and shape in-session affiliative encounters. Examples of factors that impact emotional experience and expression, given in this and earlier chapters, include racial battle fatigue, colorism, racial priming that orients a person to carry on and be strong and show no weakness, and down-regulating emotions and minimizing oneself for survival.

Linguistic differences for expressing emotion and variability in cultural expectations about emotional experience and expression inevitably impact how the fuel of emotion in Stage 2 restructuring is experienced. Liu, in an article on practicing EFT across different cultures (Dockett, 2022), provides a powerful example of working with an Asian couple and the importance of therapist flexibility to REC differences. Depth of emotional experiencing is likely to look very different in an Asian couple than in the traditional heterosexual white couple with whom the EFT model was founded. According to the EXP scale what appears as surface expression may in fact be significant depth of experiencing. Liu notes that in Asia, emotion is expressed in much more subtle and indirect ways. She alerts us to adaptations that are needed in shaping encounters in a culture where direct expressions of emotion and vulnerabilities to others are discouraged.

Emily pauses, "Slow down. Engage with deeper empathic curiosity to this client's context. What appears to be avoidance from my frame of reference, may in fact not be avoidance at all."

Since it is beyond the scope of this book to illustrate the many and varied ways that REC organize emotional experience and expression, it is important to explore your implicit biases (Jana & Baran, 2020) and expand your cultural awareness of each client in order to be the best EFT therapist you can be. When working in the deepening processes of *engagement* and *softening* change events, it is especially important to be in concert with your clients and not impose steps of change or styles of emotional deepening and vulnerable encounters which may fall outside their norms of cultural acceptability or familiarity.

Recap of Stage 2 Change

In Stage 2 with couples, partners fully access and express their attachment fears and needs and discover the motivation and courage to risk reaching congruently to the other partner to ask for their deepest attachment needs to be met. Together, they create the safety for a former withdrawer to stay engaged and for the more pursuing partner to remain soft and open. Both are pulled into supportive, connecting responses by the other's vulnerable risks and reaches. The previously more critical partner comes to show acceptance and appreciation for the other partner's more assertive and engaged position, and the former withdrawer, in a newly engaged position, shows responsiveness, engagement, and open presence to their own experience and to the other partner.

Emily finds that some couples spend longer in Stage 2 than she expects; however, she is discovering patience and trust in the model, which is both linear and circular. At times, she is pleased to see that even after a withdrawer has engaged and a softening begins, the withdrawer's engagement continues to expand. Partners have a circular impact on one another as the new positive cycle broadens and builds (Mikulincer & Shaver, 2015, 2023a). More engagement encourages more softening, and more softening encourages more engagement and connection.

Research showing that the softening change event is necessary to reduce attachment anxiety and to successfully reshape an attachment bond is cited at the beginning of this chapter. Research also validates the importance of the engagement change event for lasting change. A two-year follow-up study found that "the predictor that accounted for greater variance in relationship satisfaction across follow-up was reduction in attachment avoidance" (Wiebe & Johnson, 2016, p. 400). If a more withdrawn partner has not fully engaged, it is a likely contributor to less relationship satisfaction over time. EFT therapists need "to actively target attachment avoidance in therapy, and to monitor changes in attachment avoidance before termination" (p. 400). Many EFT therapists find that when they've reached a plateau or an impasse in shaping a softening, there may actually be more withdrawer engagement needed.

Secure attachment bonds achieved in Stage 2, function to modify the perception of threat, thereby creating a safe haven and secure base for partners to become one another's primary source of comfort, support, and emotion regulation. In the newly restructured secure bond, partners send clear messages about their attachment needs and they are able to understand and respond to one another's expressed needs. Support from recent attachment neuroscience shows that secure bonds have a significant emotion regulation function, confirming that partners are the hidden regulators of each other's physiological and emotional worlds (Coan & Maresh, 2014; Coan et al., 2006).

In Stage 2 with individuals, restructuring, as described in Chapter 9 and this chapter, also typically involves engagement before softening. Notwithstanding a greater flow between Stages 1 and 2 change in EFIT, as clients explore different relational contexts, engagement with emotional experience, internally and interpersonally, precedes a softening. The outcomes of restructuring in EFIT are effective emotion regulation strategies, new internal working models of self and other, and an expanded sense of a competent, lovable self, securely connected in relationships with optimal dependence.

An EFT therapist's contextually relevant attunement to each client – couple or individual – takes precedence. The client map of change is not linear, and the EFT therapist has as their greatest resources, the five moves of the EFT macro-intervention, the EFT Tango, to guide the process, along with the EAR of attunement (see Box 1.3):

E: Follow EMOTION as a contextual process.
A: Attune to ATTACHMENT dynamics and strategies for responding to relational and contextual threats.
R: RESHAPE view of self and other, through interpersonal encounters. All the R's here are important: Respecting REC stressors and drawing on Relational Resources to Reshape attachment strategies, views of self and other, and to create a safer world.

Get Ready… The Clients Are Coming!

Check Chapter 10 Support Material (routledge.com/9781032151335) for a summary of the key ingredients of facilitating the softening change event. There you are also guided to review the five client cases and to identify key features of each client's softenings and to prepare for how you will integrate these transformative shifts into your next sessions.

Part IV
Consolidating

11 Consolidating Secure Connection in Stage 3

> We are Homo sapiens, and we are *Homo vinculum*—the one who bond[s]—that is, the one who is truly safe and sound only when infused with a felt sense of secure connection to a valued other. (Johnson, 2019, p. 228)

We have arrived at the final stage of EFT! In this chapter, I give an overview of Stage 3 consolidation, where the therapist collaborates with clients to integrate and consolidate the changes they have made.

In Stage 3 of EFCT, therapists help couples to continue to shape and grow their relationship bonds, to find solutions to previously unsolvable problems and to seed attachment for the future. "The relationship now becomes a secure base from which to explore the world and deal with the problems it presents and a safe haven that provides shelter and protection" (Johnson, 2020, p. 84).

In Stage 3 of EFIT, therapists help individuals to expand their newly revised working models of self and other across relationships and contexts of their lives. Integrating and consolidating corrective emotional experiences helps individuals to build on their views of self as resilient and others as responsive, celebrating the present and envisioning the future, with new confidence and self-acceptance and new ways of engaging others for effective emotion regulation.

Throughout this book, I emphasize that EFT, as an attachment-oriented therapy, views health and relational and emotional distress all from the perspective that we are first and foremost relational beings, wired to be in safe and secure connection with others. By weaving couple and individual therapy together, I show that the EFT goal of shaping secure bonds is not limited to romantic relationships. Rather, it is also effective for treating anxiety, depression, grief, and trauma reactions with clients who enter therapy without a romantic relationship or a significant family or friend relationship.

As we approach Stage 3 termination, you may be thinking of some of your individual clients for whom you are their only attachment figure, and wondering if they will ever be ready for termination. You may be asking, "How do I consolidate safety and security in EFIT, when I am terminating with a client who continues to live without a supportive relationship?" The EFT model has space for these questions. As shown throughout the book, EFT has a very clear path toward shaping corrective emotional experiences of hopeful safety and security for both couple and individual clients.

Max, for example, terminates therapy celebrating change and feeling hope. He is continuing to grieve the loss of his long-term relationship, but through the emotional, interpersonal corrective experiences he had in therapy, he feels liberated from the impacts of past trauma. The familiar tightness in his chest is no longer there. He feels emotionally balanced, secure about feeling his grief, and confident and hopeful moving forward. He has achieved his initial goals to fully face his fears of his traumatic memories and to lessen their impacts on him; to openly engage with his current loss and to find emotional balance.

DOI: 10.4324/9781003242673-17

Likewise, Sahra, who continues to grapple with insecure relationships – discrimination at work, estrangement from her father, and uncertainties in her romantic endeavors – terminates therapy with new hope and strength, created through various imaginal interpersonal change events. Her initial goals to "feel lighter in my emotional life, more kindness towards myself and to be less easily triggered" are clearly in progress and are continuing to be realized.

The relationship stories of Wayne and Jessica, Sophie and Ella, and Phil and Julie, and Max and Sahra's stories of change, exemplify this newly created, safe and sound connection to one's own emotional life and to others, whether physically present or those held in the mind. This is the change that is integrated and consolidated in Stage 3. Relationship bonds are strengthening and the self is continuing to grow.

Stage 3 is a time of celebration, satisfaction, and happiness for many clients. Partners collaborate to solve pragmatic problems and, despite their differences, create ways to keep their secure bond of love alive (Johnson, 2008). Individuals describe and integrate how the shifts in view of self and other that they have made, ripple across their different relational contexts. Their emerging readiness to terminate therapy is mixed with fears of moving on. Stage 3 is also a time when clients are helped to solidify their emotional shifts into vivid stories and images. Implicit, transformative change is made explicit in couples' personally created love story or romance film and in individuals' dreams and visions of how they will build the future with the changes they have made and will continue to live fully and well. Clients' stories of how they moved from their initial distress to the present security become the basis from which they create narratives of future hopes that can be retold or reviewed at will. In a format similar to the previous four chapters, I describe what EFT therapists see and hear during this stage, what they do to help clients take Steps 8 and 9, and *how* the therapist guides clients through this stage.

What EFT Therapists Typically See and Hear in Stage 3

The prime marker indicating readiness for Stage 3 integration and consolidation is the new sense of safety and connection that clients exude and discuss. This newness has a different quality to it than the positive change seen at the end of Stage 1. It is more than a respite from the turbulence or stagnation that they experienced in their old cycles of distress. The transformation of Stage 2 "seem[s] to render future miscues and disconnections unpleasant rather than catastrophic; separation distress, when it occurs, is manageable and resolvable" (Johnson, 2013, p. 231). Following this Stage 2 change, there is a new, reliable foundation on which to build in Stage 3. I will describe the new bonding cycle between partners and then explore a similar new pattern in EFIT.

A Broaden-and-Build Cycle in EFCT

In EFCT, there are clear indications of growing safety, active engagement, and caring responsiveness between partners. Softened pursuers express needs clearly and coherently, without criticism and exasperation, and show acceptance and appreciation for their partner's more assertive and engaged position. Former withdrawers, in a newly engaged position, show responsiveness, engagement, and solid presence to their partner's distress, fears, and excitement. Partners are accessible and responsive to one another's emotional expressions, tuning in with curiosity and caring to needs expressed by their partner. As a result, despite occasional "small moments of danger" (Johnson, 2008, p. 207) when the old cycle starts to take over, the couple can repair breaches together.

A former pursuer can observe and tolerate twinges of avoidance in their partner – lovingly, with understanding and compassion. Previously, the slightest shrug of Ella's shoulder or her lack of response would send Sophie into cascades of panic and anger. Now she responds with caring and concern. From her softened position, Sophie says:

> It's as if I can feel and hear my waterfall of anxiety in the remote distance, and yet am solidly anchored in your love and I know you are staying with me, even if you seem annoyed and start pulling back just a little.

Positive cycles of interaction are seen: Partners reach and respond to each other's expressed needs, and they make mostly positive attributions about each other's responses. The clear way partners ask for their needs to be met encourages response and warmth from the other. The *broaden-and-build* cycles continue to nurture the secure bond. In Stage 3, partners describe incidents where their new bond is making it possible for them to thrive and grow without the therapist's guidance.

A Broaden-and-Build Cycle in EFIT

Sahra is clearly integrating and consolidating changes across her life as she reflects back on the journey she has traveled with Emily, "I feel like lost parts of me have come back. I don't have to hide so much of me anymore! When I had that empowering conversation with my colleague – my former friend – I knew I managed it well. I kept from getting sucked into old patterns of apologizing profusely and absorbing her jabs at me. This time I didn't excuse her by telling myself, 'It is just her pain.' I held my own and conveyed that, 'We are different. I care for you but we are too different for a friendship.' The conversation went well," reflects Sahra, "but it was not until I am sharing it with you that I can now unfreeze the part of myself that always hides when I am with her. Here, with you, I have a safe place for this emotional part. You are interested and I can share and notice my feelings. That lost part of me is with me again! It's like I carried a shameful part of me – and always hid her. And that was the same part that went into hiding with my sexual abuse! After we encountered that nasty babysitter (she shudders) and I held my own with him, I have felt different. I have that hidden part of me back and I am proud of her! You've helped me experience that survivor part as such a beautiful, strong, sensitive part that doesn't need to hide anymore!" Emily is fully attending, responding mostly nonverbally and with minimal encouragers.

"I am more balanced," Sahra continues. "My body doesn't ache with so much tension! I am not alone anymore – I couldn't have done this without you – I wasn't safe to face this all before. I wasn't even safe to take in that amazing experience with the priest, until I shared it with you." She pauses, weeping, and then continues, "These are happy tears. That healing experience with the priest – I was almost afraid to talk about – afraid it would vanish. You know how difficult it was for me to share. My tears just wouldn't stop, but the whole thing was too far away for me to really take it in until I shared it with you. When you said maybe I need to see the priest's kind, tender, caring eyes to see God's eyes, that totally struck me! They *were* the eyes of God that I have longed to see. Now I see those loving eyes and they help me survive some very difficult moments – frustrations at work, regrets over not saving my mother's life, trying times with my daughter, and disappoint-ments with men whom I've begun to date."

"Remember when you helped me tell my little six-year-old self how I want to protect her and keep her safe but that I am afraid I will let her down? (Emily nods). And you said, 'Well you might let her down again.' You helped me form a message to tell her, 'I'm afraid I could let you down again. But I want to protect you and help you feel your goodness. I want to keep you safe. I want to help you notice who is safe to share with and who is not safe to share with.' And I can tell I am doing that now."

New Views of Self and Other

With their new attachment bond, partners can discuss differences and conflicts without triggering attachment threat. Discussions now can actually be about the pragmatic issues, unlike at the beginning of therapy, where the content-focused differences triggered attachment fears and self-protective behaviors. For Sophie and Ella, an ongoing issue that was sure to trigger their pattern of Sophie demanding and Ella withdrawing was their different views regarding their summer cabin. Now, when they disagree over what to do with maintaining the cabin, they productively consider options. "I know she cares now and wants the best for me. It makes me feel calmer and more flexible to look at the practicalities with her," says Sophie. With their newly secure bond, differences about how best to repair the cabin are truly about the cabin, whereas previously the fights about the cabin were fueled by attachment fears. They were essentially fights-in-code, about, "Are you there for me?" and "Do I matter to you?" Now they can work together to deal with the issues about the cabin and about other complex matters.

Sophie continues to get triggered at times by Ella's collectivist family. Their close bonds stand in sharp contrast to her family who has alienated her since her marriage to Ella. The big difference now is that when threats arise, she is able to reach to Ella to soothe her grief and fear, instead of criticizing or pushing her away. Their growing capacity to reach, respond, and repair is strengthening their bond. Ella is relieved each time to see that her presence and her comfort make a difference for Sophie and that she is valued as a partner. "It's never draining for me to comfort Sophie" she beams. "We understand each other now. I see her grief with her family's rejection, and I am so happy she is becoming part of my family!"

With the reduced anxiety and avoidance that EFT creates, changes in automatic responses to one another are apparent (Burgess Moser et al., 2015). Internal working models of self and other, which guide expectations and reactions, are clearly shifting. Models of self as lovable and worthy, and of the other as reliable and caring, "positively reshape their unconscious blueprints for close connection with others. The new blueprint helps them to be truly present with their partner, rather than fight echoes from past relationships" (Johnson, 2008, p. 226), or from their own previous negative pattern.

In EFIT Stage 3, Sahra says, "When I have excruciating head and backaches and hear echoes of my mother telling me all my pain and struggles must be because I don't pray enough – that God might be punishing me – I shake my head. Her familiar old reverberating jabs don't cut so deeply now. I say to an image of her, 'No! Stop your jabs! I need support now. I'm in pain – I need to hear from the hidden part of you that cares about me. Then my mother's voice softens and I almost feel as though she is supporting me. I have changed. I know now that my physical ailments are not punishment from God. I know my sexual abuse was not my fault. I know it was wrong. Ever since speaking to that image of my abuser, I know I did not bring that on me! And I feel I have brought my mother onto my side now too. I feel much more resilient." Turing to Emily, she adds, "I feel your warmth and belief in me too. I feel deserving of calling in sick to work and arranging extra childcare for my daughter, when my health requires it."

Increased Celebration and Joy

In Stage 3, partners express surprise and joy as they discover that they can handle challenges on their own without the therapist's help. Couples frequently return to therapy celebrating how they resolved some longstanding difference between sessions without jeopardizing their connection. Likewise, individual clients in Stage 3 report amazing shifts in different relationships and contexts, that may not have been a focus in therapy. The change in view of self and other is opening new meanings and new behavioral options. Interactions which characterize secure engagement with others, and flexibility to follow the guidance from inner emotional experience, continue to have expansive, positive ripple-effects! For example, Sahra reports feeling empowered in her conversations with her lead doctor at work and with her colleagues. She is also feeling more peace about the ways she cared for her mother from a distance when her mother refused to immigrate with her. "I can stand up for myself now and I feel worthy of reaching out to my friend for support too."

Max reports a similar shift, saying that the tension in his chest has not returned, and he is feeling more and more like a genuine friend. His sense of being an imposter has not returned.

Wayne and Jessica come to a session filled with delight that they worked through a former hot button issue, all on their own. They describe encountering a situation that, in the past, would have been sure to lead to their *spilled milk tango*, ending in silence for days. This time, they report directly expressing their needs to each other and resolving a difference that left them feeling closer and more precious to one another. They report that they typically spend a week each summer in what they jointly call Jessica's parents' *snooty white beach community*. It means a lot to Jessica that Wayne complies with this arrangement when she knows it is not an easy time for him. He has described the times at the beach house like the movie *Get Out*, the 2017 horror film of a black man visiting the very white racist world of his girlfriend's family. This year, however, Wayne is hoping to spend this very same week with his biological father, whom he recently located for the first time in his life. Jessica is rigidly set on the annual family vacation with her family. It is a long-standing tradition. Rarely does any family member miss, and unfortunately if they do, the state of their relationship becomes a topic of family gossip and speculation.

They report that Wayne, in his newly more assertive and open manner, acknowledged:

I understand you feel this traditional summer plan is unshakeable and very, very important to you. And no matter how we describe to your family if we would miss this year, they are likely to start drawing conclusions that we aren't getting along. But, Jessica, this is the first time I can spend a week with my father and my half-sibs. I've never even met them. Only had this one Zoom chat with my father – a totally new person in my life! I hope so much you can be flexible for me, this one summer. I know it is a lot to ask–but I'd love so much if you could come with me instead of going to the beach with your family! I want them all to meet you and the kids!

Jessica recounts that this request felt like a *momentous ask*, but that she was immediately struck with how vulnerable his voice sounded and how clearly she felt his caring! She describes to Emily a surprising surge of desire to extend herself, to make it possible to meet Wayne's desires to be with his father! She tells Emily and Wayne how deeply she appreciates him asking for what he needs in this clear, vulnerable way, "Knowing you understand what a sacrifice it is for me, how difficult it is to withstand my family's questions… and knowing you'll feel especially loved by this, gives me all the motivation and determination I need to support you and have us all be with your family. Hearing you tell me what *you want* makes me want to come! I'm still shocked that my love for Wayne could pull me in this direction," giggles Jessica. "I will be in trouble with my *fam*, for sure! But I'll risk it – just for him!"

Jessica acknowledges that previously she would have "resented the obligation" and felt taken advantage of, if she had given in, whereas now she experiences joy, motivation, and certainty of Wayne's love and of her importance to him. New attributions are part of the new positive cycle.

In Max's Stage 3, his growing capacity to feel his sadness over the loss of his long-term relationship is experienced as healing and revitalizing. Engaging with his core emotions of guilt, shame, and fear in Stage 2 has lifted his shame and reshaped his fears. He can now experience what he calls, "the healing of pure grief." He is at peace with himself and his relationships, indicated in their closing therapy session as he quotes from a Disney Plus movie, "What is grief, but the persistence of love?"

What EFT Therapists and Clients Do in Stage 3 Consolidation

In Stage 3 the therapist is less directive than in the first two stages and the process is less intense. Attuning, reflecting, tracking, evoking emotional experience of the changes and heightening clients' shifts across their lives, the therapist helps clients to take two steps of change in Stage 3. These steps are Step 8, integrating the new security with the old pragmatic problems, and Step 9, consolidating change by creating a resiliency story and building rituals to nurture the secure connections. In EFCT, the therapist tunes in with engaged empathic responding to the new quality in couples' interactions that emanates from their newly shaped secure bond. In EFIT the therapist resonates with and integrates clients' growing emotional resilience and expansion of self. These shifts appear in increasing engagement with others and in an expanding sense of competency and flexibility to face existential dilemmas and uncertainties.

To help clients take Step 8, integrating their new security with their old pragmatic problems, the therapist uses Move 5 to reflect and track how important pragmatic issues and conflicts are being dealt with now. By heightening their successes in dealing with previously unsolvable issues, and validating markers of their growing security, therapists help couples and individuals to recognize how they are active participants in creating a new reality. They are integrating their new views of self and other into difficult matters. The newly secure base they have created through Stages 1 and 2 empowers them to resolve long-standing problems and challenges.

In EFCT, therapists celebrate with couples, summarizing and heightening how they are solving ongoing relationship problems, despite different views and preferences. Partners' conversations are constructive and kind, now that they are no longer code for the key attachment question, "Are you accessible, responsive, and engaged?" Therapists' concrete reflections and summaries help partners to have a coherent story of the new meanings and possibilities they are creating.

In EFIT, therapists explore and review how clients' corrective emotional experiences are playing out across their lives. They offer tracking reflections and summaries as clients' recount emerging positive views of self and new capacities to engage. Therapists heighten clients' felt shifts and new views of self and other. They crystallize clients' *broaden-and-build* cycles as their expanded sense of self is shaping and being shaped by new relational patterns.

To help clients to take Step 9, consolidating the changes they are experiencing, therapists offer empathic tracking reflections, summarize, and heighten clients' stories of their new attachment security and emotional flexibility. Together, they build a *safe and sound* narrative. With evocative questions and responses, therapists help clients to identify ways to continue this momentum and to envision a future on this trajectory.

The therapist's goal is to help EFCT partners consolidate their positive shifts so they can continue to have intimate conversations and interactions that will shore up their secure bond and foster growth in their views of other and self. Likewise, the goal in EFIT is to consolidate clients' change to ensure that the new perspectives, new behavioral options, expanded sense of self, and dependable relationships will thrive and continue to bolster their interpersonal bonds and emotional flexibility and resilience.

Broaden-and-build cycles of attachment behaviors and emotion regulation are strengthened as therapists invite clients to reflect on their emerging shifts. New meanings, new interactions within and between, and bodily felt shifts in their working models of self and other are specifically identified. Clients are invited to create their *resiliency stories* of moving from distress into continued growth on this new path. The positive cycle has its own reinforcing momentum, as the follow-up research shows. Many EFT clients continue to improve after therapy ends. Research attests to improved couple relationship and individual functioning in terms of reduced depression and post-traumatic reactions (Ganz et al., 2022; Wiebe & Johnson, 2016).

Discovering clients' readiness for Stage 3 is a milestone experience for Emily. Not all her couples and individuals progress smoothly through the stages of client change. Some seem to linger a long while in Stage 1, however, Emily and her clients continue to recognize forward-moving progress, despite apparent movement backward and recurrences of the old pattern.

There are times that brief or longer returns to Stages 1 and 2 are needed, for example, if unaddressed addictive patterns emerge. When there is a discovery or disclosure that a partner or individual client has been relying on a *faux attachment* (Flores, 2004) – of addictive substances or behaviors – the therapist assembles the process as an explicit part of the cycle to first regain stabilization, assess if additional treatment is needed, and do more Stage 2 work before Stage 3 (see Chapter 15). If a client or therapist discerns that they have missed acknowledging some key cultural difference between them or between partners in a couple, the differences are discussed and the impacts of minority-stress trauma are validated and explored before Stage 3 consolidation.

De-escalated couples, where the withdrawer has engaged and stepped assertively into the relationship, stating what they need to remain engaged, sometimes encounter an unresolved relationship injury, known as an *attachment injury*. These specific events of broken trust need to be discussed and a Stage 2 process of rebuilding trust is required (see Chapter 16) before the couple is ready for Stage 3 consolidation. EFIT clients, likewise, can have an unresolved trauma or injury that needs to be processed before they are ready for Stage 3.

Regardless of the length of time her clients take in Stages 1 and 2, as Emily continues to integrate this new model into her therapy practice, she is discovering signs of client readiness for Stage 3. She is struck with the different tone in the room. With their new attachment bond, she witnesses partners taking over more of the growth processes on their own. Likewise, Emily notices that her individual clients' growing, positive internal working models of self and other seem to be engendering much continued growth outside of therapy. Nevertheless, in this new climate, she continues to resonate, reflect, track, evoke, heighten, and to facilitate encounters. The five EFT tango moves remain salient as the therapist tracks and deepens new bonding experiences and shapes encounters to integrate and consolidate in Stage 3.

Tango Moves to Help Clients Integrate Solutions to Pragmatic Problems (Client Step 8)

The EFT therapist supports a couple, with Move 1, to explore pragmatic issues and old relationship problems, supporting the former withdrawer to stay engaged, and the former pursuer to remain receptive and open. This support comes in the form of tracking, heightening, and celebrating the new positive cycle as it unfolds in session, and as the couple reports it happening outside of sessions. Together with the couple, a therapist focuses on ways partners have found to exit their repetitive pattern. Partners are invited to explicate how they are solving problems that were previously attachment threats and triggers for the old cycle. The therapist validates their courage and the risks they have taken.

Ongoing issues that have triggered a negative cycle and are revisited in Step 8, from the perspective of a newly secure attachment bond, might include sexuality, spirituality, extended family relationships, step-children, location of residence, school choices, and many others. Partners, feeling safe and more connected, can work with the therapist to resolve the yet-unresolved issues. Here, the therapist will continue to use the five moves of EFT, reflecting emotions within and between partners, deepening core experience, structuring and processing enactments, and heightening their new capacity to remain connected while finding new solutions. Exercises such as "bonding through sex and touch" (Johnson, 2008, p. 200) can also be helpful for partners at this stage if their sexual relationship was not a key focus earlier.

Similarly, in EFIT clients are helped to translate their corrective emotional experiences into effective ways of responding to pragmatic problems and to relationships across their everyday lives. Move 1 is used to reflect clients' unfolding changes. Evocative, empathic responses and questions are used in Move 2 to access, linger with, and heighten client's reflection on changes they are making. Together, clients and therapist reflect upon their restructured attachment safety, how new views of self and other are impacting their previous pragmatic problems and how the evolution of new strategies are being reinforced by their current *broaden-and-build* cycle.

Tango Move 5 to Help Clients Consolidate Change and Build a Safe and Sound Narrative (Client Step 9)

Much time has lapsed since Johnson (2008) suggested that it is relatively new in EFT to be asking couples how they plan to hold on to positive changes. In the early decades of EFT, therapists trusted that if partners had restructured their relationships into ones that were accessible, responsive, and emotionally engaged, and the partners knew how to ask one another to meet their needs for attachment and love, that the relationship would naturally flourish from there. Couples have shown, however, that it is important to be proactive to nurture their bond and to "take the new emotions, perceptions, and responses and integrate them into a narrative that captures all these changes" (Johnson, 2008, p. 223). With Move 5 integrating and summarizing, EFT therapists help clients to consolidate change, and to envision a future by building on this change.

Johnson proposes ways for couples to consolidate and safety-proof their secure attachment bond. After reviewing three EFCT activities, I present similar means to consolidate change in EFIT.

Create a Resiliency Story. An EFT therapist supports a couple to tell a resiliency relationship story of how they moved from their former state of distress into the current bond of safety. Partners are guided to turn the corrective emotional experiences that have transformed their relationship into vivid stories and imagined movies, which they can draw on as a resource when emotional danger signals arise and attachment warning bells sound. Tracking and reflecting emotional experience, the therapist tracks how, in the face of the familiar cues, partners now perceive and respond differently. This helps to consolidate their change events. Their amygdalae are reacting differently, perceiving safety rather than danger; however, their prefrontal cortexes do not fully integrate this shift until the couple is helped to formulate it explicitly into words. Evoking and tracking how both partners are contributing to the changes in the relationship, and how they now deal with ruptures and threatening moments, can help the couple to consolidate their changes.

Evocative questions, reflections, validating interventions, and empathic conjectures are used. For example:

Let's look together at how you've moved from the distressed, almost ready-to-give-up despair you felt in your relationship when we began therapy to this hopeful, positive cycle you now have where you are reaching and responding to one another openly.

Emily says to Phil and Julie, a former withdraw–withdraw couple:

Before, you both hid from the other when you felt small, unsafe, or unworthy of showing up. And now you move close to one another when the waves threaten to pull you onto separate deserted islands. Can you describe how those moments are different? How you now feel safe to move close when you are "in doubt?"

Partners co-create their own stories of attachment behaviors. Narratives portray how they are facing problems and differences and are making repairs, time and time again. Creating these accounts nurtures the newly growing seedlings of connection and attachment, strengthening and consolidating the new reaches and responses of the positive bonding cycle. Images that capture the nuances of their unique story evoke oxytocin-producing triggers, which calm and soothe and pull them closer together. The *resiliency story* also evokes the new views "of what it means to love and to be loved" (Johnson, 2008, p. 226). The new views invariably contain a sense of the partner as trustworthy, and oneself as motivated to reach to the other in caring and daring ways. Partners are creating new neural pathways in their brains of who they are to one another, and of how they automatically reach and respond.

Phil and Julie write their resilient relationship story replete with images of crossing treacherous bridges safely together. Their love story becomes an imaginary romantic film that they watch over and over again. In the midst of a moment of danger, the old perceptions of threat and judgment arise, and Julie is about to shut down and disappear. However, she describes a new dynamic:

> Just as I am about to abandon the hike and return home alone, I look at Phil and see this guy who loves me and who will not disappear unless I go away. So, I reach out and say, "I need you. Will you take my hand? I cannot cross this bridge alone!" And he reaches back and takes my hand and walks with me over the most dangerous, narrow bridge with no railing to hold on to – only his hand. My heart melts and we cross the hazardous, creaking bridge together. And I know in my heart we have made the world a safer place.

Phil chimes in:

> That's right! I've only disappeared in the past when you got scared or were in pain because I was afraid to feel. With you, I have learned how good it is to feel – how good it is to feel you needing me and wanting me. I've come to trust that holding your hand makes us both feel safer. And we've crossed some very treacherous bridges hand in hand.

Create a Future Love Story. A therapist can seed secure attachment by highlighting how the changes in their resiliency story will help to protect and support them in the future. To help partners plant new seeds of hopes and visions for the future of the relationship, and to extend their story into the future, they are invited to create a future love story. An EFT therapist focuses on the moments that foster accessibility and responsiveness, using reflections, evocative questions and responses, and heightening to elicit couples' stories and pictures of themselves in the future. Partners strengthen their connection and sense of importance and security by hearing from each other of their hopes and longings. "Keeping Your Love Alive" (Conversation 7 in *Hold Me Tight*, Johnson, 2008) presents "a road map for taking your love into the future" (Johnson, 2008, p. 205).

Plan Rituals for Keeping Love Alive. "What you don't recognize slips away" (Johnson, 2008, p. 211). The therapist explores attachment rituals the partners might have developed, or that they would like to develop, to help maintain this positive connection. What makes an activity an attachment ritual is not the activity itself, but the meaning the activity has for the couple. The ritual is an opportunity for partners to routinely remind each other of the connection they share, typically around moments of separation and reunion.

Examples of couple attachment rituals include special ways of saying goodbye and hello each day, leaving notes for each other, sharing religious rituals, checking in with one another during the day, daily rituals of conversation or times of cuddling, or volunteering or doing hobbies together. Rituals to nurture, fertilize, and water the attachment seedlings range from tiny moments, like

Wayne and Jessica's habit of texting the other whenever they notice it is 11:11, to grander celebrations like having a ceremony to renew their vows, or Phil and Julie's simple shared glances at the rustic painting of a bridge which they purchased to symbolize their bond and trust in each other.

Consolidating Change in EFIT. Similarly, in EFIT, with Move 1 reflecting emerging shifts and Move 5 integrating, validating, and summarizing, therapists help clients to integrate new positions and strategies across relationships and contexts. The three activities for consolidating change in EFIT are similar to EFCT: Celebrate with a coherent resiliency story of how they arrived where they are today, write a future narrative, and plan rituals to build on the positive trajectory.

Therapists help EFIT clients to celebrate how they have moved from distress to resilience and flexibility. They invite clients to create a coherent *resiliency story* of how they moved from distress to positive models of self as loveable and resourceful and new views of others who are trustworthy. They elicit a future narrative, asking clients to picture the future unfolding and imagine how they will be facing life's uncertainties and inevitable existential dilemmas, with their new inner and interpersonal security. New strategies, new meanings, and emotional resources are identified and heightened across relational contexts and images of the future. Finally, clients are helped to reflect on rituals or activities that are helping them to strengthen the ways they are engaging more effectively with self and others and how they are fortifying their new sense of motivation and meaning. The integration and consolidation of Stage 3 builds on validating and heightening clients' emotional fitness, summarizing both their growing capacity to tune into emotion as a guide for meaning and action and their shifts in views of self and other, and heightening their flexible strategies for engaging with others and within self.

Sahra reflects back to when she began therapy, "I felt emotional and bodily tension all my life. Smallest things triggered me strongly." She reviews, across relationships, how her hyperactivating/numbing out patterns used to result in her dismissing her own emotions when frantic attempts to get what she needed for support were unsuccessful.

Shifts Sahra has made in her internal relationships with her deceased mother, her estranged father, her heart-broken six-year-old self, her childhood sexual abuser, her abusive ex-partner, her racist colleagues, and in her current-day friendships, all come together in Stage 3. Her revised working models of self and other are helping her to discover new meanings and new ways of relating as she continues to tune into her own core emotions as a reliable guide. She is identifying who are safe others whom she can trust. She is finding a new sense of agency and discovering interpersonal comfort. Both interpersonal and internal shifts are leading her to naturally find solutions to old problems and to seek available support when contextual barriers frustrate her or when she feels lonely. She celebrates and grieves with emotional balance.

Recalling her imaginal encounter with her abusive ex, she says, "I made a huge difference that day! I so clearly recall the relief I felt – my anger at him and my grief that it had to end this way. I felt so free as I said to him, 'I can step away from you now – I am ready to let you go – I don't trust you are safe for me or my daughter. I clearly regret ever having let you into our lives – but I am not going to change you. I am feeling free to move on, without needing your approval anymore'."

Sahra's future story is already beginning, she reveals, "Now I am living one of my key goals – to feel lighter in my emotional life. I feel more kindness toward myself, toward my own daughter and toward my own little-girl-self, all longing for loving connection. I am finding colleagues who respect me and am building on those relationships. I feel resolved toward my mother and all my attempts to help her before she died. I feel she has forgiven me for leaving Ukraine. She is safely alive in my heart now. I am free to explore if I will ever try and connect with my father – but there is no need to decide that now. Life is not fair," Sahra acknowledges, but she is strengthening her emotional muscles to see she is on a path of hope. She is building relationships in a country that she is making her new home, and building a career she enjoys.

Max's story began with feeling foggy emotional and cognitive dissonance, fearing and seeing others as hostile and unsafe, and self as guilty and disingenuous, like a *monster-in-a-box*. He tells a narrative of moving through layers and layers of fears, grief, remorse, guilt, and love, including loving connections to and from the man he killed, until he finds himself living into the self-identity he has always craved. This is an identify of being *a kind gardener of people*. As this kind gardener, he makes amends to those he has hurt, treats those who have hurt him with kindness and emotional balance, and nurtures his few friendships. He also begins to trust that he deserves to rely on others and to expand his social network. These activities are the core of his future narrative and the rituals by which he is strengthening his hopeful trajectory.

How EFT Therapists Facilitate Stage 3 Consolidation

Stage 3, like all of EFT is a collaborative process between client and therapist. In this stage, clients need less direction from the therapist, for emotionally intense exploration, and are likely to express much gratitude to the therapist. This might draw a therapist to happily take the credit offered, however, EFT therapists resist receiving praise. Instead, they share their client's joy, celebrating the successful journey they have taken together, to reach their goals. They express appreciation for the honor of taking this voyage with them.

EFT therapists help clients to notice the steps they have taken to have arrived at their chosen destination. They invite partners to identify how they began to send clear signals to one another of their deepest fears and needs and, in so doing, created an amazingly more responsive, safe relationship. Likewise, in EFIT they elicit clients' reflections on how they openly explored what seemed like unthinkable, unmanageable, unacceptable emotional experiences and shifted stuck patterns and strategies into powerful ways of reshaping their inner and outer worlds.

Person of the Therapist

EFT therapists remain emotionally engaged in the EFT *way of being* (Rogers, 1980) through to the end of therapy. The therapist's active and emotionally engaged presence and role as safe haven/ secure base continues to be important in this final stage. The empathy, acceptance, and genuineness which create a safe base for exploration remain as significant in the final sessions of launching clients on their own, as they have been throughout the entire process. "When we are safe and sound, confident and clear, then we can help our clients come home to the same place" (Johnson, 2019, p. viii).

The strength of EFT research can give EFT therapists confidence and clarity about their role in this process. Emily is tempted to question her therapeutic competence when clients express fears about the changes enduring, however, she feels reassured with EFCT studies that have measured changes within individuals, as well as changes in relationship functioning. She is reassured that she is on track with this model, when she recalls studies showing that individuals' changes in attachment behaviors persist at three-year follow-up (Burgess Moser et al., 2015). She also feels assured by the studies showing that after EFT therapy, individual brains respond with less alarm to threat as shown in brain scan studies (Johnson et al., 2013) and that EFT is effective in relieving symptoms of depression and posttrauma reactions (Ganz et al., 2022; Wittenborn et al., 2019). Having scientific support that EFT has lasting positive effects on reducing relationship distress and key emotional disorders of anxiety and depression, grounds Emily in offering a serene, engaged therapeutic presence.

Emotional Tone

One way Emily keeps herself actively engaged in the final stage is by attuning to the emotional tone – heightening joy and relief and validating hints or directly expressed fears of relapse. She stays engaged by celebrating present process, with Move 1, making clients' joys explicit and validating fears of relapse, with Move 2. She recognizes how important it is to use Move 5 to help clients be fully aware of the changes they created and to explore how these changes speak to their fears. The goals of Stage 3 integration and consolidation remind her that the power of the corrective emotional experiences which she has helped clients to create, are enhanced significantly by her taking time with Move 5 to heighten these events and to invite clients to reflect aloud on coherent stories of their progress. She grounds herself in Move 5 summaries, *tying the bow* on clients' transformative change, heightening the precious bonds that couples create with one another and that individuals shape in the relationships populating their inner, and possibly outer, worlds. When clients celebrate how good things are now, she resolves to remain emotionally engaged with the specificity of Move 5. In this way, client and therapist, alike, have a consciously formulated awareness of their path from past distress to current hope and resilience, and of their capacity to repair bumps in the road and to nurture this trajectory.

Evocative Mode

In addition to the reflecting and tracking of Move 5, evocative questions and responses are important to help clients reflect on the active changes they are integrating and consolidating. Evocative questions and responses help to elicit and deepen clients' capacity to reflect on where they are, where they have been, and the vision of where this trajectory will take them. An EFT therapist keeps the evocative mode active by picking up tones of hope and joy to ensure they are concrete, vivid, and specific, and to heighten and savor them. The therapist also attunes to any client anxieties about slipping back to the old patterns. Evoking full expression of clients' fears about relapsing, or discouragement at a recent recurrence of a negative cycle or a broken promise from a significant other, the therapist validates and normalizes clients' anxieties and concerns. Emily experiences growing certainty that it is safe and helpful to validate clients' fears and discouragement at this stage of therapy. This is a context where acknowledging anxiety or discouragement does not eliminate the leaps and bounds of change. Part of consolidating growth is discovering that when the old patterns and strategies recur, the couple or individual is able to get back on track. Quick recoveries are celebrated in Stage 3 consolidation. An EFT therapist can be confident that it is safe to evoke and reflect the precise, present moment process of clients. The impact of earlier corrective emotional experiences will not vanish but will remain a reliable resource.

In summary, in Stage 3 of EFT therapists confidently track, reflect, and deepen partners' reports of effective reaching and responding and individuals' stories of emotional fitness, expanded sense of self, and connections with others. While attuning to partners' renewed bonds, therapists elicit their reviews of how they are successfully repairing after disconnection, and help them to discuss ways to safety-proof the relationship. While attuning to individuals' resilience and freedom from emotional distress, a therapist similarly invites reflections on the new patterns and strategies to help them consciously consolidate these strategies to remain emotionally fit and prepared for existential living.

Conclusion

Distressing cycles of emotions, perceptions, and reactive behaviors are driven by working models of self and other (Bowlby, 1973). In Stage 1, EFT therapists help clients to identify and track these models and the patterns which shape their worlds, reinforce their views of self and other, and impact their intimate bonds. With the corrective emotional experiences of Stage 2, clients are helped to reshape their worlds, transforming emotional reactivity into safe and loving interactions, and restructuring working models of self and other. Finally, in Stage 3, partners and individuals are helped to integrate, across their life circumstances, the new working models of self and other that affirm lovability and competence in self, trustworthiness in other, and the value of effective dependency for emotional regulation and vibrant living.

Secure attachment bonds have a transformative impact in several ways. In a secure bond, each partner is able to remain emotionally present to the other, and thereby make a profound difference to each other's felt security. Individual and couple clients alike, experience the positive impacts of security, including strengthened capacities to retain emotional balance during times of stress and threat, to seek and receive care and support in ways that continually renew attachment bonds, and to implicitly access powerful mental and physical health benefits (Feeney & Collins, 2014; Johnson et al., 2015).

For a summary of key ingredients of change in Stage 3 consolidation, see Chapter 11 Support Material (routledge.com/9781032151335).

12 Recognizing and Following Markers of Emotion on the EFT Terrain

Tracing with your eyes the precise line where heaven meets earth, you reflect on the insignificance of your presence… At first you see what appears to be nothing more than a speck in the distance. Soon it creates a focal point… Stone upon lichen-encrusted stone, it is an inuksuk… Eventually I acquired a detailed image in my mind of a number of inuksuit and their locations. They became reference points from which I could depart and return with confidence. (Hallendy, 2000, pp. 21, 22)

Traditionally, Inuit have followed human-shaped stone sculptural markers for guidance in travel across the vast arctic landscape. I have always been drawn to the artistic variability of these markers, called *inukshuks or inuksuit*, just as I am to the variability of the information-rich micro-process markers of emotional experience and "micro-moments of interaction" (Siegel, 2012, p. 327). Although the split-second markers in a relational dynamic differ significantly from the static stone of *inuksuit*, an EFT therapist can navigate the EFT terrain with confidence, by seeking and following markers of clients' emotional, cultural experiencing and their interpersonal dynamics as reference points to guide them across the landscape of present-moment process and therapeutic change.

Before exploring markers of client steps of change on the EFT terrain in Chapters 13 and 14, I discuss signposts or markers of emotional/cultural nuances and implicit emotional experience to follow through the EFT change process. Tracking micro-markers of emotion is at the heart of change in EFT. Following these throughout the entire EFT change process will help you increase the emerging depths of clients' experiencing (Gendlin, 1961; Klein et al., 1969, 1986; see Box 12.1).

The chapter ends with a brief discussion of an EFT therapist's *felt-sense understanding. Felt-sensing* – feeling another's micro-moments of experience in one's own body as much as possible – is the link between scientific knowledge and a therapist's therapeutic artistry or creative competence.

Micro-markers of Implicit Emotion: The Heart of Change in EFT

Micro-markers of unspoken emotion are fleeting and easy for both therapist and clients to miss. They point to clients' emotional experiencing that is frequently outside of conscious awareness. Since EFT therapists know that following emotion is the route to change, they are constantly seeking to notice and follow signs of emotional experience. Johnson (2004, 2020) suggests that the territory of romantic love is replete with markers signaling to the therapist what to attend to and when to intervene. Partners are implicitly tuned in to the slightest non-verbal indications of emotion and attachment threat in the other; yet, micro-moments of emotional experience can be so fleeting that individuals frequently are unaware of their own emotional experience or of having sent any signs of internal experience. It behoves EFT therapists, across modalities, to fine-tune their ability

DOI: 10.4324/9781003242673-18

Box 12.1   Details of the Experiencing Scale (EXP)

Low Levels (1–3) Distant from emotional experiencing – *talks about events, ideas, or others* without expressing emotion. Or talks *about* emotions and thoughts, without experiencing them or reflecting on them. Detached from present-moment experience, either hyperactivating or deactivating.

Medium – Level 4 (Engaged with the *felt flow* of inner experiencing) – Experiences emotions in an alive, vivid manner in the present moment. Reflects inwardly on emotional awareness of triggers, meanings, bodily sensations, action impulses.

High Levels (5–7) New depths, edges, and felt shifts of emotional experiencing emerge. Gains an awareness of previously implicit feelings and meanings. Engages in new depths of experience and perspectives.

Level 5 – Focuses on emerging edges of vague, implicit experience – seeking to elaborate it.
Level 6 – Explores emergent experience – which is increasingly active, vivid, immediate, shifting or resolving.
Level 7 – Fresh way of knowing; expansive, trustworthy source of new meanings and actions. (Klein et al., 1986)

---

to detect makers of emotional experience as they fly by. Noticing the markers is a therapist's first step, followed then of course by incorporating these signals into the therapy process (Kailanko et al., 2022).

Various verbal and non-verbal micro-markers of emotional experiencing, listed below, signal to the EFT therapist to pay attention and to listen to what has not yet been put into words or been fully tasted. By following these markers, the therapist can help clients to explicitly experience emotion that has been on the leading edge of their awareness.

Non-verbal Markers of Emotion

Therapists who seem to have a magical ability to tune into clients' emotional experiences in their negative cycles of interaction are simply paying exquisite attention to non-verbal micro-processes. Much more is conveyed by *how* one speaks than by *what* one says (Kailanko et al., 2022; Porges, 2011, 2015). When EFT therapists attune to and comment on non-verbal markers and bodily signs of unexpressed emotional experiencing occurring in the present moment, they can bring alive greater depths of emotional experiencing in their clients (Kailanko et al., 2022).

Non-verbal markers are frequently so brief that they occur beyond participants' edge of awareness, or if there is an awareness, the fleeting emotions are probably not "tasted" or fully savored. Between partners, a soft touch or a quick glance of compassion can point to a moment of warmth and caring. With couples or individuals, tightening breath or downward-cast eyes amid much *verbal noise* can trigger a sense of attachment threat that initiates a cascade of dysregulated emotional reactions. Non-verbal micro-markers of bodily arousal might be subtle movements such as pulling back, a tightening voice, a slight shrug, or grander gestures such as a broadly sweeping arm, chopping hand movements, a deep sigh, a sudden gasp, a blank face, or an alternation in vocal tone or pace. Markers of bodily arousal indicate that the attachment fight-flight-or-freeze system is activated.

Vocal quality (Rice & Kerr, 1986; Rice et al., 1979) is another non-verbal marker of a client's engagement with, or distance from, emotional experience. A focused voice indicates emotional engagement, whereas an externalizing, detached voice with a tight seamless quality, a fragile and limited voice, or a whiny, emotional voice can all indicate distance from inner experiencing. EFT therapists make transparent observations to gently engage clients in present-moment awareness. For example, "Your voice just cracked as you said that. Did you notice? I wonder what is coming up for you."

Since in-session engagement with emotional processing is predictive of success in EFT, it is vital that therapists become skilled at tuning in and responding to verbal and non-verbal micro-process markers. Reviewing video recordings of one's own and others' therapy sessions is perhaps the best way to fine-tune an ability to be guided by process markers and to effectively weave process and content.

Verbal Markers of Emotion

Emotion implicit in clients' verbal reactions to danger cues is often hinted at in the words they use. EFT therapists listen for verbal *emotional handles* or *cultural handles, which inevitably have an emotional charge,* to open doorways into core emotional experience (see Box 12.2). In particular, words claiming lack of emotional experience or words rich with imagery can be markers of un-clear, emergent emotional experience.

EFT therapists listen to the *leading edge* (Rice, 1974) of the words. For example, "I feel noth-ing. I am just numb" probably indicates that the client has a sensation of numbness or a freeze re-sponse that the therapist can actively evoke and explore. To do so, the therapist slows the process, first with Tango Move 1 reflection of present process. For example, "Right now, as you tell me this story" … or "As your partner recounts this story, you say, 'I feel nothing. I'm just numb.'") Responding with some Tango Move 2 assembly, a therapist can evoke the cue, the meaning, the action tendency, possibly the bodily felt sense of numbness, and then link the various elements to order, create coherence, and validate the experience of numbness. What began as a *nothing* response becomes an active dynamic of *feeling nothing* to regulate intolerable or alien emotion.

Another example of a verbal hint of emotion on the leading edge is when a client says that they don't want to feel a particular emotion. "I don't want to be afraid," implies fear. The therapist re-sponds using empathic reflections, evocative questions, and empathic conjectures in the interactive context, at the leading edge of what the client has expressed but not fully put into words.

Therapist:	You say, "I don't want to be afraid" (repeats slowly), and I wonder if a little part of you isn't maybe a little afraid?
Client:	Uh huh, maybe a little bit, yes.
Therapist:	Can I get you to stay with that little bit of fear? Can you feel it here, right now? (pause). Each time your partner turns to his mother (repeating the cue) and not you, your fear of not mattering (meaning making) gets a little bigger? Is that it? (Checks in with client and tracks their non-verbal response.) Are you feeling that fear right now? (Giving the client time to check and respond; client nods.) Where in your body do you feel it?
Client:	Here (pointing to their stomach and their throat).
Therapist:	It is much, much safer to get angry and blame him for not letting go of his mother than it is to share with him your fear of not mattering, isn't it? In your typical pattern of interacting, you don't feel safe enough to share this fear—you don't even want to feel

this fear, is that it? (conjecture). It makes sense, then, that when you sense he holds back from you, you swallow your panic, get this knot in your stomach and lump in your throat, and you lash out at him (tracking).

Box 12.2   Emotional and Cultural Handles

Emotional handles are poignant words, images, or metaphors that EFT therapists discern as indicators of greater depths of experience and unclear or complex stories which may have not yet been put into words. Subtle bodily cues of emotional arousal or suppression – changes in face, posture, vocal tone, pacing, and partners' glances at one another – can also be emotional handles signaling doorways into greater depths. By repeating these emotional handles, a therapist can expand and evoke a more precise experience of a previously fragmented, vague, or inaccessible emotionally felt sense.

Cultural Handles

Similarly, a subtle hint of an REC (racial, ethnic, cultural) resource or stressor that appears in a phrase, an image, or bodily movement can be an emotionally charged *cultural handle* to take hold of, gently, to invite further exploration. Examples of cultural handles indicating that volumes of undisclosed emotional experience are likely on the other side of the door are *our people; what's happening in the news; performing blackness; always bypassed; but she's my mother; stepping back from me; being ignored; invisible; despised; can never be weak.*

Therapist Tasks in Response to Detecting a Cultural Handle

1. Notice the cultural handle.
2. Knock on the door, to evoke, rather than presume understanding. Examples: Tell me more about what performing blackness means to you. Can you say more about how the current news is impacting you?
3. When the door is not opened, indicating a client does not want to talk about it in the moment, respect their choice. Have the courage and the confidence to trust it is not only ok but important to come back to knock gently again and again (Tanisha James, personal communication, n.d.).
4. Learn about lived experiences of difference, subjugation, oppression, exclusion, and other reasons a client may not be opening a door yet, even though you are knocking.
5. Trust that gentle, repeated knocking is likely to convey the important message, "I see you! I want to know you. And I accept however much or little you are ready to open with me."

Other verbal micro-markers of implied emotion call for the therapist's attention and finely tuned response. When verbal expression contains poignancy, for example, "It's chilling," EFT therapists reflect, heighten, or conjecture about the poignant element in a client's repetitive pattern and make it explicit. For example, "It's chilling—like when you hear them say you never get it right, then a chill runs right through your body, yes?"

Markers of Distancing from Emotional Experience

Clients' retreat from emerging emotional experience is a marker signaling an EFT therapist to refocus the process. For example, in EFCT a client may interrupt when their partner gets close to vulnerable emotion, or in EFIT, a client may suddenly change the topic. Retreating from emerging emotional experience can happen rapidly and without anyone's awareness unless the therapist catches the moment, slows it down, comments on it, and finds a way to refocus and re-engage the client. It is *emotionally focused* therapy, after all, and whenever a client diverts from core emotional experience, an EFT therapist redirects back to the moment of experience.

There are various interventions to use to refocus and redirect such as tracking (making a process replay of what has just taken place in the session), asking an evocative question, and finding a metaphor to conjecture about the client's core experience. For example, "As you describe what must have been very difficult, I find myself wondering, what this must be like for you?" Or, "Several times when I have attempted to ask you how this is for you, you've kept right on talking (transparency and tracking), almost as if you're feeling an urgency to get every detail out before your story is crushed?" (conjecture based on a couple's criticize–demand, withdraw–defend pattern).

When clients begin rambling, EFT therapists respectfully interrupt and refocus on some emotional handle, or make a process replay, "I'm just going to slow you down here, alright? A moment ago, your voice quivered as you said, 'Do you really mean that?'" When clients speak in vague, general terms with flat or distant descriptions, EFT therapists use immediacy of language, shifting the vague to vivid, the general to specific, the abstract to the concrete, the global to the personal, and "then" to "now," using emotionally evocative language.

In summary, markers of verbal and non-verbal micro-processes signal to the therapist to pay attention and to respond sensitively to the tiniest slices of implicit and emerging emotion. These markers retain relevance throughout clients' steps and stages of the EFT change process in the following ways:

- A verbal or non-verbal marker indicating an alliance rupture points the therapist to respond with empathic curiosity and validation.
- A seemingly casual or factual reference to a REC experience of exclusion (e.g., "always ignored") points to an emotionally alive story for the therapist to take note of and invite more from the client, while respecting the client's inclination to disclose or not to disclose more in the present moment.
- A sudden non-verbal reaction to a partner in EFCT or to an imaginal other in EFIT indicates some attachment-significant fear has been touched, directing the therapist to slow the process, replay the moment, and refocus on the implicit emotion in the non-verbal response.
- An abrupt retreat from emotional experience points the therapist to firmly and gently explore what happened immediately prior to the exit.

Felt-sense Understanding

An EFT therapist's capacity to detect and follow markers of emotional experiencing is augmented when they listen to their own bodily responses while doing so (Kailanko et al., 2022). "Attending to the 'bodily felt sense' of a problem makes any orientation more effective" (Hendricks, 2007, p. 41) and it gives a therapist multiple sources of information about the *feeling of what happens* (Damasio, 1999). Being fully, viscerally present is an art form and it "can also be seen as the most important element of helping others heal" (Siegel, 2010, p. 1).

Adapting our attachment theoretical assumptions to REC means opening to differences with respect to emotion regulation strategies and display rules for expressions of love, affection, and other emotions (Allan et al., 2022; Keller, 2022; Liu & Wittenborn, 2011). It also means listening deeply and patiently with empathic curiosity toward others who are conveying their experience and having much patience toward self as listener, recognizing one's limitations to fully step into another's world, particularly if there are differences in power and privilege.

Empathic resonance includes listening and responding to more than spoken words. It involves tuning in to the simplest, smallest, concrete "micro-moments of interaction where attunement is crucial" (Siegel, 2012, p. 327), including voice tone, pace, breathing, posture, facial expressions, eye gaze, and other micro-movements. Tracking micro-moments grounds everyone in the room in the present moment and frees therapists and partners or individual clients alike, to be curious and open to explore what is happening.

A felt sense could be described as feeling the other's experience in one's own body. Having an implicit understanding of another's experience is something other than, though not totally separate from, understanding the other's experience explicitly or conceptually. For example, a therapist with a felt sense of how Jill's voice threatens Darius and propels him into reactive defense and disappearance, has a richer understanding than the therapist who simply conceptualizes that Darius is triggered by Jill's shrill tone of voice. Present-moment, felt-sense awareness (Stern, 2004) is sometimes described as "mindfulness," or for some, as the spiritual element of EFT (Furrow et al., 2011).

Attending to a felt sense of present-moment experience can enhance therapy in the following four ways: Felt-sensing feeds the therapist's empathic imagination; it helps a therapist to communicate empathic understanding to clients; it increases clients' depth of emotional experiencing; and it strengthens the therapist's confidence and creative competency. The Chapter 12 Support Material on felt-sensing (routledge.com/9781032151335) expands on these dynamics of a therapist's deliberate *felt-sensing*, including sensitivity to cultural differences.

Conclusion

I open this chapter by suggesting that subtle signals of emotional experiencing can be reference points in the complex emotional landscape, not unlike inuksuit, the human-shaped stone markers, guiding travelers in the vast arctic. The resource of detecting and following micro-moments of clients' verbal and non-verbal indicators of cultural and emotional experiencing combines with the resource of a therapist listening to their own inner felt sense of resonance with their clients. Together, these activities augment a therapist's capacity to attune and to help clients deepen and expand their experiencing.

13 Recognizing and Following Markers on the EFT Stage 1 Terrain

Building on the metaphor of recognizing inuksuit, stone markers, as reference points in the vast Arctic landscape (Hallendy, 2000), I explore in this chapter the value of spotting and following client markers on the terrain of therapeutic change in Stage 1 of EFT. This is your opportunity to integrate and consolidate what it means to be an EFT process consultant dancing the EFT Tango in attunement with your clients as they move through Stage 1 change. Being able to detect markers that indicate where a couple or individual client is situated on the landscape of EFT change, gives EFT therapists confidence to move fluidly with the EFT Tango, confidently returning to the client's present location on the map of change. (See Boxes 1.1 and 1.2 to review stages and steps of client change.) In this chapter, I hope to strengthen your scientific precision and knowledge of client steps of Stage 1 change and to increase your confidence in flowing artistically with the EFT macro-intervention. This review of signposts or markers to follow through Stage 1 is built on the foundation of the micro-markers of emotion, discussed in the previous chapter.

Markers and therapist questions in search of these markers begin with identifying racial, ethnic, and cultural (REC) doorways, important for alliance building and empathic understanding. This is followed by a search for markers of typical positions; markers of typical protective moves or strategies for engagement; markers of core underlying emotion; markers that stabilization is in progress and finally markers that stabilization/de-escalation has been achieved.

Therapist Questions in Search of Markers to Situate Clients on the EFT Map of Change

Markers of the EFT steps and stages orientate a therapist to where a couple or individual is on their journey toward secure connection. Since the EFT model is both linear and circular, it is helpful to clearly recognize clients' steps and stages of change, so as to flow more deliberately and fluidly with the repetitive moves of the EFT Tango. Recognizing markers of clients' steps of change contributes to therapist confidence and creativity. EFT therapists look for markers to indicate where clients are on the map of change as they help them move toward the destination of *safe and sound in relationships and in their inner worlds* (see Box 13.1).

Certain change events are prerequisites for others. For example, in EFCT, the more withdrawn partner cannot step more visibly and emotionally into the relationship in Stage 2 until after the Stage 1 change event of de-escalation/stabilization, where partners collaboratively recognize, and thus, weaken the power of their repetitive, self-protective cycle to take over their relationship. Similarly, the softening change event cannot happen until after the more withdrawn partner is accessible and has engaged the parts of self that were previously left out of the relationship. Lest this sounds like a rigid and linear model of change, let me clarify that change in EFT is, paradoxically, both linear and circular.

DOI: 10.4324/9781003242673-19

Box 13.1   Markers to Situate Clients on the Terrain of Stage 1 and Therapist Questions in Search of These Markers

1. **Markers of Racial, Ethnic, Cultural (REC) Doorways:** Can I notice markers pointing to REC doorways that might facilitate Step 1 alliance building, communication of clients' core attachment struggle, and collaborative goal setting? (client Step 1)
2. **Markers of Typical Position:** Can the client (including both partners in a couple) identify their typical, protective position of anxious pursuit, avoidant withdrawal, or fearful-avoidant *push-pull* when experiencing an attachment or contextual threat? Do they recognize their typical position/strategy for engaging? (part of client Step 2)
3. **Markers of Typical Moves:** Do the couple or individual client and therapist recognize the link between the threatening cue (*the emotional music*) and their reactive *self-protective moves*? That is, do they recognize the specific link between their experienced threat (attachment or contextual) and their automatic move to hyperactivate, suppress, or flip between anxious hyperactivating and avoidant down-regulating? *Do they own how threatening signals move them to react?* (part of client Step 2)
4. **Markers of Underlying Core Emotions:** What hints are clients sending about the core emotion that is driving their problematic pattern? Can the therapist hear or see hints of underlying emotions? (client Step 3)
5. **Markers that Stabilization Is In-progress:** Does the client (couple or individual) have some experiential awareness and acceptance that their distress stems not from self or other but from their repetitive pattern? (beginning of client Step 4)
6. **Markers of Stabilization/Readiness for Stage 2 Engagement:** Is the client (couple or individual) stabilized and can they fully grasp the pattern, own their triggers, their immediate bodily sense of threat, their automatic action tendencies, the meanings they make, and the core underlying fears driving them? Stabilization indicates readiness for Stage 2 engagement. (client Step 4)

Correspondingly, in EFIT, Stage 1 stabilization (achieved through a solid therapeutic alliance, clarification of therapeutic goals, and the recognition of the pattern as the problem) is required before the Stage 2 change event of deepened engagement with unfamiliar and frightening emotions. Also, Stage 2 engagement precedes a softening change event toward self and some others. At the same time as we have clear markers of the differences between Stage 1 and Stage 2 change, there is some fluidity between Stages 1 and 2, in both EFCT and EFIT, and particularly in EFIT as change evolves across relational contexts and emotional depths.

Stage 1 change deepens and consolidates as Stage 2 change events occur, with clarity of the old pattern becoming more and more a part of the newly emerging positive cycle. While there is a fluid boundary between stages, the basic order of change events is: De-escalation/stabilization precedes engagement, and engagement precedes a softening.

Emily remembers the early days of EFT when she would ask herself:

Where am I? Are my clients in Stage 1 or Stage 2? This distancing partner just became tearful. Does this mean we are engaging the withdrawer, or are we still in Stage 1, getting a clearer sense of how the more withdrawn partner gets sucked into the cycle? This pursuer seems so vulnerable. Are they ready to begin a softening or have we not stabilized yet? Partners are kinder to each other. Does this mean we have de-escalated? The withdrawn partner is trying harder to engage in conversation. Does this mean engagement has happened? My individual client is deeply accessing core anguish when they talk about their brother. Does this mean they are ready for a Stage 2 encounter to engage the long-suppressed pain? But wait, I have no sense of this client's basic pattern of how they typically cope with this unclear, amorphous blob of pain, with the anger, sadness and fears all jumbled together! We need to identify the pattern before rushing to Stage 2 change.

Although she used to think these questions were simply the mark of a novice, Emily has come to respect there is value in curiously asking these questions and seeking markers and signposts for guidance.

Emily often pauses to ask herself where her clients are located on the EFT map of client change. While attuning and intervening with the macro-intervention of the EFT Tango, she assesses which step her clients are taking or are ready to take, by asking herself one or more of the 11 questions in Boxes 13.1 and 14.1. In response to questions about markers on the Stage 1 terrain in Chapter 13 and questions on the Stage 2 terrain in Chapter 14, EFT therapists can discern client markers to situate them on the landscape of the EFT change process.

Question 1 and Markers of Racial, Ethnic, Cultural (REC) Doorways

Therapist Question: *Can I notice markers pointing to cultural doorways that I can knock on to facilitate clients' Step 1?* (Client's Step 1 is to form an alliance with the therapist, share their core attachment struggle, and collaborate with the therapist to set goals.)

Emily looks for emotional and cultural handles (see Box 12.2) that may point to a cultural doorway. Cultural doorways for Emily are indicators that, due to different social locations, she is limited in her capacity to walk in clients' shoes to taste and deeply experience what it must be like to live in their world (Rogers, 1957). She realizes she has limitations in her ability to enter the worlds of clients with different cultures and contextual experiences than her own and that she needs to take time to listen deeply and to be very tentative when expressing what she intends as empathic understanding. Emily ponders how crucial it is to create a welcoming space and a respectful pace for her clients to share their unique inner and outer worlds. She discovers that clients telling their personal stories and opening their world to her can create newness at several levels. Telling their story and having it held, engaged with, and valued, can give a client a fresh, coherent felt sense of their own experience, validating their strengths, despite their distress. As the therapist begins to get a visceral and emotional taste for what it is like to be this client, to be in this client's shoes, in their relationship(s) and in their world, a safe-haven connection of support and a secure-base collaboration for exploration can form between client and therapist.

Markers of REC Doorways

A therapist from a dominant culture with many advantages is at risk of overlooking some very important doorways. Brief comments that may appear to be spoken in a casual tone, such as, "It was a difficult conversation," or "I'm used to that," or "It's not too bad," can all indicate a rich, untold story of pain, exclusion, or persecution. Careful attunement to micro-markers of experience can help a therapist to detect these markers; however, cultural sensitivity to catch a glimpse of these markers of deep, untold stories, and the skill to knock on these REC doorways must be deliberately cultivated. EFT relevant resources include Allan et al. (2022), Guillory (2022), and Nightingale et al. (2019).

Following Markers of REC Handles

To follow any of these markers into a client's world and lived experience, a therapist can use Move 1 reflections, validations, and evocative questions and responses. Emily pauses to repeat Wayne's poignant phrase, "The world is like warfare." She notices her temptation to simply validate, "Yes, the world is like warfare for black men in America," implying that she understands (and thinking that, as a competent therapist, she really *should* understand). She pauses, however, reminding herself that simple, surface validation could send a message to Wayne that she is not interested in hearing *his story*. It could ring of white supremacy or power imbalance where she seems to *be telling him how it is*, rather than inviting him to tell her precisely what it is like for him (F. Villodas, personal communication, May 2022). She slows her pace, and with empathic curiosity, uses an evocative response to invite him to tell her more about how he experiences the world as warfare.

In addition to a general invitation to say more about their specific lived experiences around a cultural handle, EFT therapists can also use evocative questions and responses, with Move 2, to access the specific elements of the client's experience and deepen their core struggle. To access the trigger, a therapist will ask, "*When* does this come up for you?" To access the meaning, a therapist can ask, "What does that say to you?" To access the bodily sensations, a therapist might ask, "I hear tightness in your voice," "I see you catch your breath," or "How do you feel that in your body?" To access the action tendency, a therapist can ask, "What do you typically do or feel like doing when…?" Linking these elements together, the therapist can linger longer in the moment with the client, to deepen the moment of core experience and therapist empathic understanding. In EFCT, this will be a key moment for Moves 3 and 4 to help the listening partner to take in newly disclosed experience of which they may have been unaware.

Another way to follow markers of cultural handles and open doorways into more vivid descriptions of clients' core struggles and the impacts on their relationships is to conjecture with a *cultural disquisition*. Disquisitions are stories of "others" used to tentatively and respectfully conjecture on what the client may be experiencing (Johnson, 2004, 2020). Seiff-Haron and Calamur (2022) call this *a collective reflection* which has the validating impact of implying, "You are not alone – others share your experience." For example:

1. "Other neurodiverse clients tell me how difficult it is to sit through long, structured class presentations. I wonder if you have that experience too?"
2. "Other clients in inter-racial marriages have told me how, day in and day out, the world is unsafe, and it is lonely coming home, realizing that their spouse has no sense of the battles they have endured."

Finally, therapist transparency is another way to knock on a cultural doorway when a subtle marker of cultural pain appears. Ella sighs heavily with sad eyes as Sophie reports, matter-of-factly, that her family has never accepted her being in a lesbian relationship. Emily attempts a *collective reflection* (a.k.a. *cultural disquisition*) by saying:

Your struggle is different than my experience, but as a mother of two disabled daughters, I know the pain of feeling I just do not belong in the group of parents at school – like no one understands or cares about the challenges I face daily, and it is very lonely. I wonder if being at Sophie's family gatherings, you feel some of that sense of exclusion and loneliness as well?

Question 2 and Position Markers

Therapist Questions: *Can the clients and I clearly identify their typical positions when under threat? When attachment needs or contextual needs for safety and dignity are threatened, do they automatically take a hyper-activating (pursuing) position or a deactivating (withdrawing from needs in self and others) position or do they take a position that combines the pursue/withdraw (come here/go away) strategies?* (Client Step 2 is to identify their automatic self-protective position.)

Position Markers

Following position markers is helpful for therapist attunement in EFCT and EFIT. Common markers which point to positions of anxious pursuit or avoidant withdrawal/defense can be found in the following elements of emotion.

Cues. Behaviors in others that trigger a client can indicate what a client's typical position or strategy is. A partner who is triggered by the other's distancing, apparent nonchalance, and lack of response is likely to be in a position of pursuit, whereas a partner who is triggered by the other's critical complaints or look of disapproval is likely to be in a position of withdrawal. A partner's turning away, or angry retort could trigger distress for a partner in either position of pursuit or withdrawal. The therapist, however, needs to also attune closely to the larger context to learn how the cues are perceived and experienced by the reactive partner.

Action Tendencies. Typical action tendencies signal specific positions, but it can become complicated in that action tendencies gradually morph over time when they fail to generate hoped for responses. Pursuers typically demand closeness and push, often with criticism, for control and connection. If they are not successful in getting a response, after significant protest, they frequently pull away in despair.

Withdrawers distance, comply to keep the peace, and frequently resign in defeat when there is little reprieve from their partner's demands. Withdrawers' resignation or total distancing is frequently preceded by a blast of anger in self-defense or a counterattack to stop the partner's protests. Counterattacks or walls of silence can become the dominant behavior after the pattern is well entrenched.

Additionally, typical positions of pursuit or withdrawal are sometimes difficult to recognize from markers of behaviors and action tendencies alone. Again, the therapist needs to attune to the larger context. For example, accusatory behaviors could be a marker of a pursuer's search for closeness and connection, or they could be a withdrawer's defensive self-protection against rejection.

Attachment Meanings. Attributions that clients make are also position markers. Pursuers frequently make sense of the other partner's behaviors with attributions such as, "You don't care," "I'm not important," "I can't count on you to be there for me," "You don't have my back," or "You will leave me." Withdrawers, however, are more likely to conclude, "Nothing I do will ever please you," "You are hopelessly demanding," "You expect too much," "You drain me dry and still want more," "You are unpredictable," "You are out to hurt me or change me," "I'm failing you," "I'll never measure up or be good enough for you," or "One day you will give up on me and reject me."

Views of self and other, often emotionally charged attributions, can also serve as position markers. Hyperactivating pursuers, despite all their criticisms leveled at other(s), commonly have a negative view of self, ("I must be unlovable,") and a positive underlying view of the other, ("If only they would respond to me, I would be all right.") Suppressing withdrawers are likely to exude a pseudo-positive sense of self, ("I'm just fine on my own, thank you,") and a negative view of other, ("Others are unpredictable, demanding, and impossible to please.")

Somatic Signals. A client's bodily responses can also be a marker of anxious pursuit or avoidant withdrawal. The unacknowledged gasp, rolled eyes or tonal change, could be a client's rapid attempt to disregard their immediate response. Tracking reflections of the bodily movement or paralinguistic signal (Kailanko et al., 2022) with empathic curiosity and evocative questions will help client and therapist discover if this is anxiety or avoidance in action.

Expressions of Reactive or Core Emotions. Different emotional expressions can help to identify positions of anxious pursuit or avoidant withdrawal. There are typical differences in the emotional expressions of pursuers and withdrawers. Reactive emotions from pursuers are typically surface exasperation and frustration with other's failings and lack of response. Withdrawers characteristically express reactive frustration, helplessness, powerlessness, hurt, and numbness. The numbness may be a denial of feeling anything or insisting they feel "just fine."

When core emotions are accessed, pursuers usually express sadness, loneliness, despair, fear, and panic of abandonment. Withdrawers are initially unlikely to be aware of feeling fear; rather, they are likely to access exhaustion and pain at feeling rejected and disliked. Fear of rejection or annihilation eventually emerges at the core for withdrawers.

Identifying position markers in a withdraw–withdraw couple pattern can be complicated. Since a withdraw–withdraw cycle is often devoid of overt attacking or critical behaviors, it can be very challenging to detect different positions. One partner might be withdrawing to protect the connection, like Julie, an extremely cautious, soft pursuer. Another partner, like her partner, Phil, might be withdrawing to protect against rejection, automatically dismissing his own and his partner's attachment needs for emotional support, speaking with pride at how independent they both are. The therapist may need to assemble more of their emotional experience with Move 2, before it becomes clear.

Following Position Markers

To follow position markers, an EFT therapist will use Move 1 to reflect the basic present process as it unfolds in session. Most examples above relate to pursue–withdraw couple dynamics, however, similar positions markers of hyperactivating pursuit or down-regulating, deactivating withdrawal, are also found in EFIT clients. Recognizing the markers can help therapists attune with increased empathy to clients' anxious or avoidant attempts to cope with threat and discomfort. When the therapist makes Move 1 reflections of these typical positions and strategies of either *upping the anté* or *turning it down,* clients and therapist alike deepen their empathic understanding of the repetitive, problematic pattern that has them stuck.

It should be noted that position markers in complex patterns with trauma survivors are frequently unclear. Emily is finding that the more she recognizes the markers of positions just described, the better she can attune to trauma survivors who frequently flip between hyperactivating and deactivating. She recognizes that fearful-avoidant strategies have survival value in situations where the very persons who should be safe and responsive are also the ones who cause hurt and oppression. She understands *come here/go away* patterns were resourceful survival strategies in the past for her trauma-survivor clients, even though these strategies in the present day are often not helpful. She knows Sahra's fearful-avoidant strategy has helped her survive numerous traumatic events, particularly her abusive and neglectful relationships. In Stage 1, she uses Move 1 to reflect how these patterns continue to play out in other relational contexts.

Emily also recognizes the impact of socio-cultural context. Avoidant and fearful-avoidant strategies that play out in intimate relationships are more than a dynamic attributable to the couple's interpersonal patterns. She is sensitive to the impact of the larger cultural and racial contexts of her clients such as Wayne, who survives daily discrimination and threats due to his Black skin color, and Ella, who endures Asian-hate and LGBTQ+ discrimination. She includes these factors in her Move 1 reflections and weaves them into Move 2 assembly as well.

In summary, using Move 1 and some Move 2 assembly, an EFT therapist follows markers of anxious hyperactivating or avoidant deactivating to help clients take Step 2 of recognizing their typical positions and strategies in their self-protective patterns.

Question 3 and Markers of Typical Moves

Therapist Questions: *Do the couple or individual client and I recognize the link between the threatening cue (the emotional music) and their reactive self-protective moves? That is, do we recognize the link between the threatening emotional music, like an alarm, and their reactive moves to that music?* (This is a search for a marker-in-action; happening in the moment.) *Can we identify active markers of this link between danger cues and reactive moves?* (Client Step 2 includes identifying automatic self-protective positions, strategies, and moves as reactions to signals of danger.)

Looking for markers of moves entails looking for the rapid link between the emotional music (the attachment/contextual threat) and the protective dance move (strategies of down-regulating or hyperactivating). Threatening alarms trigger some to withdraw, defend, and move away, and others to become exasperated, critical, and to push forward.

Markers of the Link between Danger Alarms and Reactive Moves

The self-protective pattern or negative cycle can frequently be seen playing out in session. Four common markers of the protective dance moves (reactions to a danger cue) occurring in the present moment in session are:

1. *A couple replays their last fight.* Partners reactively recount their last fight, as though looking for the therapist to choose sides or to solve the problem. Attachment themes, such as fears of loss or rejection, can be heard on the leading edges of each one's account.
2. A *recurring pattern is heard in stories shared by an individual client or a couple.* Pivotal moments or sore points might have obvious significance for one partner yet seem unimportant or confusing to the other. An individual's stories may seem, initially, to be detached stories about others, until the therapist and client recognize markers of their repetitive, reactive, rigid moves.
3. *The cycle is ignited in session, between partners or between a client and therapist.* Moments when partners pull each other into reactive behaviors and emotions are opportunities to curiously attune to the links between cues and reactions. Likewise, the moments an individual client gets knocked off balance emotionally are moments to attune to the link between the behavioral reaction and the trigger.

4. *A positive cycle* occurs in session or is discussed and is *suddenly interrupted or minimized by a partner or an individual client*. This is another marker of the self-protective moves which automatically take over and block clients from safety and security.

Following Markers of the Typical Moves in Action

To follow these markers of the self-protective pattern playing out in session, an EFT therapist uses Move 1 to reflect the moves in reaction to a danger cue, and Move 2 to assemble elements of emotion that make up this pattern.

In EFCT, partners frequently pull each other into the cycle. Emily has learned to reflect the pattern as it gets triggered between partners. When Wayne says, "Things are going well between us," Jessica grimaces and slowly shakes her head, and then Wayne throws up his hands and tosses a puzzled look. Emily reflects this quiet version of their typical pattern, where Wayne's expressed hope that Jessica is happy with him, and that, "Things are going well between us," triggers Jessica's criticism and disappointment, which, in turn, triggers his sense of futility and turn-away response.

Similarly, with fine-tuned listening, Emily can detect and reflect markers of an individual's repetitive moves in session. Sahra's accounts of distancing and dismissal from others sets her on a rapid *fearful-avoidant* pattern of judging others, sensing others judging her, judging herself, and feeling unsafe and lonely. With Move 1 reflection and some of Move 2 assembly, an EFT therapist will make links between cues and action tendencies and may include obvious bodily reactions and expressed meanings (views of self and other). In response to any of these markers of typical moves in a repetitive pattern, a therapist can identify one link at a time in the unfolding dynamic of emotion.

Of particular importance in following markers of the moves is to reflect the triggers and action responses. Link the cue – the alarm bell of attachment threat – to the automatic action tendency, such as, "I see the look on her face and I run for cover." Exploring the clients' experience of this link engages clients to *experientially* understand their self-protective pattern. Experiential understanding, gained by reflecting on cues and moves in the present moment, engages clients more fully than a cognitive description from the therapist. Experientially exploring the danger cues and moves sets the stage for recognizing and owning, "This is me – this is what I do under threat." Tracking the surface links of the pattern (danger cues – reactive moves) also helps to validate self-protective moves, without getting caught in the trap of explaining the reasons for behaviors. Examples of following danger cues and moves include:

1. With Move 1, track the moves in brief, concrete, specific ways that match each client's moment-to-moment experience, checking for accurate understanding with each tracking reflection.
2. With Move 1, in EFCT, clarify how the behavior of one partner is the cue that triggers the other into a compelling and hurtful response. In EFIT, identify the perceived interpersonal cues that trigger the self-protective moves that get them stuck and feeling alone.
3. When the pervasive impact of trauma and shame blocks couples or individuals from seeing their cues and moves in action, use images to capture the pattern with Move 1. Triggers, action tendencies and underlying meaning-making readily emerge from images. Sahra felt responsible for everything and everyone and saw no repetitive moves until she found the image of herself as an empty, broken pitcher. The image brought to life her pattern of giving, always giving to others. She sees others in need of a drink (cue), and having no water left in the pitcher, automatically chips off parts of the pitcher to give to others (action tendency), continually ignoring her own struggles and exhaustion.

This is a simple yet very poignant image of the link between danger cue and reactive move. Her danger cue is *seeing others in need*; her reactive move is *to give and give and give until exhausted and broken.*

Wayne began to recognize the moves in his pattern of avoidance and distancing from his own experience and from Jessica, with the chilling image of surviving in the world by stepping back after knocking on a door, to keep from "getting caught in the crossfire" when someone sees he is Black. In his marriage, if Jessica looks upset or tired (danger cue), he automatically steps back emotionally (his reactive move) to keep safe from hearing her complaints (another danger cue) that feel dangerous, like crossfire, to him. This, of course, leads to more complaints because he is distancing from Jessica who longs to see more of him.

4. Using Move 1, reflect moments of positive contact, between partners in EFCT or with another in EFIT, to give hope and put the negative cycle in context. Heightening positive contact consolidates the secure base from which to collaboratively identify the self-protective moves that can so quickly take over and block positive connection.

5. Explore, specifically, what happened in a moment just before connection was abruptly broken. An EFT therapist evokes the trigger for the distancing move and the negative attachment meaning that interrupts the connection. For example, in EFCT, to Julie, Emily says, "I noticed that when you said, 'I am unbearably lonely!' Phil put his hand on your knee and you turned away. Can you tell me what happened inside just before you turned aside?"

In EFIT, for example, to Sahra Emily might say, "For a moment, your face softened as you said, 'I trust my dad did love me and I deserved better.' Suddenly your face fell and tears started to flow. Can you tell me what came up for you just before your face fell?" Again, the therapist is using, primarily, Move 1 tracking reflection of present process, mixed with a little of Move 2 assembly of the meanings and bodily reactions linked to the cues and action tendencies.

In summary, to follow markers of the links between danger cues and reactive moves, the therapist uses Move 1 tracking reflections of the present process and some Move 2 assembly. This helps clients to take Step 2 and to get an experiential felt sense of their moves under threat in the repetitive pattern that is imprisoning them.

Question 4 and Markers of Underlying Core Emotions

Therapist Questions: *What hints are clients sending of the core underlying emotions that are driving the pattern? Do I hear or see hints of underlying emotion?* Core emotion needs to be discovered since it contains agency and motivation towards change. (Client Step 3 is discovering underlying core emotion.)

Emily is aware that the common core fear for pursuers is fear of abandonment, for withdrawers is fear of rejection or annihilation, and for those caught in complex moves of fearful-avoidant push-pull dynamics, is a conflictual, mixed fear of being abandoned and/or rejected and hurt by others. Despite this awareness, she knows she must foster clients' discovery of their own unique, granular experience and expression of their fears and longings. She also recognizes that implicit emotions on the edge of client's awareness must be evoked and assembled before clients can fully grasp the core attachment fears that are fueling their ineffective strategies for emotion regulation. Below are five markers of emotional experience that an EFT therapist can follow to engage clients in discovering a felt sense of their core emotion that is frequently outside of their awareness. Each marker is followed by a discussion of how an EFT therapist uses mostly Move 2 to follow this marker to access and deepen client's awareness of the core emotion which drives their self-protective pattern.

Markers of Underlying Core Emotion and How to Follow Them

Hints of underlying core emotion that a client may not be fully aware of, can be detected in several ways. Each of the following is a marker of core emotion in action: The manner in which a client describes an event; attachment distress attributed to a deficit in a significant other; expression of powerful, conflicting emotions; a sudden exit from emotional experience; and a partner's an interruption.

1. **The Manner of Describing an Event.** The first marker of underlying core emotion is the manner in which a narrative is shared. Three different examples of this type of marker and how to follow them are:

   Strong Reactive Emotional Responses Interrupt a Story. A client tells a factual story and suddenly expels a non-verbal "Ughhhhh!" while clenching her fist. To follow strong emotional reactivity as a marker of implicit core emotion, an EFT therapist reflects and validates the reaction, assembling elements of emotion. "Something big just came up in your voice and in your fist (reflecting bodily signals of emotion), as you spoke about riding in the back seat while his son rides in the front seat with him (naming the cue), almost as if you feel left out of his inner circle (conjecturing at the attachment meaning), as if you are *starving* to matter to him, yes?" (Conjecture at a bodily felt longing). With Move 2, the therapist validates the reactive action tendency of the fist-clenching "Ugh!" and links this reaction to the cue, attachment meanings, and bodily arousal. This opens the door to accessing the attachment meaning of "not mattering," and the core fear of abandonment. The therapist accesses the underlying core fear and longing by following the bodily signals of implicit emotion, linked to the danger cue.

   A Client Is Incongruently Unemotional. When a client appears nonchalant while recounting a story with a seemingly powerful emotional impact, an EFT therapist sees this as a marker to follow toward accessing core emotion. To follow incongruence between the words and expressed emotion as a marker of implicit core emotion, reflect and be curious about the client's emotional detachment (action tendency), and the incongruence between the intensity of the words and the lack of apparent affect. Use empathic curiosity with Move 2 to assemble and deepen the implicit emotion signaled by this marker.

   Ella: (Matter-of-factly.) All my actions are driven by fear — fear that she wants to destroy me.

   Therapist: I'm curious, you speak about your fear as though you were reporting a simple fact (action tendency). But I can't help but wonder how very, very terrifying it must be to sense that she wants to destroy you (attachment meaning).

   This conjecture of terror can evoke the underlying fear. Conjectures are most effective when therapists first attune to understand, validate, and match the intensity of the reactive emotions before offering a conjecture. If a conjecture about an underlying emotion is too far on the leading edge, it will not fit for a client. "Your goal is to get as far ahead of the client as you can but have the client recognize what you say as part of what she or he meant" (Martin, 2016, p. 26). Empathic conjectures convey accurate understanding when a client recognizes your words as precisely matching the experience for which they did not have words.

   Emotionally Intense Attributions or Rigidly Held Appraisals Stated as Facts. When clients adamantly state their attributions as absolute facts, an EFT therapist sees a hint of some unaccessed core emotion. For example, "He never knows how I feel, and I know he doesn't even care." Rigidly held assumptions are not truths to be reflected as facts but are part of how one partner in separation distress interprets a negative interaction.

To follow rigid appraisals stated as facts, as a marker into core emotion, first, reflect and frame these statements as, "What you say to yourself, is ___?" or, "Your best attempt to make sense out of your pain, loneliness or fear is to explain it as___." Second, evoke and link the elements of emotion to assemble into a coherent whole. For example, "When he is silent and says he has nothing to talk about (cue), you explain it as meaning that he just doesn't care or isn't interested in you (attachment meaning), your heart goes cold (bodily response) and you feel so lonely that you have begun to give up trying to reach him" (action tendency). After verifying that this assembly fits for the client, help the client engage in owning their core attachment fear, likely some nuance of abandonment.

2. **Attachment Distress Is Attributed to Another's Failing.** A second marker pointing to implicit core emotion is seen when a client identifies attachment distress as the result of another person's failing. Doing this, they convey a marker of core underlying emotion that an EFT therapist wants to follow. For example, comments such as, "The problem is that they can never be counted on. Can never be on time!" or, "The problem is my mother – she is never satisfied!" evade all personal agency and engagement. Pointing to the problem as *residing in another*, leaves a client helplessly frustrated, without access to their core emotion or awareness of their participation in this emotional dynamic.

To follow *the problem attributed to another person's failing* as a marker of core emotion, assemble the process with Move 2. Link the cue (what the other person does, such as arrive late), to meaning-making (view of other as the problem, as in, "They can never be counted on. There is nothing I can do about it."), and action tendency (stew in frustrated helplessness). Assembly may evoke the core fear from the client. Alternately, the therapist can conjecture after assembling the links of perception-feeling-meaning-action.

EFCT: "Your partner arriving late (danger cue) says to you that they cannot be counted on and that you must be unlovable (meaning-making). This leaves you stuck in helplessness and lethargy (action tendency/bodily response) about doing anything to improve your relationship. It sounds like you almost give up in fear that you've already lost them, yes?" (conjecture at fear of loss)

EFIT: "Having your mother send endless demands and criticisms your way (danger cue), pulls you into this *exhausting mission-impossible cycle* of trying to please her (action tendency; bodily exhaustion). You say, 'She can never be satisfied or appreciate my efforts' (meaning-making). Sounds like you long for her appreciation, yet live with a constant fear of failing her, yes?"

Both examples validate the links between the danger cue of another's behavior, meaning-making of how the problem is the other's behavior, bodily responses, and action tendencies of reactivity and helplessness. Move 2 assembly is used to empower clients to discover the active process of emotion – danger cue, body, meaning-making, and action tendency – as doorways into their own core emotion. Core emotion empowers and motivates new action tendencies and new meanings.

The main difference between the EFCT and EFIT examples above is that in EFCT, the attachment figure is in the room, to also take responsibility for how they impact and are impacted by their partner, to name the core emotion driving their reactivity, and, together with their partner, to shift this pattern. In EFIT, the attachment figure is present in the client's inner world and may never engage in participating to shift the pattern and transform their core attachment fears and views of self and other. Nevertheless, with both couples and individuals, an EFT therapist begins with naming the threatening cue (in this case, another's hurtful or unreliable behavior), which sets in motion the client's cascade of perception-feeling-meaning-action responses that need to be assembled and "owned." Tango Move 2 is used to help each client assemble and *own* their action steps of emotion, by which they process their attachment threat, until the core fear is discovered, distilled, and deepened, and then disclosed in Tango Move 3.

3. **Powerful, Conflicting Emotions.** A third marker of underlying core emotion is conveyed by a client expressing powerful, conflicting emotions. There could be intense anger mixed with twinges of core fear, or futile helplessness combined with shame. Clients frequently report feeling hurt, which, as detailed in Chapter 5, is a complex blend of anger, sadness, and fear of loss (Vangelisti, 2009).

To follow conflicting emotions as guideposts into core emotion, an EFT therapist stays in the present moment by first accepting and validating the emotional reactivity. With gentle Move 2 assembly, the therapist uses evocative questions, reflections, validations, and conjectures, to slowly move with a client into their more vulnerable, core emotion.

With hurt, validate what is most accessible, such as the anger, and evoke or conjecture about another part, such as sadness or fear of losing. First validate, "I get the part of you that flares up in anger when you see her shut down." Then conjecture, "I wonder if perhaps there is an edge of fear too in your heart as you say, 'There she goes – she just shut down! Will she ever let me back in?'"

4. **A Sudden Exit**. A fourth marker of underlying or implicit core emotion is a sudden exit from emotionally engaged exploration. Sudden exits are clear indications that, like touching a hot burner, a client briefly experienced core emotion and then rapidly fled from it.

First, an EFT therapist, following sudden exits as markers leading into core emotion, uses Move 2 to redirect the exploration and continue assembling emotional experience. The therapist will link the danger cue that was being discussed, to the sudden non-verbal shift and the action tendency of rapidly exiting. For example,

> "Can we just go back; you were exploring something very difficult there and then suddenly your body shifted. You stopped your tears, and said, 'What's the use?' Can we please go back to see what happened as you were saying, 'I have this wall – without this wall it would hurt too much!'"

The therapist is also likely to conjecture at a briefly felt sense of danger or fear. "It seems almost like, suddenly, it feels too dangerous to stay with the fear of letting down your wall, am I getting it?"

Second, persist with curiosity. Use a playful voice or smile and show your willingness to be puzzled when a client dips into the vulnerable emotion and quickly exits. "You just touched that dreadful fear of not being able to get it right with her, and when I repeated that, you say, 'It's not a big deal.'" Track the moment-to-moment process. Evoke emotional experience. "What just happened inside as you crossed your arms and said, 'Not a big deal'?" Conjecture about possible discomfort: "Is it almost too painful to stay with this sense that your survival seems to depend on being enough for them?" Allow time and space for the client to reflect and organize their inner experience.

Third, move toward this core attachment fear to keep it in the clients' awareness and deepen it. Engage with the fear despite the discomfort it evokes. Normalize and validate the difficulty. For example, a client cannot engage with vulnerable core emotion when shame has the upper hand, so validate the immediate impulse (action tendency) to want to hide. "It makes sense you'd just want to hide if you fear she'll reject you when she sees how much you struggle in silence." Then, to deepen exploration, evoke, "Can you say more about what you imagine might happen if she sees you do not feel like the confident provider you think she wants you to be?" Alternatively, conjecture about the fear or pain and sadness embedded in that shame. "It must be so exhausting to _____." Use RISSSSSC (repetition, images, simple, soft, slow pace, specifics, somatic signals, and clients' words) to maintain exploration of the bodily felt sense of the fear or pain, and link it to the automatic, self-protective attempts to regulate these unbearable emotions.

5. **Partner's Interruption**. A fifth marker of underlying emotion appears in EFCT when the observing partner interrupts the experiencing partner's emotional exploration. The therapist can frame this as *moving in to protect the other* or *finding it difficult to accept* what is being shared. In couple therapy, partners are frequently more closely attuned to one another than the therapist is to each one, and thus when a partner touches on core emotion, they might get triggered by this depth before the therapist recognizes what is happening.

To follow a partner's interruption as a marker indicating the other partner is touching a new level of vulnerable core experience, an EFT therapist gently and firmly blocks the interference while validating how foreign and difficult it must be to hear what the partner has hidden for so long. "It is very hard to hear this! I do want to hear your experience. In just a moment, I will come back to you." Continue to direct the process and deepen the experiencing partner's exploration. This marker appears in EFCT, but of course not in EFIT. In EFIT, interruptions come from the client themselves as described earlier in "sudden exits."

In summary, five key markers to follow to access and deepen core emotion are offered above. This task of client Step 3 accessing and deepening previously unaccessed and unexpressed core fears is pivotal since core emotion contains agency and the motivation toward change.

Question 5 and Markers That Stabilization Is In-progress

Therapist Question: *Does my client (couple or individual) have some experiential awareness and acceptance that their distress stems not from self or other but from their repetitive pattern?* (Client Step 4 begins with: Identifying that the real problem is the pattern.)

Markers of Initial Grasp of the Pattern as the Problem

A first marker that Step 4 is in-progress yet incomplete is that clients acknowledge that there is a recurring pattern but continue to hold the view that the real problem resides in their partner (EFCT), in another person (EFIT), or in the general system. They do not sense that the repetitive internal/interpersonal coping strategy in which they participate is the actual prison blocking them from reaching safety, security, their unmet longings, and therapeutic goals. A second marker that Step 4 is in-progress yet incomplete is that clients have an intellectual understanding of the cycle but feel distant from grasping how it pulls them in. A third marker that Step 4 is in-progress yet incomplete is that clients have an intellectual understanding of the cycle but are unable to access the core fear driving their action tendencies.

In EFCT, Emily asks herself if partners grasp how their actions have an impact on one another's deepest fears which, in turn, triggers their self-protective actions in a repetitive and self-reinforcing way? Can they see, "The problem is not you or me, it is our recurring pattern of 'the more you_____, the more I_____ and the more I _____ the more you_____'; and underneath we are both struggling and doing our best to protect ourselves and our relationship?"

In EFIT, she asks herself if clients sense with emotionally engaged knowing how their inner processing patterns reflect and are reflected by their interpersonal patterns, in a cyclical, reinforcing manner? Do they see, "The problem is not me – it is my stuck pattern of best attempts to avoid experiencing 'frightening, and/or alien and unacceptable' emotions and urges (Bowlby, 1988, p. 139) that are blocking me from connection, support and personal confidence?"

Following Markers of the Initial Grasp of the Pattern as the Problem

To follow the markers of clients taking a partial yet incomplete Step 4, therapists use Move 2 assembly and deepening, and shape Move 3 encounters to access and bring to life the missing link(s) of the imprisoning pattern. By assembling and deepening client's emotion, therapists guide clients to engage more fully in seeing and owning the pattern as the real problem and one over which they are no longer powerless. They guide clients to deliberately linger with: (a) assembling affect and specifically owning their **action tendency,** thus gaining agency as participants in the pattern; (b) identifying **the trigger** that pulls them off balance and into the cycle; and (c) accessing a felt sense of **the core fear** driving their action tendencies. Then, with Tango Move 3 they shape relevant encounters to heighten this engagement by disclosing the distilled, deepened emotion to a relevant other.

Wayne and Jessica can quite readily name their typical cycle. They recognize that Wayne holds back to avoid upsetting Jessica, and Jessica pushes Wayne to let her in more and to trust her to support him. They each continue, however, to see their distress as rooted in what the other needs to change.

Wayne dreads getting hurt and being rejected. Jessica fears being abandoned and left emotionally alone. They don't, however, fully grasp how their own core fears are triggering and getting triggered, and driving them to do more of what is distressing their partner. Wayne, muses, "The more you push, the more I hold back. I am very self-sufficient and have no need to have your support. You just need to relax and see I will always help you." He does not yet grasp how his self-sufficiency is a danger cue for Jessica.

Jessica retorts, "Yup – and unfortunately, the more you hold back, the more I push or walk away and stew in silence. I just wish you'd open up more. I am living with a stranger most of the time! I know you are stressed but you won't let me help!" She does not yet understand how her pushing him to open up is a danger cue for Wayne.

Move 1 reflection of their distancing dance is accurate but not sufficient to help them fully engage with how their fears and distress create and are created by their cycle of interaction. Emily deepens their experience with Move 2, first with one and then the other. With Wayne, she assembles his emotion as they have done before, this time deliberately more slowly, pausing with each response to check if he is engaged. He sees a look of fatigue on Jessica's face, he feels his gut tighten, he disappears into his computer, wishing she didn't push herself so hard. This time as Emily assembles his emotion, Wayne can touch the tightness in his stomach and hear what this tightness says (his core fear), "I'm just not quite what she wants or needs. I'll never make her happy. It's a lonely place. I tell her to take better care of herself; I never ask her to care for me – that is my job."

Emily shapes an encounter for Wayne to disclose his core sense of rejection and loneliness, particularly wanting to protect Jessica and feeling he constantly fails to protect her and keep her safe from exhaustion and overwork, and to own that he does indeed hold back from her. In this encounter, he adds that taking care of his own needs and being guarded is simply his lifelong survival strategy as a Black man in a white-dominant society. Emily's Move 3, slowly shaping an encounter from Wayne to Jessica, deepens their grasp of their cycle. Though still unhappy with the distance between them, Jessica is beginning to grasp how his holding back is not abandoning her. She trusts, just a little more, that he is totally committed to her and holding her in his heart. Together they are grasping more clearly how their core distress comes from "the more you, the more I" pattern of pushing and stepping back/stepping back and pushing. Emily also assembles Jessica's emotional reactions with Move 2, followed by a Move 3 encounter where Jessica discloses to Wayne her vulnerable fear of "not mattering" that drives her into her agitated pushing and gloomy silence.

When a therapist sees a marker that partners in EFCT are in the process of stabilizing yet do not fully own or recognize how they contribute to the pattern or how they get pulled into it, they repeat Moves 2 and 3. There is value in doing this rerun of Moves 2 and 3 in slow motion to help each client, in turn, share what it is that threatens them and triggers them to get pulled into the cycle, to own their action tendencies in the cycle, and to share the underlying fears driving their moves, at a deeper, more emotionally engaged manner in an encounter with their significant other. In this *rerun* of assembly, deepening, and direct encounters, partners access a deeper felt sense of this dynamic cycle as the real problem. With Move 4, the therapist helps them to process and linger in this deeper acknowledgment of their cyclic dynamic.

Analogously, in EFIT, a therapist may see a marker that a client is *stabilizing*, yet does not *fully recognize at an experiential level* (a minimum of Level 4 on the EXP scale) *how* their processes of emotion regulation "prime and maintain their symptoms (e.g., depression, anxiety, traumatic stress) and how these recurring patterns shape their inner emotional worlds and prototypical patterns of engagement with others" (Johnson & Campbell, 2022, p. 124). The therapist then follows this marker with Moves 2, 3, and 4 to bring this process into fuller awareness and engages the client to experience themselves as an active participant in this pattern, thereby evoking hope and agency.

Emily uses Moves 2, 3, and 4 to expand Max's initial grasp of the pattern as the problem. Max recognizes that his pattern of avoidance leaves him "trapped in dissonance." He describes, "My shame compels me to say one thing to look good, but I know I am the one who drove the street-racing car when Léo was killed." His chest tightens at the image of his dead friend at the scene of the accident. He wants to wipe it from his memory, as he has done for decades. Emily shapes an encounter for Max to tell his deceased friend, Léo, "I have spent decades downplaying my responsibility, to keep from feeling the absolute anguish that what I did resulted in your death and my trauma of going to jail." Helping Max to own this action tendency in an encounter with Léo helps Max to engage more deeply with his automatic pattern of suppression and denial, moving more fully toward grasping how his pattern of avoidance is the problem.

Question 6 and Markers of Stabilization: Readiness for Stage 2

Therapist Question: *Does my client (couple or individual) fully grasp their pattern as the problem, by owning their triggers, their immediate bodily sense of threat, their automatic action tendencies, the meanings they make, and the core underlying fears driving them?* (If so, this is client Step 4 stabilization. Client Step 4 is the gradually evolving Stage 1 de-escalation /stabilization change event where client(s) identify their specific repetitive pattern as the problem. It is a marker of readiness for Stage 2.)

Markers of Stabilization

In EFCT, markers of stabilization (detailed in Box 8.2) are more specific than getting along better and being kinder and softer with one another, although that is part of it. In stabilization, partners have a felt sense of how their distress stems from their self-protective pattern which has become automatic and rigid. They have an experiential grasp of how their actions threaten their partner, triggering self-protective actions that threaten them and set in motion a repetitive and self-reinforcing pattern of danger fuelled by specific attachment fears of abandonment or rejection. They grasp their typical protective pattern and are ready to begin Stage 2.

In EFIT stabilization, a client is emotionally balanced and open to explore more of their frightening, unfamiliar and/or unacceptable inner and interpersonal emotional experience. They are more aware of how their self-protective patterns fuel more fear and distress, and more ineffective responses from others. (Markers of stabilization in EFIT are detailed in Box 8.3.)

Sahra describes a growing sense of calm and hopefulness:

> I feel like I am starting to get myself back again. My lethargy and darkness seemed to come out of nowhere and I felt anxious and weighed down most of the time. Now, I've made sense of how hard I have worked to ignore my trauma and losses! I see that they were not all my fault. I see there is not something wrong with me as much as that I am grieving – and angry too at Fahrhad (her former abusive partner). I know I need more [imaginal] conversations with him but just having had that first [imaginal] conversation has left me feeling so much better!

Following Markers of Stabilization and Readiness for Stage 2

To follow these markers into Stage 2, a therapist will use Move 5 to integrate, heighten, and celebrate this Stage 1 change, remembering that stabilization/de-escalation "is only halfway home. ... [U]nless a positive cycle of bonding is created, then the risk of relapse remains high. De-escalation is the essential precursor to the second stage of EFT, restructuring attachment" (Johnson, 2020, p. 146).

Using Move 5, the therapist repeats the emerging new views of self and other, linking them to the newly accessed vulnerable, core emotions that had previously been hidden in the self-protective cycle. The therapist also describes the value of staying in therapy to restructure attachment, so that in EFCT, partners together can calm each other's fears and meet one another's needs, and in both EFCT and EFIT, clients can create a positive interaction pattern that will build cycles of growing safety and security.

Conclusion

In this chapter, I examine markers that situate clients on the ever-evolving terrain of Stage 1 change and how EFT therapists can follow these markers with moves of the EFT Tango. After EFT therapists, see clear markers of stabilization, they are on the lookout for doorways into Stage 2. In the next chapter, I point to markers to follow into Stage 2 and to continue to situate your clients on the landscape of Stage 2 change.

14 Recognizing and Following Markers on the EFT Stage 2 Terrain

Client markers of change through the transformative change events of Stage 2 are outlined in this chapter. These markers are built on the foundation of the micro-markers of emotion, the heart of change in EFT, and the markers of Stage 1 change, outlined in the previous two chapters. The art and science of EFT (Johnson & Brubacher, 2016) lies in practicing the attuned micro-skills of the EFT Tango through Stage 1 stabilization and the empirically validated Stage 2 steps that lead to lasting change.

To further build on the metaphor of inuksuit across the vast arctic, these Stage 2 markers leading to lasting change could be likened to a special kind of inuksuk, known as *inuksuapik,* found at

> places where people have waited...It's at the waiting places where you can sometimes find an *inuksuapik,* ... the most beautiful kind of inuksuk. It is built with the greatest care, and its shape, as well as the color or texture of the stones, causes it to stand out from all the others. (Hallendy, p. 27)

I present client markers on the terrain of Stage 2 change and therapist questions in search of these markers (Box 14.1), beginning with a therapist's search for markers to follow to enter Stage 2. A discussion of the micro-elements of Stage 2 change precedes four more therapist questions in

---

Box 14.1   Markers to Situate Clients on the Terrain of Stage 2 and Therapist Questions in Search of These Markers

Markers of Emotional Handles for Entry into Stage 2: What emotional handle can be used to open the doorway into Stage 2? (Stage 2 begins with client Step 5.)

Markers to Shape Encounter to Disclose Core Fear: What indicates that the client is ready to disclose their clearly distilled core fear and longing or need from a place of deep engagement? (client Step 5)

Markers to Promote Acceptance from the Recipient of Their Partner's New Position and Newly Disclosed Fear or Longing: What indicates it is time to promote acceptance from the recipient of a partner's new position and newly disclosed fear or longing? (Recipient, is the partner in EFCT, and in EFIT is the one to whom the core fear or longing is disclosed. (Step 6)

Markers to Shape the Unique *Request Encounter*: What indicates a client is ready to make the unique Step 7 reach-and-request to meet attachment needs? (Step 7)

Markers to Invite a Response to the Step 7 Reach/Request: What indicates it is time to process the Step 7 request by facilitating responding and receiving?

DOI: 10.4324/9781003242673-20

search of markers of readiness: (1) to shape an encounter for a client to disclose their core fear; (2) to promote acceptance from the one to whom the fear was disclosed; (3) to shape the unique *request-encounter,* the apex of Stage 2; and finally (4) to invite a response to this request. The Stage 2 markers are as beautiful and as tenderly shaped as *inuksuapik,* standing out as markers of newly emerging safety and security.

Question 1 and Markers of Emotional Handles for Entry into Stage 2

Therapist Question: *Can I find a marker of core emotion on the leading edge – an emotional handle to open the doorway into Stage 2?* (Client begins Step 5 by experiencing, distilling, and deepening core fears and longings.)

To guide a client into Step 5, the beginning of Stage 2, the therapist confirms the client's decreased reactivity and emotional balance, and then looks for markers of the core fears identified in Stage 1. Following are the three markers pointing to core emotion on the leading edge as doorways into Stage 2.

Markers of Emotional Handles and How to Follow Them into Stage 2

A first marker of core emotion on the leading edge is *a client's expressed readiness to terminate therapy.* A de-escalated partner might say, "Things are better than ever. I think we can end therapy." This can, but need not, be a discouraging marker for a new EFT therapist. Couples are typically pleased to reach de-escalation, and sometimes not very eager to return to exploring their attachment panic. Individual clients might appreciate the stabilization and prefer to leave the *frightening, and/or alien and unacceptable* emotion in the background.

To follow the marker of suggested termination, an EFT therapist normalizes and processes the comment, savoring the moment with them, and exploring their hesitancy to continue. With Move 1, in EFCT, a therapist will validate and evoke how a couple has changed their relationship, or in EFIT, how an individual has decreased their symptoms. Reflecting how hard they are working to avoid getting sucked back into old patterns, the therapist paints a clear picture of their specific story and the strategies they are employing. Frequently, this will include some variation of a withdrawer accommodating much of what the pursuer wants and the pursuer striving to be softer and more tolerant. While engaging in some Move 5 summary and celebration of their much-improved relationship, the therapist also describes that it might be effortful to maintain, and that without deeper shifts to their underlying fears, the old pattern is likely to resurface. The therapist can also remind them of the underlying fears which they identified but have not yet shifted, such as a withdrawer's fear of letting their partner down again and a pursuer's fear of having such enormous needs that might eventually push their partner to leave them.

The therapist lets them know that they can continue this path forward and come to an even safer and more stable place. She plants the seeds of a secure bond, where partners are freer to be themselves, perhaps more of the persons they initially fell in love with, freer to make mistakes and to be vulnerable and imperfect, freer to give and receive comfort and care without holding their breaths that this current good place might vanish. This discussion frequently opens the door into Stage 2, but if it does not, the therapist respects a couple's choice to terminate and keeps the door open for them to return later.

Analogously with EFIT clients, a therapist validates the growth and stability which a client has achieved, while also planting seeds of the possibilities of traveling further on this path of change, toward their initial goals. The therapist describes moving beyond symptom reduction to a more resilient, competent sense of self and more secure and meaningful interpersonal connections.

A second marker of core emotion is slightly paradoxical. This marker is *the absence of core emotion in a more withdrawn partner* in EFCT, or in EFIT, *a down-regulating individual's flat affect*. To follow this marker, the therapist can comment directly with Move 1 tracking and conjecture. "That old familiar pattern of going blank or feeling nothing that often shows up to protect you, seems to be taking over just now." The therapist can also seek to evoke an emotional handle by reviewing clinical notes to recall words and images that the avoidant client used earlier to describe their core emotion. Recalling these images and emotional handles can prime the therapist to be finely tuned to the verbal and non-verbal micro processes and bodily cues of emotion to track, reflect, and evoke in the present moment. If core emotion cannot be evoked through repeating images or tracking somatic cues, a therapist can make an explicit invitation, such as, "Can we go back to that dread you expressed last time?" To evoke that dread, the therapist can replay the typical *trigger* for a partner's typical withdrawal and defense or an individual's automatic strategy of minimizing and suppressing. Replaying the trigger is likely to evoke the felt sense of dread and panic expressed in previous sessions.

Recalling previously felt core emotion, a therapist says, "Last session, I asked if we might come back to the fatigue that you described around trying relentlessly to be enough, and the rock in your gut, heavy with the fear that one day you will wake up to find there is nothing left of you? Can we go back there?" After bringing the withdrawing partner's or stoic individual's core emotion to life again, the therapist will engage and expand the experience with Move 2, entering a doorway into Stage 2.

A third marker of core emotion for a doorway into Stage 2 is a *withdrawn partner or avoidant individual hinting at or touching briefly on their core emotion, and then suddenly exiting or being interrupted* by their partner in EFCT. The core fear identified in Step 3 that typically drives the automatic action tendencies of withdrawal, defense, or minimizing is so briefly expressed that it is easy for a therapist to miss, but a partner notices. Frequently, this core emotion is some variation of fearing rejection or annihilation, often including exhaustion from striving to keep the peace, to avoid accusations, and to gain approval or appreciation.

Emily nearly misses a hint of Ella's core fear before Sophie interrupts her. In de-escalating their cycle, Sophie has heard how exhausted Ella is with trying to second guess her demands and is being much kinder. Ella, who has acknowledged she does get secretive at times to avoid upsetting Sophie, timidly ventures, "It is still hard to tell her when I talk with my sister." Emily misses that hint of Ella's core fear of "being annihilated and having nothing left of me" before Sophie reacts with a harsh outburst. Sophie reacts to Ella's hint of fearing her getting upset faster than Emily realizes that Ella is hinting at her own fear. She steps in to catch the bullet of Sophie's reaction. Since the couple has stabilized, Sophie also sees what happened and sits back and chuckles at the drama. "She is afraid about my getting harsh and squashing her down and I just did it! Voilà – the dance!" With some Move 5, Emily summarizes what just happened, heightening their capacity to see and stop the cycle. She then returns to the emotional handle of Ella's hint of fear, and with Move 2, assembles and deepens this fear of upsetting Sophie. They move into Stage 2, where Ella deepens and discloses her fears and grief, and assertive anger about living in this relationship where she is constantly guarding herself from Sophie's explosions.

For a client living in a context of oppression and marginalization, the threat of annihilation and exhaustion at trying to stay safe is an ongoing reality. Sahra's fearful-avoidant strategy has helped her survive numerous traumatic events, including her abuse from her father and an ex-partner, and the ongoing *subtle acts of exclusion* (Jana & Baran, 2020) as a black immigrant woman in the workplace. Her highs of anxiety and lethargy of depression are stabilizing, and she is finding emotional balance. As she describes her joy at a senior physician requesting her opinion and expertise, she makes a quick reference to "all those other times!" and starts to wring her hands and look down, then smiles at Emily and says, "This physician is so great to work with!" To follow this brief hint of core emotion into Stage 2, Emily engages with Move 2, tracking Sahra's quick smile after a briefly pained face and twisting hands. With Move 2, Emily assembles Sahra's meanings, the bodily felt sense, and the emerging action tendencies of the painful core emotion in "all those other times" when colleagues have dismissed her expertise. Cruel messages of being called "that girl" and questions about whether she is a real doctor re-surface and she is flooded with outrage! Emily assembles her pain – the core anger, deep sadness, dread, and fears. In particular, Emily attunes to this core anger in her social pain of discrimination and exclusion that Sahra is quick to dismiss.

As with Sahra, in EFCT there is likely to be some core (non-reactive) assertive anger mixed with vulnerability as a withdrawn partner brings themself more fully into the relationship. The therapist will linger with the core emotion – moving around in it and heightening the felt experience – working on the leading edge of the partner's experience, reflecting, evoking and conjecturing to expand the felt sense and meaning of this core fear or pain.

In summary, to move into Stage 2, when clients are stabilized, therapists can follow one of the three markers of core emotion discussed above: Expressed readiness to terminate therapy; client's flat affect or absence of emotion; or a brief expression of core emotion followed by a rapid exit or interruption. These three markers are emotional handles to turn to open the doorway into Stage 2.

Stage 2 Micro-elements

Before describing markers to follow through the Stage 2 engagement and softening change events, I briefly comment on the nature of Stage 2 change. Stage 2 change events contain "set steps or microelements" (Johnson, 2019, p. 33; see Box 14.2). These micro-elements of Stage 2 change in EFCT are also referred to as two rounds of client Steps 5, 6, and 7 (Johnson, 2019, 2020), with the more withdrawn partner in a pursue-withdraw dynamic taking the lead. The engagement change event precedes a softening change event; however, there can be some reciprocal flow between partners in the early part of Stage 2. Thus, it is important to prioritize being responsive to the clients' processes and being flexible. Increasing openness from withdrawn partners, at times, elicits softening moments from typically critical partners, and softer openness from typically demanding partners encourages more engaging from a more withdrawn partner. Steps 5 and 6 exploration and encounters may be intertwined between withdrawers and pursuers; however when it comes to the final change-event reaches of engagement and softening (EFCT Step 7), the engagement change event from a withdrawn partner needs to precede a softening.

Concomitantly, in EFIT, a client needs expanded intrapsychic engagement with their own emotional experiencing before participating in a softening change event. For Stage 2 EFIT encounters, engagement and assertive reaches precede softenings toward self and toward select others (Johnson, 2019).

Emily knows of the importance of Moves 2, 3, and 4 to assemble, shape, and process corrective emotional experiences in Stage 2. Each client needs to be guided to assemble and linger more deeply with their core underlying fear to discover the core attachment need embedded in that fear and to ask directly to have that need met by their attachment figure or relevant other (a partner in EFCT or an imaginal other, part of self, or the therapist in EFIT). A response from the one to whom the request is made is processed immediately, followed by processing the client's reception and integration of that response.

Box 14.2   Micro-elements of Stage 2

As detailed in Part III, Stage 2 change events "contain set steps or microelements" (Johnson, 2019, p. 33). The micro-elements of Stage 2 in EFCT change are also referred to as two rounds of Steps 5, 6, and 7– (Johnson, 2004, 2019, 2020).

Step 5 – Distill, Deepen, Disclose (experiencing partner): In the first part of Stage 2, using Move 2, the therapist guides one partner at a time to engage deeply in *experiencing* the most intrapsychic part of the model and to take the client's Step 5 of the EFT change process (to distill and deepen engagement with core emotions and disowned needs and parts of self). Then with Move 3, the therapist shapes an encounter for the *experiencing* partner to disclose these core fears and needs clearly to the observing partner.

Step 6 (observing partner): After core fears and longings are shared, with Move 4, the therapist processes with the experiencing partner, how it was to share this, and with the observing partner, how it was to receive this new message. Then with Move 3, the therapist invites a response from the receiving partner, helping them take to their Step 6 of processing and responding to this newly formulated expression from their partner. Genuine responding is facilitated, acceptance is encouraged, and authenticity, if acceptance is weak or absent, is validated.

Step 7 – Reach and Request (experiencing partner): The therapist will use Move 2 to help the experiencing partner access needs from within their core emotion and to risk asserting needs and making a request to their partner. Reaching toward their partner to ask for their attachment needs can be an assertive reach from a previously withdrawn partner (the engagement change event), or a vulnerable reach from a pursuing partner (the softening change event).

The authentic Reaches to Request, Respond, and Receive between partners culminate in the engagement and softening change events. They are shaped with the interventions of Moves 3 and 4, and integrated and solidified with Move 5.

In EFIT, these micro-elements are less distinct, just as the boundaries between stages of client change are somewhat more fluid in EFIT than in EFCT. In both modalities, stabilization is needed for the deeper Stage 2 work; however, additional Stage 1 change can occur during Stage 2 change. Additionally, in EFIT, restructuring happens across multiple relationships. Stage 1 exploration (within/between/in context) potentiates further restructuring. Although patterns across relationships frequently share parallel dynamics, all Stage 2 restructuring does not generalize to all relationships, and clients may benefit from some revisits to Stage 1.

Question 2 and Markers to Shape an Encounter to Disclose Core Fear

Therapist Question: *What marker indicates a client is ready to disclose their core fear from a place of engagement?* (Client Step 5 is distilling and deepening engagement with formerly disowned core fears, longings, needs and parts of self, and disclosing this in an engaged encounter.)

Markers of Readiness to Disclose Core Fear

Non-verbal markers and expressed bodily felt sensations and images are key markers that granular, expanded core emotion is alive, fully felt in the present moment, and ready to be disclosed. The other marker of readiness to choreograph a Step 5 encounter is that the core emotion is fully distilled and coherently meaningful. (Research suggests that for these Step 5 encounters of sharing core fears, the depth of emotional experiencing is at a minimum Level 4 on the EXP scale for withdrawers and at Level 5 for pursuers. See Tables 9.1 and 10.1.)

Following Markers of Fully Alive, Clearly Distilled, Core Emotion

To follow markers of core emotion being online and distilled, therapists use Move 3 to sharpen a message with the client to share this fear. Then they heighten the bodily felt sense of the fear, help the client to anticipate the experience of disclosing it, maintaining safety and a sense of risk at a high level of emotional experiencing, and direct the client to present the message of this core fear while it is alive and fully felt. Chapters 9 and 10 describe and illustrate these encounters. There are likely to be numerous encounters for clients to take Step 5, as the therapist helps them to deepen, bring to life, and disclose clearly distilled and formulated fears, longings, and needs.

Question 3 and the Marker to Promote Acceptance from Recipient

Therapist Question: *What indicates it is time to promote acceptance of a new position and a newly disclosed fear or longing and to help a receiving client to take Step 6?* (Client Step 6 is expanding ways of relating and accepting or struggling to accept this "new person.")

Marker of New Position

The marker to promote acceptance of a newly disclosed position is rather simple. It is a partner or individual client taking a newly assertive or softened position and disclosing their core attachment fear and longing or need (a Step 5 disclosure). This disclosure marks a tangible felt shift in the room. A formerly withdrawn partner or individual client asserts previously hidden parts of self while exuding a newly engaged, congruent presence. A formerly critical, pursuing partner or hyperactivating individual authentically and vulnerably expresses core emotions and needs, conveying a new, soft, openness.

Following the Marker of a Newly Disclosed Position

Following this marker of a newly disclosed position, with Move 4, the EFT therapist validates the newly disclosed position, processing with the discloser how it was to share and with the recipient how it was to receive this newly expanded, assertive, or vulnerable disclosure of fears and longings. The therapist seeks to promote acceptance in the recipient of this newly disclosed position, thereby helping the recipient to take Step 6. The recipient in EFCT is the partner, and in EFIT, is the one to whom the core fear and longing or need was disclosed. The therapist is also prepared to offer empathy for disorientation or difficulty accepting "the new" and to validate them for their authenticity and nonacceptance.

Some partners and imaginal others will be accessible, responsive, and comforting, while others may be hostile or dismissive. When a recipient responds with negativity, disbelief or disorientation, an EFT therapist will use the tracking and reframing micro-intervention of *catching the bullet* in Move 4 processing. In each case, with partners in EFCT and in EFIT with imaginal others or part of self, a client's connection to the other is explored and emotion is expanded. New meanings and ways of interacting evolve. For example, in EFIT, when an imaginal parent responds negatively, this "enables a client to move into asserting their need, accepting their loss, and taking a new position with this internalized parent. Asserting an emotion with another also deepens engagement with this emotion and allows it to be integrated" (Johnson & Campbell, 2022, p. 83).

With couples and with individuals, the encounters in Stage 2 can have many repetitions with increasing levels of depth, from Levels 5–7 on the EXP scale (Klein et al., 1986). After processing with Move 4, the therapist will typically, with Move 3, shape an encounter for the recipient to respond. Growing warmth and affiliation with others emerges through a series of encounters. In EFIT, when an imaginal other does not respond with kindness or is an unsafe other from whom no response is evoked, the client develops increasing confidence to discriminate others who can be trusted, from those who cannot be trusted and must be kept at a distance.

Examples of New Position and Following this Marker

A Withdrawer's Newly Assertive Position. In his Step 5, Wayne offers a clear expression of the pain and exhaustion of hiding and holding back, and the fears of falling short of the mark and hurting Jessica. He says:

> I am exhausted with tiptoeing and trying to be good enough for you! I want to stop feeling so inept in your eyes. Exhausted from holding back — so afraid to count on you because I am so certain I will lose you, and then I don't know what I'd do!

After processing with Wayne how it was to share this with Jessica, Emily follows the marker of his new disclosure to explore Jessica's experience in hearing this (Jessica's Step 6). She asks, "Jessica, what happens inside when Wayne speaks up to share his exhaustion and fear of losing you?" Then she supports Jessica with Move 3 to share her authentic response with Wayne.

A Pursuer's Newly Vulnerable Position. After Wayne completes Step 7 and steps courageously into the relationship, Jessica offers a vulnerable disclosure of her fear of disconnection and abandonment. "I am afraid he'll disappear again. I get into a sheer panic, and then I lash out, before going silent! So afraid he will disappear again!" (View of other.) Her fear of reaching shifts to unworthiness and shame. "I am desperate for you to reach out for me. I am so ashamed of how much I need you! I have this embarrassingly huge need for closeness. I feel ashamed, humiliated!" (View of self.) This Step 5 disclosure of her distilled fear and shame is a marker for a Step 6 exploration of the observing partner's experience.

To follow this marker, Emily elicits Wayne's experience, "What happens for you to hear Jessica's fear that you will disappear again?" and later, "How is it for you to hear Jessica's humiliation at owning how much she needs you?" This processing (Move 4) helps Wayne take his Step 6 of sharing how he is experiencing this "newly-disclosed Jessica." Emily shapes an encounter for Wayne to respond directly to Jessica.

An EFIT Client's Newly Asserted Position. Sahra vulnerably and assertively addresses an image of her estranged father:

> I am terrified I wasn't enough for you! That we lost a place in your heart as your precious ones. You stole all my safety the day you left! You broke my heart. I deserved to have you in my life! How dare you to have left the way you did?

After evoking how it was for Sahra to disclose this to her imaginal father, Emily evokes, "Sahra, how do you imagine your father responding to you as you share your broken heart and assert,

'I deserved to have you in my life. You had no right to leave like you did!'?" She may also invite Sahra to respond as if from her imaginal father - in his voice."

Additional examples of facilitating responses to these newly disclosed positions are detailed in Chapters 9 and 10.

Question 4 and Markers to Shape the Unique *Request* Encounter

Therapist Question: *What markers indicate it is time to shape the Step 7 reach and request to have attachment needs met?* (Client Step 7 is reaching to make a specific request for attachment needs to be met. Step 7 marks the big change events of engagement and softening: Risking reaching and requesting what they need to meet their attachment needs.)

Markers of Readiness to Shape the Unique Request Encounter

Therapists new to EFT frequently find it challenging to take the directive stance of shaping an encounter for a client to risk making a direct request of another to meet their core attachment need, thereby facilitating clients to take Step 7. Familiarity with the markers of readiness for Step 7 can lend confidence to therapists to direct this important step. Included here are three markers of readiness to persist with inviting the Step 7 reach/request. Many of the examples given are EFCT, though a similar process of requesting to have attachment needs met is followed in EFIT.

A Lack of Awareness of Needs. The first marker to follow is *a lack of awareness of needs* in the experiencing partner or in an individual client. The client might express their core emotion from Step 5 (e.g., fear of rejection, of being annihilated, of abandonment, of loss), but have no present-moment felt sense of their attachment needs and longings embedded in that fear. There might be no sense of how their partner or relevant other could help to soothe this fear.

Micro-interventions to Access the Need. Heighten and savor the core emotion until awareness of the need emerges. Since core emotion is a reliable source of information about needs, the therapist ensures the core emotion is "online," and then evokes the longings and needs embedded in that emotion with evocative questions, reflections, heightening, and empathic conjectures, as exemplified below.

A therapist's capacity to evoke longings and needs is enhanced by having a comprehension of the longings frequently embedded in core emotion: Fears of rejection and being found inadequate imply longings for reassurance and acceptance. Feeling unwanted can evoke a longing for reassurance that one is wanted, desired, needed. Shame and emptiness can call forth a longing for acceptance and assurance of worth. Fears of abandonment and unworthiness imply longings for comfort, reassurance, and connection.

Examples of Micro-Skills to Access Needs with a Withdrawer.

- Evocative questions: "Feeling the tightness of that fear right now in your chest, what do you long for?" or, "How could your partner help you with that fear?"
- Reflection: "You said, 'I am afraid to look in their eyes. I am afraid they will judge me.'"
- Conjecture: "Almost as though you are longing for their acceptance or reassurance that it really is *you* they want, is that it?"

- A *seeding attachment* conjecture can also be used to heighten attachment fears and to evoke and heighten the unmet longings for a safe response from the partner: "You couldn't imagine reaching and finding that they want you totally, just as you are! It feels so foreign to let them see how crumbly and imperfect you feel when you've lived so long thinking that they just wanted you to be a superhero? You can't imagine them welcoming the real you!"

Examples of Micro-Skills to Access Needs with a Pursuer.

- Heightening is used to bring the attachment fear to a *boiling point* (Bradley & Furrow, 2004), and from this most intense fear (EXP Levels 5–7), the needs are accessed.
- Evocative question: "In that place where you feel so small and unworthy…" (Therapist touches their own heart, the place where the pursuer has located this bodily felt sense.) "What do you long for from them? How can they help you with that fear of being unlovable?"
- Conjecture: "Almost as though you are saying," (in proxy voice) "'I get terrified at how big my need is. I long for you to hold me and assure me I am a good person, worthy of your love.' Is that it?"

After a partner (withdrawer or pursuer) accesses their attachment need, the therapist heightens it and then prompts the partner to risk asking their partner to meet this need. Similarly in EFIT, a request is made to a potentially responsive, imaginal other, to a part of self, or to the therapist.

A Clearly Expressed Attachment Need or Longing. A second marker to follow to invite the Step 7 reach and request is a clearly expressed attachment need or longing. To follow this marker, the therapist repeats, reflects, and ensures the emotional experience is fully *online*, and then explicitly invites the experiencing partner to directly ask their partner to meet this need.

Examples of Inviting the Reach/Request with Withdrawing Partners. Heighten the growing sense of entitlement and longing to have a place in this relationship; to be seen and heard and truly wanted. While this core emotion is *online*, invite the client to step toward their partner or significant other, and to ask to have their needs met. To a withdrawer who has identified needs for acceptance and appreciation, from their female partner, the therapist might inquire:

Can you ask her to help you – to stop berating you and show you appreciation? Can you ask her to reassure you that it is safe to depend on her? That despite all your slip-ups and fears of letting her down, it is really *you* she wants?

To a withdrawer who has identified needs from a male partner, the therapist might say:

Can you tell him, "I long to be enough for you. Can you assure me that I deserve you? I need to know there is some margin for error. I want to feel safe committing to you and to know you won't give up on me!" Can you turn and ask him for this reassurance?

Example of Inviting the Reach/Request with Pursuing Partners. Heighten the fear, and when the fear is *at a boil*, invite the reach for example by saying:

So afraid he won't find you acceptable if you show who you really are. So afraid that you look pathetic and needy, and he won't want to comfort you. Can you risk it? Can you see he is leaning towards you just now? Can you take the leap, right now, to ask if he can accept you like this?

Examples of Inviting the Reach/Request with an EFIT Client. With an adult longing for her mother's acceptance, the therapist might say:

> So terrified that she wanted a different daughter, that you were never quite the one she wanted. You are trembling just now. Can you ask her, can you ask her if she can accept you for you? Can you ask her if she truly loves you as you are to-day? Can you take the risk to ask her?

With a trans individual who has identified needs to an imaginal parent, the therapist might ask:

> Can you look at this image of your father and can you tell him, "I need to know you see I am worthy of your love! I have a right to have a father loving me and believing in me! I know you are disappointed with my transitioning, but this is the real me! Can you see that I am your worthy and competent child? Can you please welcome me home?"

A Tentative Reach for Support. A third marker to follow to invite the Step 7 reach is an experiencing partner or individual client making a *tentative* reach for support or reassurance. The therapist's task in response to a tentative reach is to track, reflect, and validate the hesitancy. Heighten the courage it takes to make this reach. Validate the bravery required to take the leap of faith that the other will respond. Encourage them to repeat the tentative request, validating the courage, and the significance of this very important new step of risking to reach and to ask for what they need to meet their attachment need. This is also a good time to seed attachment to encourage and heighten the longings for a warm and supportive response.

The above three markers of readiness to invite the Step 7 reach are offered, recognizing that therapists and observing partners alike might wish to save the client from this vulnerable moment. An observing partner might introject, "It's all right—you don't need to ask. I get the message." Knowing, however, that risking to reach and receive an engaged response is the transformative antidote to a client's greatest fear, an EFT therapist is careful to block such interruptions and to insistently and supportively prompt the reach. This interpersonal risk to reach and receive the needed response (Client Step 7) creates the supreme bonding moments of EFCT.

Analogously in EFIT, the direction to request a specific attachment need from a safe, imaginal other, a part of self, or the therapist, creates a transformative corrective emotional experience as exemplified in Chapters 9 and 10. Risking to ask is empowering precisely because so much is at stake. Being caught when in free-fall is life changing.

Question 5 and Markers to Invite a Response to the Request

Therapist Question: *When do I choreograph a response to the Step 7 reach?* (Client Step 7 is completed with Move 4 to help the client process and integrate the response they receive from their partner or relevant other.)

Marker to Invite a Response to the Request

The basic marker to invite a response to the Step 7 reach, if it is not offered spontaneously, is very simple. The reach itself is the marker that an immediate response is needed. The other marker is the momentum of emotion. The risk to reach and request what vulnerable, fully alive, core attachment emotion tells a client they need from this significant other is akin to being in free-fall. An attuned therapist can feel the urgency of this emotional risk calling for an immediate response from the partner in EFCT and from the *other* in EFIT. Of course, when the imaginal other in EFIT is an unsafe other, then the request will be an assertive boundary to stay at a distance and a response will not be elicited.

Following the Marker of the Request

Stay with the momentum of emotion and immediately invite an emotionally engaged response from the partner in EFCT, and in EFIT, to invite the client to describe the imagined response they are experiencing. If an EFIT request was directed to the therapist, the therapist will respond. For example, with soft, direct eye contact, Emily says to Max:

> Yes, I am eager to assure you that I also see your kind gardener heart. I am touched that you took the risk to ask me for this assurance. I have great respect for your honesty and how you have survived so many years, feeling like a monster-in-a-box without access to your kind gardener heart. Your kind heart is a big part of who I experience you to be and the place from which you are relating to your ex-partner amidst all your grief.

In EFCT, a client's Step 7 encounter can look different coming from a withdrawing partner or a pursuing partner. A withdrawer steps into the relationship with assertive vulnerability and asks for what they need to remain engaged, typically for acceptance and less judgment. A pursuer reaches from a newly vulnerable position to ask for what they need to feel safe and secure in the relationship, typically for reassurance of the other's continued presence and assurance of their own goodness in their partner's eyes.

Moves 4 and 5 are used to process and heighten this new bonding moment for each partner in EFCT, or the shifts to newly experienced safe and secure views of self and other in EFIT. Markers of readiness to move into Stage 3 (Chapter 11) will emerge as these key change events are summarized and integrated.

Conclusion

Emily is increasingly valuing these simple 11 questions in search or markers of client change in Stage 1 (Chapter 13) and in Stage 2 (this chapter). She recognizes with increasing ease how this rich set of markers reliably orients her to where on the map of EFT change her clients are and how her flowing with the EFT Tango and its micro-skills will continue to guide her couple and individual clients along this path toward secure connections and emotional fitness. The additional element supporting her to follow the EFT model is that of expanding her capacity to spot client's somatic signals and other markers of emotional experiencing, together with deepen her own bodily felt-sensing (Chapter 12), bringing her experience of EFT to be one of an artistic, empathic, attuned flow – repeating and adding steps like a Tango dancer.

In this and the previous two chapters, the process of EFT as a scientific and artistic endeavor coalesces. Together, micro-markers of emotional experiencing and markers of the steps and stages of client change can be reference points in the complex emotional landscape, like *inuksuit,* the human-shaped stone markers in the vast arctic. The markers explored throughout these three chapters orient EFT therapists to clients' multi-dimensional emotional landscape and precise moment-to-moment experiences, so that, like Hallendy in the arctic, they find that the more clearly they recognize these markers of emotion and change processes, the more reliable they become as "reference points from which [to] depart and return with confidence" (Hallendy, 2000, p. 22).

The EFT resources reviewed in Chapters 12–14 are: following micro-moments of clients' cultural and emotional experience; listening to the therapist's inner felt sensing; situating clients on the EFT map of change; and fine-tuning facility with the EFT macro-intervention (the EFT Tango) and its micro-skills. To practice the art and science of EFT, an EFT therapist draws on: A culturally humble, curious, and creative capacity to resonate with a felt sense of the clients' present moment experience; knowledge of the steps and stages of client change; and a grasp of how to attune and shape change with the EFT macro-intervention and its micro-skills.

Part V

Commonly Experienced Impasses in EFT

Introduction to Part V

Commonly Experienced Impasses in EFT

While mastering the basics of the EFT model, you are likely to discover that it can be challenging indeed to face the many different nuances and complexities that each couple or individual brings to therapy. Two specific issues that frequently create complications and can block relationship repair in EFCT and impede progress in EFIT are addictive processes and relationship-specific injuries, defined as attachment injuries. Both create relationship trauma and pose a serious threat to the security of a couple's attachment bond, and to meaningful connections and a sense of belonging for individual clients. They make Stage 1 stabilization very challenging and block Stage 2 restructuring.

Consistent with earlier sections, EFCT is presented first, followed by parallels to EFIT when relevant. An EFT therapist seeks to be attuned for potential signs of addictive behaviors or attachment injuries that are likely to create an impasse in therapy if they are left unaddressed. I hope to increase your awareness and comfort with assessing for and working explicitly, first with addictive behaviors as *faux* attachments (Flores, 2004) in Chapter 15 and, second, with relationship-specific attachment injuries in Chapter 16.

The manner in which an EFT therapist works with the challenges of addictive processes and the resolution of attachment injuries is similar to all EFT work, together with the additional sensitivity required for working with trauma. Given the likelihood of trauma in the background of addictive processes (Giordano, 2022; Maté, 2010) and the traumatic nature of attachment injuries, the therapist needs a clear focus on being empathically attuned with unconditional acceptance. There is no separate chapter devoted to EFT and trauma in this book, essentially because as Johnson maintains, EFT therapists do not work differently with trauma; however, they work more slowly, simply, softly, and more sensitively attuned to the client and to their window of tolerance (Johnson, 2002).

An EFT therapist needs the genuine acceptance of a collaborative stance combined with curiosity and skill to track how specific action tendencies or turning to *faux attachments* (such as substances, pornography, or gambling) might be part of a pattern of turning away from attachment relationships for comfort and support. The goal in EFCT is to facilitate non-judgmental safety for each partner to explore how the action tendencies of addictive processes or specific relationship injurious events are continuing to have an impact on the relationship. Similarly, for EFIT clients, addictive processes and relational attachment injuries are explored for their impact on emotion regulation and strategies for engagement. In all EFT therapy, clients are invited to explore contextual trauma, whether racial, ethnic, or cultural for its complex and ever-present impacts.

DOI: 10.4324/9781003242673-22

15 Addictive Processes as Substitute Sources of Connection and Emotion Regulation

"What you said about hating yourself and feeling sorry for yourself. What if you were to replace your harsh judgments with some genuine curiosity…What if you use drugs because you're afraid that you can't bear the pain without them? You have a reason to feel hurt after all you've been through. It's not a matter of 'fucking up.' You just haven't found any other way to cope." Dr. Gabor Maté, speaking to a heroin and cocaine addict, pregnant for the fourth time and dressed to attract potential customers on the street. (Maté, 2010, p. 351)

EFT offers a compassionate, empathic attachment frame for addictions as one's best attempt to cope with unbearable emotional pain and isolation, in the realities of their socio-cultural context. It is a paradigm shift for many clients and therapists alike to replace a judgmental stance toward people suffering from addictive processes with a validating lens that sees their human goodness and needs. Addiction is viewed in EFT as a disorder of attachment and emotion regulation (Barlow et al., 2018; Flores, 2004; Maté, 2010; Walant, 1995). "No one ever escapes their need for satisfying relationships, and the degree to which we are unable to form healthy interpersonal intimacy determines the degree to which we are vulnerable to substitute substances [and addictive behaviors] for human closeness" (Flores, 2004, p. 53). Those with emotion regulation difficulties are at higher risk of addictive behaviors and substance addictions (Estevez et al., 2017), including sex addiction (Cashwell et al., 2017; Katehakis, 2016) and social media and internet gambling (Girodana, 2022). Experiences of marginalization and systemic oppression need also to be considered for their impact on emotion regulation strategies when exploring the emotion regulation function of addictive processes (Giordano, 2022). Additionally, substance use disorders (SUD) and other addictive behaviors are more frequent in survivors of trauma and oppression, along with the accompanying risks of interpersonal violence, self-harm, and suicidal ideation. This chapter's opening quotation from Maté encompasses the need for compassionate curiosity, to validate that, without sociocultural safety and secure attachment to regulate emotion, addictive behaviors can appear as the only viable relief from pain.

Initially considered a contraindication for couple therapy, addictive processes are now approached as an attachment-related problem that, if acknowledged, can be worked with in EFCT. Substance use and addictive processes are nonjudgmentally tracked as action tendencies in the recurring pattern with Move 1 and assembled with Move 2 as part of the unfolding process of emotion. If the impact of an addictive process is not recognized by a client initially, an EFT therapist is curious, as always, to form an alliance with them and explore their longings and goals for change and their patterns of interaction that may be blocking them. This may lead a client to discover and own the negative consequences of the addictive process and to move to a position of acknowledging the unwanted effects of this action tendency.

DOI: 10.4324/9781003242673-23

Consistent with reported findings (Hogue et al., 2022) on the benefits of involving concerned significant others in treatment for SUD EFT therapists welcome the opportunity to work with couples where at least one partner is acknowledging a struggle with some addictive process and, if needed, is concurrently participating in specific treatment for addictive behaviors. When partners reach outside of their relationship for emotion regulation (for reward, comfort, pleasure, or relief from pain), they block accessibility to, and emotional responsiveness from, their partner. Their relationship is a latent resource that is also in peril.

EFCT takes center stage in this chapter, because of the benefits of involving significant others in treatment (Hogue et al., 2022) and the value of interpersonal connection as an effective antidote to addiction. EFIT is effective for individuals struggling with the negative consequences of addictive processes and I include it for the situations where couple therapy is not an option.

When an individual client struggling with addictive processes wishes to engage in EFIT, an EFT therapist will hold a non-judgmental, respectful stance, by framing the addictive processes as attempts to regulate difficult, overwhelming emotion (Barlow et al., 2018) in the absence of an accessible, responsive attachment figure, real or representational. To provide safety, mitigate risk, and maintain professional integrity, the therapist will discuss collaboration with specialists in addiction or psychiatric care as indicated. Individuals with no secure other to turn to for comfort and care to meet their essential human need for connection, may find that some addictive processes and patterns help them deal with overwhelming negative experiences in the short term but in the longer term, these *faux attachment*s are unsatisfactory and have negative long-term consequences. It is important in EFIT, as in EFCT, to assess the clients' tolerance for emotional intensity and to be mindful of pacing and containing so as not to overwhelm them and trigger their addictive patterns.

Addiction Defined

Alexander (2022) presents an *adaptive paradigm of addiction* which "denotes human beings struggling desperately with unmet needs" (p. 5) in a society characterized by isolation, loneliness, and dislocation. This is a perfect fit with the attachment view of EFT. Addictive processes can encompass a range of addictive behaviors, including substance use (alcohol and drugs), online gaming, gambling, compulsive activities such as overeating, shopping, pornography and cybersex, non-suicidal self-injury, compulsive sexual behaviors, work addictions, and others. Giordano (2022) refers to the "evolving definition of addiction" as she reviews the range of behavioral addictions that are now widely recognized, including compulsive use of substances and an extensive array of addictive behaviors, that are compulsively engaged in, despite their negative consequences. Online and offline "behavioral addictions affect individuals worldwide, and there are no signs that these addictions are subsiding" (p. 1).

The American Society of Addiction Medicine (ASAM) defines addiction as

a treatable, chronic medical disease involving complex interactions among brain circuits, genetics, the environment, and an individual's life experiences. People with addiction use substances or engage in behaviors that become compulsive and often continue despite harmful consequences. Prevention efforts and treatment approaches for addiction are generally as successful as those for other chronic diseases. (ASAM, 2019)

There remains an ongoing debate about how to conceptualize addiction (Heather et al., 2022). Is it a brain disease, a matter of individual choice and morality, or a societal problem of disconnection and dislocation? Some overlap in the divergent views can be found, and there are multidimensional biopsychosocial efforts to unify the brain disease model of addiction with the social view without suggesting that addiction is one or the other (Kelly et al., 2022). Conceptualizing addiction and patterns of turning to addictive substances and behaviors as a combined neurobiological, psychosocial process, supports an EFT therapist from getting caught in definitions of addiction. The "bio" or genetic or disease part of the biopsychosocial model, can also promote unconditional positive regard and guard against therapists searching for causality in negative relationship experiences or morality. Most people who work in the addiction field acknowledge that a portion of addiction is attributed to genetics (A. Giordano, personal communication, August 2023). Individuals with a genetic predisposition to addiction are more vulnerable to a drug or an addictive behavior becoming their most important relationship, to the detriment of other attachment relationships. Most importantly, for effective EFT therapy, therapists need kindness and unconditional regard – a non-judgmental view of individuals using addictive processes and the perspective "that people act to survive hardship in the most promising way that is available" (Alexander, 2022, p. 4).

Addictive Processes: A Search to Regulate Emotion and Find Connection

Difficult, overwhelming emotions are at the core of all disorders claim Barlow et al. (2014), suggesting that people use addictive behaviors toward substances and other processes to cope with alienation, disconnection, and loss of belonging and meaning. Barlow et al. submit that attempts to avoid or dampen the intensity of difficult emotions ultimately backfire and contribute to the maintenance of the symptoms. Addictive behaviors take one's mind off emotions in the short term but have negative consequences long term.

As social beings, we need nurturing, comforting, human connection for survival; however, in the face of a lack of attunement or explicit neglect or abuse, an insatiable hunger for connection can interfere with the normal development of a child's nervous system (Hari, 2015, 2018; Maté, 2010). Throughout life, a lack of a safe and secure attachment bond with at least one other human being will foster a craving for relief from the pain of social isolation and will frequently motivate a person to seek non-relational addictive behaviors for relief or reward. Individuals can be surrounded by seemingly available attachment figures yet become stuck in a pattern of isolation. Take Jean-Guy for example, a fellow in his early forties who is stuck in a pattern he has used all his life. He is the "good guy," never complains, routinely put others' needs ahead of his own. Though he feels daily pressure and stress at work and some growing agitation at what he calls "unfairness," he anesthetizes with daily whiskey. The greater his agitation and stress, the quieter he gets at home, sharing none of his struggles with his partner, who longs to support him. He doesn't reach to his partner and his partner experiences him to be unreachable.

Affective neuroscientists claim that separation distress can promote addictive processes and depression. In turn, addictive processes to alleviate the pain of social loss can deplete the desire to seek connection and promote further alienation and depression (Panksepp et al., 2014). Addictive processes are a *secondary substitute* in the face of alienation and unmet needs for connection (Walant, 1995).

As an enthusiastic new EFT therapist, Emily is excited to embrace the challenge of seeing addictive processes in an attachment frame. In the past, she held an individualistic view of addictive behaviors and referred individuals struggling with addictions to an addiction specialist before working with a couple with one such individual. EFT is expanding her perspective on addictive behaviors, with its attachment base that validates the human need for connection and holds that addictive processes are attempts at regulating emotion.

At times, she finds that compelling content threatens to derail her from the EFT model: She feels pulled in the direction of taking sides and labeling "the addict." She feels sorry for a partner whose spouse is rarely sober in the evenings and who essentially feels alone in the relationship. She wants to challenge the partner who insists that their compulsive use of online pornography has no impact on their ability to engage with their partner, in spite of his wife's suggestion that they engage in increasingly rough sex to entice him into enjoying sex with her. "Do I know how to handle all this?" Emily wonders. She feels compassion for the individual client with a history of adversity and trauma, struggling to curb their substance use or addictive behaviors without any sense of belonging and human connection.

Emily now follows the EFT model, focusing first on building a safe alliance and, in EFCT, collaborating to name the predictable sequence of negative interactions or cycle that perpetuates distance between partners. In EFIT, she helps clients identify the pattern that constricts them from accessing their emotional experience and helps them find enough balance to begin listening to their emotions as a guide. She understands addictive processes as an attachment disorder, and works from EFT's non-judgmental, systemic stance, rather than from an individualistic, deficit model. She maintains a focus on how each partner has an impact on the other. Viewing addiction as an adaptation to alienation and psychosocial dislocation and as a client's best attempts to cope with difficult and/or foreign and unacceptable emotion helps Emily to remain curious, open, attuned, and respectful of each client. Despite her best efforts, however, she does feel the occasional pull to pathologize the behavior of a "user" and to single this client out for addiction treatment before exploring couple therapy as a highly feasible option for these clients. Indeed, additional addiction treatment may be indicated, however, Emily is beginning to understand the power of EFCT to provide clients with sufficient support to validate the "using" partner's compulsive need to move away from the spouse and find comfort, regulation, or relief by other means. This process can calm the couple sufficiently to allow for further assessment of the need for additional treatment while engaging in Stage 1 awareness and stabilization.

Couple therapy can work well alongside treatment for addictions. When one or both partners use addiction or disease labels for themselves or their partner, Emily continues to assemble each partner's emotional experience to make sense of compulsive behaviors while also processing the impact of these behaviors on the relationship.

With EFIT clients struggling with addictive processes, Emily refers to additional specialized addiction treatment where indicated. She is also prepared to work alongside the addiction treatment to stabilize and create corrective emotional experiences for clients coping with adversity and overwhelming experiences, and to help them identify their unmet needs.

Emotional Starvation

Attachment theory holds that humans are primarily motivated to seek proximity to an attachment figure when under stress, and when comfort and safety are not accessible, they resort to secondary strategies to regulate emotion. In an attachment frame, then, addictive processes are seen as emotionally motivated. When individuals are emotionally starved of human connection, addictive processes can temporarily fill a hunger for positive emotion (reward) or relief from negative emotion. Drug and alcohol use, eating disorders, and many other addictive behaviors are all responses to the normative human hunger for connection. Maté (2010) describes persons struggling with additive processes as "hungry ghosts" who can never fill the emptiness on the inside.

Paradoxically, addictive processes are a response to emotional isolation, yet addictive, compulsive behaviors also emotionally isolate individuals. Addictive substances and behaviors imprison individuals in a pattern of avoidance – distancing them from themselves, from others, and from a sense of meaning and purpose. Addictive processes increase relationship distress and heighten depression and anxiety. In turn, distress and distance increase vulnerability to turn to an impersonal, non-rejecting, rapid "feel-good" source of relief from pain.

Addictive Processes Involve Repetitive Cycles

When a person is in need, in pain, or under stress, the immediate "go-to" will be toward that to which she or he is most devoted. When a partner discovers they are repeatedly not the first one their partner seeks for comfort, they are likely to experience a sense of threat. Attachment alarm bells ring. Devotion to a substitute source of comfort, evidenced by a compulsion to turn to someone or something else before their partner for positive affect is certain to put the security of a couple's attachment bond at risk. The more an avoidant partner routinely turns away to something other than their partner, the more anxious, demanding, and critical their pursing partner is likely to become. Correspondingly, the more an anxious partner turns to an addictive process for comfort, the colder and more withdrawing and avoidant their more avoidant partner is likely to become. The more one partner demands and criticizes, or dismisses and distances, the more attractive the addictive process becomes to the other partner.

A characteristic of how people pursue substance use or other addictive processes is that preoccupation and obsession persist in spite of accumulating adverse consequences. EFT therapists recognize that, despite the negative consequences, the addictive patterns become self-absorbing and reinforcing. The real impact of addictive behaviors is the cyclical impact that the *trauma of addiction* (Love et al., 2016) has upon an intimate relationship bond and the impact that the relationship dynamic has upon the addictive pattern. Addictive behaviors become part of the negative circular feedback loop in relationships.

The circular nature of addiction is also what is known as the reward cycle, or the "dark side of addiction," which recognizes that as addictive behaviors trigger changes to the brain, individuals' capacity to feel pleasure and happiness is reduced and an increased need for stimulation from the addictive behavior occurs. Giordano (2022) describes it thus:

> Known as the 'dark side of addiction' (Koob & Lemoal, 2008, p. 38) the down-regulation of the reward system in response to overactivation is presumed to lead to negative emotional states marked by malaise, loss of motivation, stress, and irritability. (p. 27)

The *positive incentive theory* of addiction (Pinel, 2015) holds that it is the preoccupation with anticipating the reward of the addictive substance or behavior that becomes the problem. The addictive behavior or substance releases a flood of endorphins in the reward center of the brain, resulting in elation and euphoria. The element that becomes so addicting is the anticipation of this dopamine rush. Whether the addictive process involves substances such as alcohol or drugs, or the use of online pornography, or high-risk gambling practices, or non-suicidal self-injury, or eating disorders, users of addictive substances or behaviors become caught in a cyclic web of expectation—coming to expect and crave the high or the fix (Barlow et al., 2014; Giordano, 2022; Johnson, 2013; Landau-North et al., 2011). The addictive behavior compromises key relationships because it becomes the most important activity in a person's life (Griffiths, 2005).

As individuals turn away more and more from their partners, and interpersonal supports, they become preoccupied with anticipating the next fix. This web of expectation of the next fix is triggered by relationship distress and relationship distress is triggered by the addictive process, thus perpetuating the relationship distress cycle (Landau-North et al., 2011). Something other than the partner becomes the primary source of comfort, soothing, and emotion regulation. The using partner engaging in addictive processes becomes less and less available to their partner for comfort and care and the addictive process provides a quicker and more intense fix than naturally occurring sources of pleasure, such as beautiful scenery, small achievements and pleasant social interactions.

In EFCT therapists track the cycles of this *web of expectation*. Tracking the increasingly constrictive patterns in which partners become unwillingly caught, they seek to identify the triggers for *when* a partner is pulled toward the addictive process and *how* the other partner responds. They link the addictive processes into the cycle, and then access and expand the unexpressed underlying, more vulnerable, emotions of each partner. It is inevitable that addictive behaviors create relationship-specific trauma and cause one or more *attachment injuries* (see Chapter 16).

In EFIT, therapists also track patterns in which clients get caught. Jane (not her real name) is puzzled about her cycles of using. She has periods of sobriety, followed by dangerous patterns of using cocaine and alcohol. Working with an EFT therapist, alongside her self-help groups, she is able to recognize her patterns for coping. In Stage 2 she reprocesses emotional experiences and trauma that she had been avoiding. She frees herself from the weight of guilt she has carried for her husband's suicide and grieves the death of her beloved pet. In reshaping her sense of self as worthy and loveable, she is free to commit to her current relationship and to discover a new zest for life. A video session of this client is available at steppingintoeft.com

Effective Dependency/Secure Connection as an Antidote

The EFCT focus on substituting a *faux attachment* with a relationship attachment as a source of pleasure, comfort, and relief from pain can be a very effective recovery activity, in combination with additional addiction treatment, if needed. Effective dependency, which can be created through EFT, is the true antidote for the need for substances or addictive processes (Johnson, 2013). "In successful couple therapy partners change each other and the moments of deep connection between partners seem to offer us the best healing arena for and natural antidote to the compulsive behaviors of addiction" (Landau-North et al., 2011, p. 213). The best treatment approaches for addiction recognize the importance of working with the family and the social system (Hogue et al., 2022; Landau-North et al., 2011).

EFT holds that "addiction is a negative, costly, compulsive behavior that constricts a person's life and behavior" (Johnson, 2013, p. 96). In Stage 1, EFT therapists help clients to discover how their addictive behaviors are the best attempts to cope with overwhelming emotions. They are helped to own the repetitive behaviors and patterns they are caught in and to discover and acknowledge the costs of these repetitive patterns to themselves and to their relationships. In EFCT, therapists delineate negative cycles that include addictive process(es) and compulsive turning away from the other partner. Partners are also helped to discover and own how the addictive behaviors are wounding their partner.

EFT can be very helpful in Stage 1, while working with a harm reduction model. The harm reduction movement certainly aligns with EFT, in that it replaces stigma and shame and an authoritarian decision about what is best for another person with kindness. The non-judgmental humanity inherent in harm reduction is rooted in seeking to *stop the harm rather than to stop the high* (Maté, 2010; Szalavitz, 2021).

After helping clients to stabilize their pattern, an EFT therapist helps a couple to begin Stage 2 creation of positive bonding cycles— a powerful antidote to the need for substances and addictive behaviors. It is very promising and encouraging for couple therapists to know that the attachment perspective and research show that secure connection protects against the negative consequence of addictive behaviors and can be the antidote to addictive patterns.

What an EFT Therapist Sees or Hears When Addictive Processes Are Present

The first two items I present here are discussed in relation to couples, however, they are also relevant for individual therapy. The cyclic relationship in couples between addictive processes and relationship distress is often some form of pursue–withdraw, where one partner turns away from the relationship to addictive processes for comfort or relief and the other partner protests the growing distance. The cycle with addictive processes is typically complex and extreme. Two partners are caught in a negative cycle, with an additional competing source of comfort and relief (be it substances or some other online or offline compulsive behavior).

Numbing and Emotional Absence

An EFT therapist considers the attachment significance of any addictive process to be the most significant aspect. The attachment significance is not the amount of anything; rather, it is the degree to which something outside the relationship is a compulsion or an obsession and how much it leads to emotional absence and an inability to be accessible, responsive, and emotionally engaged.

In the expectation of a release and an intense dopamine high as a means to regulate affect, a partner becomes progressively emotionally absent. With pornography, for example, the planning, secrecy, anticipation, and the *quasi*-persistent state of arousal leaves a partner progressively and chronically more emotionally absent. A partner engaging in cybersex or substance use becomes increasingly distant and the other partner becomes increasingly disappointed, lonely, and angry. Chronic and progressive emotional absence erodes an attachment relationship.

Acknowledging or Dismissing the Impact

An EFT therapist looks and listens for clients' acknowledgment of the impact an addictive process is having upon their relationship. Frequently there is some acknowledgment of addictive processes, but often one or both partners will minimize the impact. "I know I can stop it if I want to." Other times, there is denial that the addictive process is having any impact on the relationship, on oneself, or on the other partner. A compulsive online gambler, for example, protests, "I am sitting right beside her all evening while she prepares her classes for tomorrow! What more does she need?"

Anxious or Avoidant Orientation in the Client Engaging in Addictive Processes

Addiction as an attachment disorder can be linked to anxious or avoidant attachment orientations. It has been suggested (Ein-Dor & Doran, 2015) that people who typically use anxious and fearful avoidant attachment strategies are more likely to develop *internalizing disorders*, such as anxiety, depression and PTSD, whereas people who habitually use avoidant attachment strategies are more likely to develop *externalizing disorders* such as substance use and other addictive behaviors and conduct disorders. Hundreds of studies, however, link anxious and avoidant attachment orientations to multiple emotional disorders. Mikulincer and Shaver (2016) argue that substance abuse and behavorial addictions can be encouraged by both avoidant and anxious forms of insecure attachment. They suggest that avoidant individuals can use substances to avoid distress and painful emotions and self-awareness, whereas anxious individuals can use substances to block distressing ruminations and memories.

Briefly, Emily finds herself slipping into pigeon-holing people in attempt to understand what to expect of them, however, she stops and reminds herself, "As in all of EFT, culturally humble attunement and fully present engagement with each client and their stories of their significant others is where my priority lies." There is no simple formula for which attachment orientation leads to which disorder, given there are multiple factors at play, including genetics and environment. Ein-Dor and Doran (2015) in concert with the UP model (Barlow et al., 2018) and Johnson's (2019) focus in EFIT, present a *transdiagnostic model of attachment insecurities* to help explain "why a different attachment disposition leads to different disorders in different people or to different disorders within the same person over time" (2015, p. 354).

Supportive Community Connections

Connection and attachments are an important part of addiction recovery, whether that is with a peer support group (SMART Recovery or a 12-step group), connection in faith communities, or connection with family and friends, however these connections are sometimes experienced by a partner as a competing attachment and a significant trigger for a negative cycle. There are many Alcoholics Anonymous (AA) slogans (e.g., "stick with the winners" "we are only as sick as our secrets") that emphasize connection and warn about secrecy and isolation. A quote from the *Big Book* of AA illustrates the focus on connection as part of the solution in the self-help addiction recovery community:

> We are people who normally would not mix. But there exists among us a fellowship, a friendliness, and an understanding which is indescribably wonderful. We are like the passengers of a great liner the moment after rescue from shipwreck when camaraderie, joyousness and democracy pervade the vessel from steerage to Captain's table. Unlike the feelings of the ship's passengers, however, our joy in escape from disaster does not subside as we go our individual ways. The feeling of having shared in a common peril is one element in the powerful cement which binds us. (Alcoholics Anonymous, 2001, p. 17)

It is not hard to see how these close bonds can pose a potential threat to the relationship bond in couple therapy. An EFT therapist may hear complaints such as, "My partner is still turning to the group more than me. It hurts to see I am less important than them. I feel left out!" If one partner's close bonds outside a couple relationship are experienced as blocking the security of the couple's bond, that threat needs to be explicitly explored as part of de-escalating their cycle and creating safety.

What an EFT Therapist Does When Addictive Processes Are Present in EFCT

Alliance Building and Assessment

When an addictive process is explicit at the outset of EFCT, the therapist engages a couple to assess its impact on the relationship. Leading with Move 1 reflecting present process and Move 2 assembly and deepening, an EFT therapist helps clients to take their Step 1 of building a relationship with the therapist and collaborating in assessment. Whether or not any formal assessment tool is used, an EFT therapist tracks the addictive behaviors as action tendencies playing out in the couple's negative cycle and delineates how they lead to emotional disconnection.

If a partner is, or becomes willing through this exploration, to acknowledge the problem and is open to additional individual or group treatment, if needed, an EFT therapist can work with a couple without requiring total abstinence. If a partner is unwilling, however, to acknowledge that the addictive process is having any negative impact, the therapist needs to consider if it will be helpful to continue working with them while this active addictive process continues. Sometimes EFT couple therapy is helpful while addictive behaviors persist because Stage 1 EFT can be part of the process of partners recognizing the impact of the addictive process on their pattern of interacting. The person with an addictive behavior can identify their habitual turning away from the partner when under stress and together they can stabilize their pattern.

The following three situations are likely to indicate to an EFT therapist that couple therapy is contraindicated until after the partner using addictive processes engages in addiction-specific treatment:

1. A partner cannot engage in the therapy process because he or she is totally shut down or numbed out.
2. A partner remains unwilling to recognize the impact of his or her behavior on the relationship, despite therapeutic exploration.
3. Safety cannot be created in session.

In such situations, confirming they are continuing to hold the attachment cycle frame and have not become caught in a pathologizing negative cycle themself, an EFT therapist needs to be transparent about why couple therapy seems inappropriate at this time. They will offer referrals for individual and/or group treatment, with an open door to return for couple therapy later.

Stabilize: Help Clients to Move through Stage 1

An EFT therapist identifies the cyclic pattern between addictive processes and relationship distress. For example, in EFCT, as one partner turns away from the relationship to addictive processes or cybersex for comfort and pleasure, the other partner protests the growing distance. The therapist tracks how relationship distress increases vulnerability to turn away from their partner to other sources (such as addictive processes) for comfort and emotion regulation. With Tango Move 2, the therapist evokes partners' exploration of how a particular addictive process might increase the distress and distance they are experiencing. Partners are encouraged by the therapist's empathic reflections, tracking, and evocative questions to engage in exploring how their distress increases their vulnerability to turn to an impersonal source of comfort or relief from pain that carries no risk of rejecting them. The repetitive pattern is delineated with the addictive process in it. Stage 1 encounters are shaped and processed with Moves 3 and 4 for partners to disclose to each other ownership of their action tendencies in their cycle, as well as the core underlying emotions they are experiencing. This helps both partners to begin to see themselves and the other in a less negative light, even though their basic pattern has not yet changed.

If partners are reluctant to discuss the addictive process, the couple's cycle can be framed as the problem that is making it too difficult to discuss this competing source of comfort. The therapist can validate and track how one partner attempts to raise the issue and the other partner dismisses its significance. This is how their pursue-withdraw feedback loop keeps them both stuck in loneliness and pain. As the therapist continues with Move 1 reflections and validations, framing this repetitive pattern as the problem, partners can gradually move toward owning action tendencies and positions. With Move 2, assembly, each one's emotional experience in this stuck pattern is clarified and stabilized. Reliance on a competing attachment erodes the trust in the bond. Stabilization requires specific naming of how the addictive process is a dominant force in a couple's negative cycle or an individual's imprisoning pattern.

Restructuring Attachment Bonds and Working Models of Self and System (Stage 2)

Using Tango Moves 2, 3, and 4 to help clients to reprocess emotion and restructure the relationship bond is similar to EFT as usual. There are the added complexities of expanding attachment fears and needs related to the addictive process and resolving attachment injuries created through the trauma of addictive behaviors. Engaging the withdrawer or burned-out pursuer is likely to include accessing and reprocessing shame, with negative views of self and frightening attachment meanings such as feeling like a rat, unlikable, and disgusting; feeling helpless saying, "There's nothing I can do"; feeling unworthy as in, "I'm never enough—never right"; feeling exhausted, "My partner's unhappiness drains everything in my body." There is likely to be considerable shame, negative views of self and other, and fear of abandonment on the part of the pursuer or the partner not engaged in addictive processes. Relationship trauma and specific attachment injuries triggered by the addictive processes, will need to be resolved with the attachment injury resolution model (AIRM; Chapter 16) before partners can complete Stage 2 and participate in Stage 3 integration and consolidation. The earlier EFIT example of Jane, who is in EFIT alongside her 12-Step groups and the EFIT case of Lyndon, presented below, illustrate stabilizing and restructuring in EFIT. Addictive processes as part of the client's strategy are explicitly assembled as attempts to regulate foreign and/or, frightening, unacceptable emotions. New views of self and other emerge and new strategies are shaped for effective emotion regulation.

EFCT Case Example with Addictive Processes

An EFT therapist is steeped in the perspective that addictive behaviors are best attempts to regulate emotion; to escape negative emotion, especially the pain and anxiety of disconnection; or to create some positive emotion in an empty existence. Jazz "enjoys" online gambling and alcohol. Casey complains of feeling isolated despite Jazz's physical presence in their home.

Jazz: I don't see what the problem is—I like to have a little fun. I'm home all the time, in fact. What's the big deal?

Casey: (Interrupts.) Jazz is home, true, but on the computer—it's like he's in another world. I can't find him. Jazz only grunts when I try and talk with him, or tells me, "Be quiet—I'm winning, don't interrupt me!" Like the time the dishwasher leaked all over the kitchen floor—Jazz refused to even listen to me calling for help. It's not a big deal—I can handle home maintenance, but it was the fact that Jazz gets so wrapped up that if I need him, he's not there! And add to that—weekends you are out all night drinking with your friends, and I'm alone at home, terrified you'll die in a car crash.

Jazz: My gambling world is fun—it's thrilling in fact, and I like the comfort of being home. This is just the way I am. I like to have a little fun—and I make money for us—and I am home—nearly every evening—so close to you! Don't you see?

Emily: (Move 1, reflecting, validating, and tracking.) So, help me know if I am getting how this goes for you. Casey, you want to talk with Jazz about how much you are missing him and how lonely you feel in the relationship, and how from your perspective Jazz's gambling is taking over the relationship and keeping you from *finding* him and being able to connect with him. And Jazz, when Casey begins to talk about how lonely he is and how hard it is to find you, and how much he resents all the time you spend online gambling, you immediately hear—what did you say—"barbs and threats of suffocation" and so you fight back and say, "It's not so bad! It's my fun. Leave me alone." And the more you push Casey away, the more Casey panics that he's already lost you—is that it?

After receiving confirmation from each of them that she is understanding their stuck pattern, Emily continues.

Emily: This is the pattern you get stuck in when you try to discuss your different feelings and attitudes about Jazz's online gambling. Right now, it's almost as though this hot topic is impossible to touch without igniting the cycle, is that right?

Jazz: You think you've lost me? You miss me? I never feel that. You just seem fed up with me all the time!

Casey: Yes, I do miss you! And I've nearly given up that I'll ever find you again!

From the perspective that the addictive behavior is the *faux attachment* (Flores, 2004), Emily helps the partners to assemble this emotional process and to identify their automatic pattern of interaction, which takes over and blocks Casey and Jazz from discussing together how fragile their relationship bond is.

With Move 1, Emily uses evocative questions and responses, followed by many reflections and validations to identify the specific moves in the dance. She attends carefully to see and make explicit their repetitive pattern playing out in the room. With Move 2, she attunes for implicit emotion in images and bodily signs of emotional experience. She helps each partner identify their triggers for the cycle.

Emily: Jazz, *when* are you most likely to turn to online gambling? (Evocative question.)

Jazz: (Shrugging.) Any time. I'll do it just about any time. It's a lot easier than dealing with Casey!

Emily moves in to catch the bullet of aggression. She makes an attachment reframe, validating that Jazz's gambling is easier than facing Casey being unhappy with him. "Dealing with Casey being upset is very difficult for you, Jazz," Emily validates, heightening the attachment frame of how important Casey is to him.

Emily also lingers with Jazz's shrug and words "It's easier" to make the vague cue ("any time") more vivid and concrete and to help Jazz own his inner process and action tendency, "You shrug and say it is difficult to know *when* you are likely to turn to gambling. It feels easier to turn to the gambling thrill than to turn to Casey, whom you sense is unhappy with you? Is that it?" (To confirm the conjecture that a specific trigger for Jazz, in their repetitive cycle, is his perceived attachment threat that Casey is unhappy with him.)

Addictive processes create relationship trauma. Emily validates the current trauma of emotional isolation in view of the addictive process, tracks the cycle that is blocking the partners from being each other's safe haven and secure base, identifying how each one is pulled into reactive behaviors. She names and brings to life the underlying core attachment fears and longings, the background musical beat that is moving both of their feet and blocking Jazz from turning to Casey at this particularly vulnerable time. It is a shaky time, for Jazz who is doing all he can to dampen and dismiss any feelings of grief and loss over his father's recent, tragic death, Emily assesses for specific attachment injury events between Casey and Jazz, for additional earlier trauma, intimate partner violence, depression and anxiety, all of which are commonly associated with addictive processes. She discovers that in addition to the relationship-specific trauma of Jazz's addictive processes, there are ghosts of trauma in the relationship between Jazz and Casey and unspoken grief for Jazz in his family relationships. Jazz's mother had committed suicide when Jazz was five years old, and Jazz's father, who meant the world to him, had died suddenly within the last year, just after Jazz and Casey had a big argument, leaving Casey cold and nonresponsive to Jazz during that time. Casey' unavailability to Jazz at his critical moment of need was a trust-shattering moment for Jazz – *an attachment injury* – that shattered his last fragments of trust and hope in the relationship bond. Similarly, Jazz's ongoing addictive process is eroding the trust Casey used to have in their bond.

When the interactions between Jazz and Casey become much less hostile, Emily recognizes markers that the couple has stabilized: Jazz enters an addiction day-treatment program and each partner acknowledges what they do in their cycle. Casey acknowledges that he criticizes and makes forceful demands, while Jazz acknowledges blowing up, shutting down, and more and more frequently numbing out with alcohol and online gambling. Jazz also describes feeling uncomfortable with closeness and conflict and finding alcohol or gambling more "relaxing" than talking while feeling stressed. Both partners disclose their core emotions underlying their negative dance. Casey acknowledges his fear of not mattering, of being all alone; Jazz touches on his fears of having "blown it," of not being wanted at all by Casey, and of being "totally inadequate in his eyes." Each recognize how they affect and are affected by the other, and how the drinking, gambling, relational distress, and Casey' coldness at Jazz's moment of need all trigger and maintain each other. At the end of the stabilization change event, Emily continues with Move 2 to reflect and track the negative dance, while linking it to cues/triggers, attributions (meanings), and action tendencies, and validating the underlying core emotions and fears.

Following the map of client change events, Emily helps Casey and Jazz to reshape their bond. They enter the second change event of engaging the more withdrawn partner as Emily uses Move 2 to further assemble and deepen Jazz's loneliness that he touched earlier. Emily heightens and expands his fears and shapes an encounter (Move 3) for Jazz to express them directly to Casey. Jazz dissolves in tears in this encounter while disclosing to Casey, "I miss you when I shut you out. I'm terrified you've given up on me and are just disgusted with me now. The bar and gambling are my escapes from this dark place."

After processing the encounter with both partners, Emily flows with more of Moves 2, 3, and 4, distilling, deepening and guiding Jazz to disclose his loneliness and core fears of losing Casey. Ultimately, she supports Jazz to ask Casey for what he needs to feel safe to step closer. Jazz asks for Casey's acceptance and assurance of love even if he blows it and lets him down. He expands on how Casey can make it safer for him to come close. This is Jazz's assertive reach into the relationship: Asking for his attachment needs to be met. This marks the engagement change event, a key part of restructuring the attachment bond.

Casey reassures him, "I have always been *in*—but it has been so lonely with you leaving all the time and being so far away even in the same house, but you are not seeming so angry anymore, and the other evening," tossing Jazz a warm smile, "you even joked a little with me while we cleaned up from dinner." In Casey's softening change event, he vulnerably shares his loneliness. Shaking with fear, Casey reaches to ask Jazz to move much closer and to assure him that he is more precious than his gaming and drinking friends. Casey expresses needs for constant reassurance that Jazz is staying involved in the addiction treatment program as well. Together, they heal several attachment injuries, including the moment Casey failed to respond to Jazz at the heart-breaking loss of his dad. Jazz and Casey move from increasingly rigid and negative affect regulation patterns to becoming effective sources of comfort and affect regulation for one another.

EFIT Case Example of Acknowledged Addictive Processes

Lyndon, a successful chartered accountant, enters therapy caught in addictive processes and a heavily depressed state, unable to work, having resumed substance use and prescription medication to calm his anxiety. He swings between frequent, intense unwanted emotions of overwhelming anxiety, combined with fearing the anxiety and judging himself harshly for these emotions. He makes elaborate efforts to avoid any emotional experience. In addition to having resumed his long-forgotten addictive patterns with substances, he is caught up with compulsive behaviors toward rescuing feral and stray animals. He is adopting an increasing number of animals from the local animal shelter and driving through the city at night looking for animals in need. Fuelling his patterns is a sense of meaninglessness with his accounting career, and despair at nearing his fortieth birthday as a "lonely bachelor." With Emily's Moves 1 and 2, empathic engagement and gentle tracking of his patterns of coping with a series of significant losses, Lyndon identifies his automatic pattern of harsh criticism toward any persistent feelings of sadness and pain and then very successfully dampening down his emotions. Lyndon has what Barlow et al. (2018) summarize as the main features of emotional disorders, "frequent intense, unwanted emotions; aversive reactions or negative beliefs about emotions; and efforts to avoid emotions" (p. 44) with his addictive processes. The final feature of avoidance is the kryptonite for emotional disorders. Damping down and avoiding emotions are precisely what addictive processes are helping Lyndon to do. The effectiveness of EFIT is that he comes to engage fully with the previously avoided emotions and restructures his sense of self, reshapes his capacity to engage with others, and discovers a new coherent sense of self, fully alive and able to deal with the vicissitudes and inevitable disappointment of life.

Following his movement through the EFT stages of client change, we see that as Emily uses Move 1 to track Lyndon's patterns of emotion regulation, explicitly including his substance use and obsessive behaviors regarding animal rescue, he discovers his problematic pattern: He sidesteps his core grief and sadness by hyper-activating fears of his own death, showing compulsive concern for abused animals, frantically adopting pets from the animal shelter and turning to substances. Historically, his reaches to others for support were disappointing. He begins to recognize that he rarely makes clear reaches for his own needs; rather, he recruits volunteers for the animal shelter and lives very self-sufficiently. He isolates himself emotionally from others since their responses never reach the core, numb and sometimes aching place deep inside

As Emily validates Lyndon's avoidant pattern as his "best attempt at coping with the enormity of his losses," he begins to discover unknown depths of grief over the loss of his first and only romantic relationship. Emily shapes some Stage 1 encounters for Lyndon to speak to several imaginal others – Ana, his long-lost love, his dog, and his sister. The encounters are life-giving and full of deep sobs. "It's like I was frozen for 25 hears! I never imagined I could speak to them again. Something in me is coming to life!" exclaims Lyndon.

He opens to compassionately experiencing his intense grief over his lost love, Ana, his beloved dog, Griffin, and his cherished twin sister, Stephanie, who drowned in a boating accident, while Lyndon was driving the boat. New emotion emerges such as the huge weight of judgment and guilt that he carries, from his parents for Stephanie's death. He also discovers new unmet longings to hear Stephanie's voice and to feel Griffin jump into his lap.

In Stage 1 Lyndon more clearly recognizes and owns his avoidant pattern of ignoring his shame and losses by focusing outward on animals in need and using substances. After stabilizing his pattern of avoiding dangerous and unacceptable emotions he opens to experiencing and processing previously blocked core emotions. With Emily's help, as she uses Tango Moves 2, 3, and 4, he distills, deepens, and discloses messages of grief and fear underlying his patterns.

The more clients are helped to formulate their emotional experience in a highly distilled and discreetly described manner, the less vulnerable they are to excessive drinking or aggression (Barrett, 2017). Barrett found that formulating emotion with a higher level of granularity or specificity is a more effective way to regulate emotion than the two popular modes of regulating emotion – cognitive reappraisal or distraction.

Identifying his core patterns and unacknowledged core emotions, Lyndon completes his Stage 1 stabilization and opens the door to Stage 2 restructuring. Flowing with Moves 2, 3, and 4, Emily shapes numerous imaginal Stage 2 encounters for Lyndon to engage in empowering dialogues, creating corrective emotional experiences. He grieves the depth of his losses and recovers "lost" parts of himself. Through these encounters he reshapes his sense of self regarding the deaths of his sister and his beloved dog, restoring a bond with the deceased Griffin, and bringing to life the nurturing bond he had known with his sister.

Emily shapes encounters for Lyndon with his imaginal mother and his imaginal father, helping him to reprocess his models of self and other and become "less under the spell of forgotten miseries and better able to recognize companions in the present for who they are" (Bowlby, 1988, p. 137). Emily helps him to step fully into his grief and loss at being single and afraid to date, reprocessing the self-blame and guilt he has continued to carry for getting Ana pregnant and being rejected by her. He reshapes his sense of self as deserving of the parental support he never had and worthy of having a loving, romantic relationship again. Together, they fully experience and transform these emotions, listening to the messages of present-day longings and needs embedded in his core sadness and loss.

He discovers a worthy, competent, and lovable sense of self. He restructures his automatic patterns of turning to substances and saving animals in need, to the more effective and gratifying patterns of reaching to relatives and friends for support and for opportunities to give and receive care. Reshaping his attachment pattern, he is able to experience joy at nurturing and being nurtured through the growing bond with his yoga group, who meets for breakfast each Saturday. He discovers the motivation and health to return to work and to build on the meaning and relational benefits of interacting with colleagues on projects that are coming to have meaning and purpose for him again.

The power of working with the flow of Moves 2, 3, and 4, assembling and deepening precise emotional experience and then disclosing and processing the experience of explicit imaginal dialogues never ceases to amaze Emily. She is pleased to be reminded of its relevance of putting emotion into finely distilled words, together with the interpersonal process of reaching and responding, for overcoming addictive patterns.

In Stage 3, they revisit the shifts Lyndon has made, moving from views of self as disgusting, unlovable, fearing terminal medical diagnoses, and of others as unresponsive and dangerous, to a revitalized sense of self as worthy, lovable, and full of life, and some significant others as supportive and caring. In their closing session, with Move 5, Emily helps Lyndon review his new cycles of emotion regulation. In place of his dependence on substances and his compulsion to adopt more and more stray animals, he is sending clear messages of need for support to reliable others and celebrating his experience of himself in relationships. He enjoys his pets now, with a connected sense of calm in place of the previous agitation and anxiety. He is building relationships that have a mixture of supporting him and being a meaningful opportunity for him to also be offering caring to others. He has a coherent story of how he has moved from despair to passion for life, describing how the previous "surges of anxiety" now bubble up as "fuel and energy" for life.

Emily is under no illusion that her EFT successes with Jazz and Casey, and Lyndon will be enough for everyone. She acknowledges the need to collaborate with addiction-treatment experts while also having much to offer as an EFT therapist to clients struggling with addictive processes. There is no end to the need for humility and collaboration in this field, she muses as she reads Maté's words, "No matter how hard I try, I have found out that I may never fully defeat my [own] addiction-prone tendencies. And I have also learned that this is alright" (p. 350). She is pleased to have a model that is compassionate toward herself and her clients. She need not be a perfect therapist, but she is energized to have the EFT model that is helpful for harm reduction and restructuring attachment bonds and views of self in interaction with others and their system.

Conclusion

EFT can be effective with couples and individuals struggling with addictions and addictive processes. If needed, to stabilize the addictive behavior, treatment for addictions can be done prior to or concurrently with EFT therapy. EFT offers a depathologizing approach to addictive behaviors by framing them as adaptive responses to unmet needs for connection. It is an interpersonal change process based on utilizing the power of emotion within the client to create corrective emotional experiences through real or imaginal dialogue with another. The change process creates lasting change and acts as the antidote to addictive processes.

A key challenge for EFCT therapists seeking to work with an attachment frame is that of tacitly seeing one partner in a couple as largely responsible for the relational distress. This challenge presents itself very boldly when addictive processes are present. Likewise, when working with individuals coping with addictive processes, it can be challenging to hold the attachment frame that views addictive behaviors as temporarily adaptive responses to regulate overwhelming emotion in the absence of adequate supportive connections. Notwithstanding the option of referring for additional individual treatment when indicated, and in spite of some features of dysfunction, mental illness, compulsions, or addictive processes in one or both partners, an EFT therapist will continue to work within a non-pathologizing attachment view. This means helping a couple or individual to delineate the cycle that is keeping them stuck, validating the addictive processes for their adaptive function, and acknowledging the cost to individuals and their significant relationships. This attachment view of addiction as an attachment disorder can support an EFT therapist to keep from being sucked into a "find the bad guy" (Johnson, 2008) mentality. This perspective helps an EFT therapist to work in darkness and ambiguity with patience, open-mindedness, and explicit honesty.

The attachment perspective enhances an EFT therapist's empathy and compassion for experiences common to individuals affected by addictive processes, including shame at violating one's core values. Negative views of self or rigid, pseudo-positive views of self are viewed kindly, in an attachment frame, as attempts to find the safe haven/secure base of secure connection. Needs for comfort or relief from pain and stress, and needs for nurturing to feed existential emptiness are seen as basic survival needs that, when unmet by interpersonal connections, leave one vulnerable to addictive processes.

The attachment frame of addiction as an attachment disorder frees an EFT therapist: (a) to expand their capacity to see the positive survival intentions in every pattern of behavior; (b) to work with the recurring, self-reinforcing cycles without invalidating or shaming anyone; (c) to reshape attachment bonds for partners to become each other's primary source of comfort and support, and for individual clients to reshape their sense of self as valuable and competent to form secure connection with others. As Maté (2010) says, the only way to treat addiction is through compassion.

EFT offers an antidote to using addictive processes to regulate emotions. Notwithstanding that genetic predisposition and insecure attachment from current relationship distress and/or from adverse childhood experiences (Felitti et al., 1998; Maté, 2010), leave individual clients vulnerable to seeking out pleasure or comforting pain with addictive processes, and couple clients susceptible to turn away from their partner to addictive processes for comfort, secure attachment bonds are an antidote. Created in Stage 2 of EFT and consolidated in Stage 3, secure attachment bonds increase flexibility, broaden response repertoires, and put less focus on regulating emotion and more focus on growth and learning. This, of course, contributes to more resilient coping and less need for addictive processes.

16 Forgiveness and Reconciliation with EFT's Attachment Injury Resolution Model

A common impasse in repairing distressed relationships has been identified as an *attachment injury* (AI). An AI is a specific event that shatters the trust and profoundly injures an attachment bond. The injurious events can range from infidelity to physical or emotional absence during a critical moment of need. After discussing the construct of AI, I explore three common ways AIs can emerge in EFCT. I discuss working in Stage 1 when an AI is openly present, and then describe EFT's empirically validated attachment injury resolution model (AIRM) for reconciliation and rebuilding trust in Stage 2 EFCT (Makinen & Johnson, 2006; Zuccarini et al., 2013). The EFT model of AI is also a useful guide for resolution in EFIT and I illustrate this with a case example to end the chapter.

Congruent with the themes of diversity and EFIT throughout this book, several additional case examples and transcripts of AI repair are available in Chapter 16 Support Material (routledge.com/9781032151335). The first example in the support material illustrates EFCT's AIRM as *a culturally informed couple healing modality* (Comas-Días et al., 2019) and the second shows how the AIRM is an effective map for transforming injuries from abusive or neglectful others in individual therapy (EFIT).

What Is an Attachment Injury?

The construct of an AI was first used by Johnson and colleagues to define a specific relational incident, where one partner is inaccessible or unresponsive to offer comfort and caring in a particular moment of need, thus shattering the bond of trust between intimates (Johnson et al., 2001). Vulnerable moments of need frequently occur at times of life transitions. Examples include *a parent's death and dying; a child hospitalized; receiving a medical diagnosis; a crucial job interview; a miscarriage; moving to a new country; increased hostility toward Asian immigrants during the COVID pandemic.*

Johnson and colleagues created the term *attachment injury* to make sense of a recurring theme they were noticing among couples who had significantly improved in therapy but were not recovering from distress. In particular, the couples were reaching an impasse in the softening change event. They discovered a reappearing dynamic of couples who, having completed the first two change events of de-escalation and withdrawer engagement, could not complete a softening. In the precarious moment when a more pursuing partner was about to make a vulnerable reach toward their partner, sudden trauma reactions appeared (see Box 16.1). They observed flashbacks, dissociating, disorientation, and expressions of, "No, no, never again! Never again will I risk trusting this person," was a theme repeated across couples. Suddenly an event, not previously discussed by the couple, from 2, 6 or even 30 years earlier popped into the pursuing partner's memory and

DOI: 10.4324/9781003242673-24

Box 16.1   Post-Trauma Reactions Following Attachment Injuries

An Attachment Injury Is a Relationship Trauma

Attachment injuries emerge in therapy "in an alive and intensely emotional manner, much like a traumatic flashback, and overwhelm the injured partner" (Johnson et al., 2001, p. 145). They are abrupt, shattering, life-changing moments that redefine the safety of the relationship and the internal working models of self and other.

Reactions Are Similar to Post Trauma Symptoms

- **persistent re-experiencing:** as though the event were happening in the present moment;
- **avoidance and numbing:** feeling oneself freezing; going numb; disorientation, detachment; feeling distant or removed from others around
- **hyperarousal:** startle reflex, jumpy, hyperalert; intense fight, flight, freeze reactions

In assessment (Chapter 7) an EFT therapist invites EFCT and EFIT clients to reflect on pivotal moments that may have changed everything for them and for their relationship. Emily asks herself when working with each distressed couple, "Is there an attachment injury that has had *a sudden shattering* impact on their attachment bond or is the couple presenting with relationship distress where their connection and trust has *gradually eroded* from a repetitive destructive pattern?" Similarly with individuals, "Do they identify a pivotal moment that changed everything?"

Some Common Markers of an AI Are Portrayed in the Following Elements of Emotion

Triggers: Triggers bring the injurious event alive in the present moment, "as though it were yesterday" or "that take me back to day one." Examples are: An expressionless look on his face like when I discovered the betrayal; his cell phone; her computer case; the doorbell ringing; the bank statement; the tone in their voice.

Body: Can't stop shaking, stab in my back, clutching my throat, cannot breathe, stomach churning; heart throbbing, head pounding, face tensing, arm twitching.

Meanings: Obsessed with the affair; obsessed with the moment he told me; can't stop thinking of the moment; I have lost everything now; I don't know any more who she is; he has become a stranger; Who am I now? I am totally lost; I am stained by this; He is forever marked by this; Now I am one of those, dirty, pathetic women; I'll never, ever be enough; something is wrong with me; what is wrong with them?

Action tendencies: Explanations, defense, accusations, distancing, pleading, weeping, yelling, calmly, logically making plans. (Lafontaine et al., in preparation).

---

stopped them in their tracks. "*Never again can I trust who I thought we were.*" Partners were typically taken off guard – having totally forgotten or dismissed the presence of this invisible *ghost of an AI,* in spite of rumbling echoes of broken trust.

The discovery of this recurring process brought to life a dynamic that is discussed in the early literature on attachment theory in adult relationships: Events in which one partner responds, or fails to respond, at times of urgent need are found to unduly influence the quality of an attachment relationship and to redefine the security of the relationship (Simpson & Rholes, 1994). *Attachment injury* became a most fitting description for a specific event that had the power to shatter the trust in the attachment bond. It became synonymous with a *never again moment.* These injurious events are pivotal, moment-in-time events that shatter the attachment bond and redefine the relationship as unsafe and untrustworthy. From that moment on, the shattering event continues to be the standard by which one partner measures the dependability of the offending partner (OP). This can be the case with seemingly minor incidents, such as a hurtful comment at a key moment of need, or the prototypical AI of infidelity. Unless an AI is resolved and trust is rebuilt, partners are unable to move beyond de-escalation and will most likely relapse once therapy is terminated (Makinen & Johnson, 2006).

Trauma expert Herman (1992) calls abandonment and betrayal at a crucial moment of need a violation of human connection. This violation is a *relationship trauma*, creating or exacerbating existing insecurity in an attachment bond and inducing overwhelming fear and helplessness in the injured partner (IP). There is a life-and-death nature to these traumatic moments. Emotions associated with the event tend to linger and trauma reactions ensue. The IP is likely to vacillate between numbing withdrawal and experiencing flashbacks and hyperarousal that is manifest in accusations toward their partner. The OP's unreliability and untrustworthiness become a recurring theme and creates an impasse that blocks relationship repair. In response to this relationship trauma, both partners typically experience emotional pain and shame. The IP feels shame and a diminished sense of self. The OP also feels shame for the injury they caused, helplessness to repair the damage, and anger or impatience for their partner to *get over it.*

The attachment significance of an event is what gives it the power to rupture a relationship and redefine its security. Attachment theory explains what makes up the defining moments in relationships and tells us what is likely to strengthen a bond or to shatter it. When a partner is accessible and emotionally responsive in a moment of need, the attachment bond is nurtured and strengthened but abandonment or betrayal at a critical moment of need violates the expectation that the partner will be there to offer comfort and care in times of danger and distress. It is not the content of the event, but, rather, the life-and-death threat of abandonment or rejection experienced during the event that gives it the power to tear an attachment bond to shreds. "What matters most to Pain Central is not the philosophical category a slight belongs to *but the level of jeopardy it threatens* ... like a shattered knee or a scratched cornea, relationship ruptures deliver agony" (Lewis et al., 2000, p. 95, italics added). An actual affair can be less injurious than the OP's defensive or emotionally absent response in the moment of the discovery of the affair. The crux of the injury – what gives it power to shatter the attachment bond – is that at a moment of urgent need, one's expected source of comfort is unavailable or unresponsive. Herein lies the relevance to EFIT, discussed at the end of the chapter. When an attachment figure, one's expected source of comfort and support, whether it be partner, parent, or trusted friend, is mis-attuned or accusatory during an individual's moment of need, a sense of connection and positive sense of self and other are shattered.

What an Attachment Injury Is Not and Why that Matters

Beginning EFCT therapists sometimes confuse an AI with recurring hurts and disappointments in a couple's life or with traumas external to the couple's relationship. There are two defining features of an AI that EFT therapists should know. First, an AI is a rupture created by *a specific event*, as distinguished from the regular ups and downs of a relationship. The slow erosion of relationship trust from repetitive negative interaction patterns does not have the cataclysmic proportion of an AI. A negative pattern slowly erodes relationship safety and trust, whereas an AI shatters the most basic assumption of an attachment relationship ("You will be there when I need you") in one identifiable moment (Johnson, 2013). Assumptions of the other's reliability and one's sense of self as lovable and precious to the other partner are shaken to the core in one specific incident. For AI repair, the specific incident needs to be named and its impact explored.

Second, an AI is a rupture *within* the couple's relationship, as distinguished from traumas external to the couple's relationship. One partner's traumatic experiences, for example, childhood abuse or neglect, a parent's suicide or mental illness, operational stress injuries, military service, a motor vehicle accident, and ongoing REC trauma and other minority stressors are not attachment injuries specific to this intimate relationship bond, although they are likely to contribute to relationship distress and to the complexity of AI repair. EFT therapists distinguish between trauma within the relationship and contextual trauma. For AI repair, EFT therapists explicitly name both the relationship-injurious event and the impacts of contextual trauma, working simultaneously to rebuild trust in the intimate relationship. The case example of Leon and Liliana (Chapter 16 Support Material, routledge.com/9781032151335) portrays the process of AI resolution in the face of racial trauma.

Attachment Injuries Appear in Three Discrete Ways in EFCT

One of the main markers that signals to a therapist that a couple is being impacted by an unresolved AI is "a sudden increase in the emotional intensity of the couple's interaction" (Johnson et al., 2001, p. 147). There are three basic ways this increased emotional intensity may be seen. I present case examples of each one. The first is when an AI, like a gaping wound, is a dominant, escalating focus in Stage 1. The second is a subtle indication of an AI appearing like a ghost peeking tentatively out of a closet in Stage 1 or 2. The third is when an AI, like a ghost roaring out of a closet, suddenly and unexpectedly emerges in Stage 2.

A gaping wound is visible from the outset of therapy with Gail and Paul who are stuck in time, unable to recover from the relationship wound of Paul's affair. Nearly every moment of therapy is punctuated by Gail's frantic protests of, "How could Paul have done this?" followed by Paul, on the edge of his chair, wringing his hands, repeatedly offering the same shame-faced apology. (This case example is expanded in the next section illustrating EFT in Stage 1 with an AI.)

A ghost of an AI peeks out of the closet when a gay couple, Jon (the withdrawer) and Kareem (the pursuer) mention an event in early assessment, which they report is "over now." It is rarely mentioned and does not block Stage 1 de-escalation; however, as they begin Stage 2, it is hinted at again. Jon's eyes mist over while discussing "that argument" when Kareem stormed off for dinner with his family. "You'd think I'd be over it by now," he says rather nonchalantly, but his eyes fill with tears. A subtle hint of a "never trust him again" moment begins to emerge. An EFT therapist zooms right in to attend to the wound and to pave the way toward naming and repairing the relationship rupture. They also acknowledge the additional minority-stress of this gay couple and fold it into the couple's pattern that is blocking Jon's engagement and repair of the AI. (See Brubacher & Johnson, 2017 for an expanded example of a similar case.)

A ghost of an AI comes roaring out of the closet as partners Aida and Eric are becoming increasingly vulnerable with one another in Stage 2. Just as Aida, the more pursuing partner is invited to risk and make a vulnerable reach toward the now-engaged Eric, a "Never again!" limbic alarm bell rings and she freezes. A memory of a traumatic relationship event from 40 years ago – a moment of intense need when Eric was emotionally unavailable – floods through her being and she halts. This example is expanded in a later section, illustrating the use of the AIRM to resolve an injury in Stage 2. First we explore validating and stabilizing with AIs in Stage 1.

Stabilizing/De-escalating with Attachment Injuries in Stage 1 EFCT

When the gaping wound of an AI is apparent from the outset of therapy, the therapist needs to attend to the wound and stabilize the present pattern that is blocking partners from repairing the broken trust.

The Gaping Wound: Working with a Visible Attachment Injury in Stage 1

Emily listens as Gail and Paul describe the event that prompted them to seek couple therapy. The event was clearly a sudden snap of the bond of trust they had shared. "He was my hero," says Gail twisting a tissue in her hands and speaking in a fragile voice:

> I knew I was his precious one and I trusted him with my life. We struggled together to success-fully raise our sons, one having many special needs. We had lovely times travelling with our children and he was always there for me. And then—at the rawest moment of my life, when my mother died—I found a receipt for a pearl necklace he bought for his office assistant. I knew at that moment I wasn't his true love any more. He has never bought me a piece of jewellery in my life!

She hesitates, "I lost my hero!" Gasping for breath and in a sudden mix of tears and rage, "I never in a million years thought he would do it, you know!" Paul reaches in, "I know—it was wrong. I've told you I'm sorry. It was so wrong of me. I've told you I am so sorry!" Emily catches her breath. The open wound of this AI dominates the session.

Emily is briefly tempted to guide Gail to share her vulnerable pain with Paul to help him under-stand how deeply he has hurt her and to invite Paul to respond with enough remorse that will heal this injury. Suddenly, she jolts herself into remembering the importance of identifying and stabiliz-ing the negative cycle before attempting the resolution process which can only happen in Stage 2. She refocuses. Attuning to the process of what is before her, she sees an escalated couple: Paul in a gently defended, placating, withdrawer position and Gail in a fragile, critical pursuing position. Emily reminds herself that she is working in Stage 1 and that first she needs to help them to as-semble their experiences and to stabilize their recurring pattern of interacting. She needs to track the negative interaction cycle, including the gaping wound, playing out in the room.

She begins with naming and validating their typical moves and meaning making in their imprison-ing pattern that may have set the stage for the AI and is certainly the interactive pattern that is keeping the hurt alive. Gail pushes to talk; Paul apologizes and wants her to feel better. Emily speaks softly:

> Gail, I am noticing that the more you share your pain and your anger that he could turn to someone else when you needed him most, the more you, Paul, apologize profusely and then get impatient when you cannot make her feel better.

Emily continues to track the process of emotion in the negative cycle, evoking and reflecting at-tachment meanings created when triggers occur. Triggers for Gail are Paul's time at his office and the receipt she discovered for the pearl necklace. Opening a doorway into Gail's emotion process, Emily asks, "What do you tell yourself, Gail, about his time at work? What does the jewellery receipt say to you?" A big trigger for Paul is Gail's unhappiness, so Emily asks, "What do you say to yourself when you see she is unhappy, and you cannot get her out of her depression? And now, when you see her pain and anger, what does it say to you?"

She validates the reactive emotions of each partner: Gail's anger and Paul's impatience and helplessness at not being able to make Gail feel better. Paul's impatience and helpless reactions extend back through years of Gail's struggles with depression and are especially alive now that he has hurt her so badly. Emily catches bullets where necessary.

Gail: I don't think he really thought he had a problem. I asked him to get therapy. I said he needed it.

Emily: (catching a subtle bullet) That was your way of saying let's break through this trap we're caught in—this repetitive trap where the harder you try to pull him close, the more he seems to disappear; the more he disappears, the more you point out the dangerous distancing, yes?

Then Emily, with Move 2 assembling and deepening, evokes and makes sense of the underlying emotional music that drives the dance: Loneliness, pain, fears of rejection and abandonment, and negative views of self ("I'm unlovable and despicable,") and other ("He is unpredictable and unreliable," and "She will never give me another chance!") Finally, she reframes their distress as the familiar dance that is blocking them from having a healing conversation about the injury. That is, the dance of Paul withdrawing, placating, and defending and Gail pushing, protesting, and crumbling in despair, blocks them from repairing the shattered trust. When they cannot turn to each other and share, the distress and fears are exacerbated.

Emily reflects what has happened as a tragic moment that broke the bond between them: Paul's turning to another woman shattered the trust between them and nearly, but not totally, banished him from being Gail's hero. While reassuring the couple that she knows the path to help them repair this broken trust, she validates that it makes total sense that Gail cannot trust him yet, and that Paul still gets stabs of fear each time he sees her pain, wondering if he will ever again be her hero.

Key Elements for Responding to an Attachment Injury in Stage 1

Of course, not all OPs are as penitent as Paul. Some are cold and dismissive or well defended with excuses and counterattacks. Nevertheless, stabilizing the pattern that is blocking a couple from having a healing conversation needs to precede the resolution process. When an AI is alive from the outset of therapy, current cycles of raging and defending or apologizing and distancing need to be tracked, and emotions need to be assembled. The pattern needs to be framed as the problem blocking them from discussing the bleeding wound and mending the shattered trust. The cycle that needs to be stabilized at this time is the current cycle which is blocking healing conversations about the injury and aggravating the wound. This cycle could be similar to or different from the original cycle that predates the injury, but the EFT therapist works with the current pattern.

When EFT therapists identify one or more attachment injuries in Stage 1, they refrain from getting sucked onto a problem-solving carousel, focusing instead on the process and the ways an AI is part of their current interactive pattern. They do this by boldly naming the injurious incident and evoking and validating its ongoing impact on their interactions. For example:

Scott, ever since you discovered Diane texting your best friend, Alec, when your mother was dying, your heart burns with anguish and you desperately demand she not leave your sight. Diane, the more he makes demands on you, the more you shut down inside, and the more you shut down, the more he makes demands.

If the couple presents multiple AI events, they are made explicit in the cycle in Stage 1. For example, if Diane adds that her heart has been on ice ever since Scott left her alone with the new baby, this event of broken trust will also be made explicit in the current pattern. The therapist continues to offer slow, gentle, relentless validation to the differing positions of criticism or shut down, turn away, or turn against, and to empathize and validate differing experiences of anguish, rage, remorse, or hopelessness.

To understand how the Stage 2 AIRM (Box 16.2) can provide some guidance for working in Stage 1 with AIs, it is important to note that the model evolved by observing how de-escalated

Box 16.2   AIRM Steps: Client Tasks and EFT Tango Moves

Cycle De-escalation Related to the Injury

Step 1

Injured Partner (IP)'s Task: Articulate the injury and impact of the trust-shattering event.

Therapist's Intervention: Move 1 to process injured partner (IP)'s account of the incident of injury and its "never again" impact.

Step 2

Offending Partner (OP)'s Task: Respond to the IP; is likely to discount the incident and move into a protective stance.

Therapist's Intervention: Move 1 to validate and support OP to hear the attachment significance of the event.

Step 3

IP's Task: Access attachment fears, shattered trust, and longings associated with the injurious event.

Therapist's Intervention: Move 2 to support the IP to stay in touch with the attachment significance of the injury.

Step 4

OP's Task: Hears the attachment significance of the event as importance to their partner, not defective. Expands on how it evolved, to become predictable again.

Therapist's Intervention: Move 2 (and some Move 4 to process) supports OP to assemble their emotional reactions, to become accessible to the attachment significance of the incident, and to how the incident evolved.

New Cycles of Emotional Engagement: Forgiveness and Reconciliation

Step 5

IP's Task: Shares core pain of the shattered bond in one traumatic moment. A more vulnerable expression of the loss and broken trust.

Therapist's Intervention: Move 2, to process the IP's core emotion of the injury. Move 3, to direct the IP's vulnerable expression of pain, loss, fears and longings to the OP.

Step 6

OP's Task: Emotionally engaged, accesses a "felt sense" of partner's pain; visibly moved. Express empathy, regret, remorse, and responsibility.

Therapist's Intervention: Move 2, to process OP's core emotional responses (sadness, remorse, regret, empathy for IP) and facilitate a "felt sense" of partner's pain. Promote responsibility, empathy, regret, and remorse. Move 4, to shape and process encounters. Move 3 encounters for OP to disclose empathy (feeling the other's pain), responsibility, and remorse.

Consolidation of the Restored Bond

Step 7

IP's Task:	Risk asking for attachment needs to be met.
Therapist's Intervention:	Move 4, to process and Move 2, to assemble and deepen IP's accessibility and responsiveness to partner's expressions. Move 3 to invite and support the IP to ask for what they need to rebuild trust.

Step 8

OP's Task:	Respond with caring, creating antidote to the trauma. Relationship is redefined as a safe haven.
Both Partners' Task:	Create new narrative of event.
Therapist's Intervention:	Move 5, to integrate and summarize partners' reaching and responding; evoke new narrative. Heighten interpersonal repair.

This model is validated in outcome and process studies (Makinen & Johnson, 2006; Zuccarini et al., 2013). See Chapter 16 Support Material for more details on client tasks and Emily's use of the EFT Tango to shape each task (routledge.com/9781032151335).

couples resolved AIs that emerged as the impasse blocking Stage 2 change (Johnson et al., 2001). De-escalated couples, facing a newly discovered AI needed to stabilize/de-escalate again, this time specifically around the injurious event. Thus, the de-escalating phase of the AIRM provides some guidance for working in Stage 1 with AIs that are apparent early in therapy.

In some Stage 1 couples, the injury is a bleeding wound needing to be addressed first and foremost. In other couples, the injury may lie quietly in the background, peaking out subtly from time to time. Regardless of how explicitly the couple addresses the injury, an EFT therapist boldly names the injury and its role in their current pattern of interacting, while working with the couple to stabilize. The repetitive pattern may be dominated by attempts to talk and/or avoid talking about the AI. The AIRM guides therapists not to rush into trying to heal or prematurely rebuild trust, nor to provide insight into *why* the injury may have happened. Rather, the focus is on helping the couple to stabilize, with the injury in full view and openly named. Stage 1 discussions of AIs are oriented toward creating sufficient safety for partners to openly name their moves in the pattern that is blocking healing conversations and to begin to safely disclose raw emotions. De-escalating the pattern around the injury makes it possible to move into the Stage 2 resolution process.

Flowing with Moves of the Tango to Stabilize/De-escalate with an AI in Stage 1

The de-escalation phase of the AIRM is a helpful guide for how to weave in the specific content of the injury and to validate two perspectives of a flaming *hot potato incident* that feels untouchable in Stage 1. The model gives a therapist courage to name the injurious event and to validate and make room for partners' two very different perspectives. It also guides a therapist to help clients through two crucial steps of AI de-escalation; (a) helping the IP to pinpoint the attachment significance of the injury and (b) helping the OP in the context of hearing the attachment significance (their importance to their partner), to become predictable again by acknowledging how the injury evolved. Stabilization and engagement change events that embrace an AI lay the foundation for Stage 2 resolution.

When an AI is blatantly in the open in Stage 1, an EFT therapist attunes and responds with EFT Tango moves to stabilize the pattern that is preventing a couple from having a healing injuries conversation. Some stabilization around the injury will happen as the therapist explores how a couple gets stuck in trying to discuss or avoid discussing the event. The crux of the injury and the deepest pain each partner carries from the injury, such as fears, anger, shame, regret, and other complexities of emotional pain, as well as their present cycle around the injury, will be delineated and validated. The attachment significance of the injury will also be made clear. Examples of using the moves to stabilize follow.

Move 1 Reflecting Present Process. Reflect triggers and action tendencies in the present process with Move 1. A typical stuck pattern in Stage 1 is some version of one partner, usually but not always the IP, pushing to constantly discuss the event and the other partner avoiding these discussions, suggesting, "It's over. Let's move on."

With Move 1, a therapist explicitly names the event and empathically tracks how each partner is triggering and getting triggered to avoid or pursue conversations about the AI event, "The more he pushes you to talk about your affair, the more you pull away from him; the more she pulls away from you, the more harshly you go after her." A therapist includes contextual stressors and triggers when relevant. For example, to a white woman in a biracial couple, having discovered her husband's affair, a therapist says:

> You say that you don't mean to put him in danger, yet you admit that you can just get so angry at him that you totally forget you are a small white woman fighting with a black man in public and that what you are doing could be deadly for him.

Explicitly naming the injury can be challenging for a therapist who struggles with directly stating something that could have an aura of shame or disgust, such as the discovery of a partner's affair, gambling activity, or dismissal at a moment of grave need. A therapist might resist repeatedly naming the injury for fear of triggering shame for the OP or heightening the IP's pain. It is actually calming, however, to boldly name the injurious event and explicitly track how the event of broken trust is part of the current cycle. Explicit naming contains the unspeakable and begins the process of stabilizing the current cycle that blocks partners from effectively discussing the injurious event. Naming tames. What is shareable is bearable.

Move 2 Assembly.

Injured partner (IP):   I can tell he doesn't want to talk about it, so I never bring it up—I just poke him to punish him sometimes.

Offending partner (OP):   I don't want to talk about it—I've said I'm sorry! It's time to move on!

A therapist assembles each partner's experience with Move 2, linking triggers (partner texting), bodily responses (hurts like a stab in the back; voice gets shrill), action tendencies (scream, yell, freeze), and meanings of the injury ("He is not who I thought he was!") and the current fallout from the shattering event. In the assembly, reactive emotions and defensive actions are validated.

Move 2 Deepening. The therapist pinpoints and validates the nub of the injury and deepens the underlying core pain, fear, or resentment that is blocking trust. For example, an IP says:

I know he didn't mean to hurt me, but it hurts worse than anything I've ever known. The moment I first saw that text is burned into my mind. When I read that text, my heart sank through the earth! I flashback to those sweet words he wrote to her and I feel like I have an elephant on my chest. I can barely breathe. I'm terrified I'll never be his precious one again!

It is important to identify the bond-shattering moment (when IP saw the text) and the crux of the injury that needs repair (*those sweet words to her, mean I'll never be his precious one again*).

Moves 3 and 4 Shaping and Processing Encounters. The therapist shapes encounters where the IP discloses the *attachment significance* of the injury (AIRM Step 3). *Attachment significance* means that the IP is hurting because of how important their partner is to them and not because their partner is defective or inherently bad. Articulating this core of their hurt as related to their partner's importance pulls for a deeper level of vulnerability and emotional engagement. In the following examples, attachment significant terms are in italics:

- It shatters me because you are the one I thought would never do this to me!
- My stomach churns every time I relive that scene of *you walking away from me*!
- I could accept the affair, but not *your cold reaction to me* when I found out!

A highly escalated couple will need much containment and support. When the IP can communicate the attachment significance of the injury and this is integrated by the OP with Move 4 processing, the therapist shapes an encounter for the OP to expand on *how* (not why) they were able to take this injurious action (AIRM Step 4). It is fundamentally important to confirm that an OP grasps their significance to their partner, and is emotionally engaged in the relationship, before posing this question. It is not a *why* question, but a genuinely curious, supportive question about *how* it was possible that they could have done this injurious action.

To invite an emotionally engaged reflection about this event being catastrophic precisely because they are so important to their partner, a therapist can ask, "When your partner is clearly so important to you, can you say something about *how* you were able to do this?"

OP: As horrible as it sounds, I was so caught up in feeling useless and guilty, that I was able to tune them out and stop caring.

An OP's disclosure in response to *how* they could have done what they did is frequently not a pleasant answer, but it is genuine and believable to the IP. This is a crucial part of stabilization/ de-escalation because it begins to make the OP predictable again. It is important to use Move 4 to help the IP to process the OP's disclosure about *how* they were able to this action which has shattered their bond. For example, "How is it for you to hear your partner admit that they so caught up in feeling useless and guilty, that they tuned you out and stopped caring?" The partner who became a stranger through the event that ruptured the trust is once again whom the IP knew them to be!

In contrast, if the OP were not sufficiently engaged, they may offer a response such as, "I have no idea how this happened. I feel so badly! I won't do it again." This lack of awareness will not make them predictable to their partner; nor will it help the couple to stabilize.

Move 5 Integration. With Move 5, the therapist helps partners to validate and integrate this stabilizing work where their view of self and other are shifting, even though the trust is not yet rebuilt.

The frame of the pattern as the problem that has been blocking them from repairing the injury, is consolidated. The couple's stabilizing work is summarized as paving the road toward lifting their respective shame and transforming hurt (anger, grief and fears) into restored trust.

Move 1 Reflecting Present Process. We have come full circle in reviewing the moves but are revisiting Move 1. Repeating Move 1 helps to build and maintain *task alliance*, with transparency about the process. During stabilization, when partners or therapist become impatient for *instant trust* to emerge, the therapist assures the couple that even though the trust is not rebuilt *yet*, they are *en route* toward trust. Normalizing the progress and seeding attachment, a therapist can say:

> Before rebuilding trust, we need first to name clearly how you currently get stuck in automatic behaviours that send messages of danger, hopelessness, and more hurt or shame to one another. I know how to guide you on this pathway, to help you to step fully into this journey, to truly share the pain, and to reach and respond with the comfort you need to rebuild trust.

The training video *After the Affair* at www.steppingintoeft.com illustrates the profound impact of helping an IP openly share the attachment significance of the injury ("I'm devastated because you are the one, I thought would never do this!") in contrast to aggressive criticism ("What's the matter with you?") Stage 1 encounters identify and stabilize the repetitive pattern around the injury and begin to make the OP more predictable. REC impacts on the attachment bond are identified and explored.

Box 16.3   Stage 1 EFT Tango Moves to De-escalate/Stabilize with Attachment Injuries

Move 1 Reflection of present process:
    Boldly name the injury in the current cycle
    Track the moves and triggers. Validate two accounts of the event.
    Catch bullets.
    (AIRM Steps 1 and 2)
Move 2 Assembly: Add *meanings* and *bodily reactions* to the cycle, validating broken trust.
Move 2 Deepening: Access both partners' underlying pain/hurt. Distil the nub of the injury.
Move 3 Shaping encounters of safe connection: Help IP to disclose the attachment significance of the injury. (I am hurting because of how important you are to me." (AIRM Step 3).
    Help OP to hear the attachment significance ("I am important, not bad.") and to expand on how the incident evolved (AIRM Step 4).
Move 4: Process encounters
    Help OP to hear the attachment significance (importance to partner, not defective) before expanding on how it evolved.
    Help IP to process OP's disclosure on how the injury evolved.
Move 5: Summarize and integrate growing safety and balance with a clear description of the pattern blocking repair. Validate the unresolved fears, hurt, and mistrust that remain. Seed hope for repair.

The Attachment Injury Resolution Model for Restoring Broken Bonds in Stage 2

The AIRM is a validated blueprint for AI repair (Makinen & Johnson, 2006; Zuccarini et al., 2013). It is a mini-model within the larger EFT model. The eight-step repair process (Box 16.2) specifically addresses the injurious incident in a series of responsive dialogues (encounters) between IPs and OPs. The conversations of reaching and responding create an emotionally engaged apology that offers reparative comfort and reshapes the attachment bond. This Stage 2 process has the transformative elements of a softening (Greenman & Johnson, 2013). As with a successful softening, partners need to have stabilized/de-escalated in order for the pursuer to be sufficiently open to participate, and a withdrawn partner needs to have engaged so as to be accessible to join in the healing conversation.

Emily notices that she and her colleagues are initially mystified that the Stage 2 process of AI repair includes client steps of de-escalation, when de-escalation/stabilization is a Stage 1 process. Then she remembers that the model was developed by observing couples who had already stabilized but reached an impasse in Stage 2. When injuries that were not visible in Stage 1 surprisingly emerge in Stage 2 after a couple has already stabilized, there will, of course, need to be de-escalation of the cycle around the injury before the couple can deepen into the vulnerable forgiveness and trust-building dialogues. Having previously explored how the de-escalation portion of the AIRM can be helpful with attachment injuries in Stage 1, the following description pertains to AIs that suddenly appear in Stage 2.

The first outcome study (Makinen & Johnson, 2006) validated the effectiveness of the model as a map for the forgiveness change process. It was conducted with 24 couples who experienced an AI. Sixty-three percent resolved the injury, forgave the injuring partner, and reshaped the attachment bond. A three-year follow-up study (Halchuk et al., 2010) showed that increase in relationship satisfaction and forgiveness in the resolver couples was maintained. In 2013, Zuccarini et al. examined the process of change following the steps outlined in the 2006 study. They delineated the specific therapist interventions and client tasks or steps that promoted successful AI resolution and further validated the change process identified in the earlier studies.

Two Key Dialogues in Attachment Injury Resolution

Although there is much exploration and many encounters through the repair process, the AIRM, presented as eight steps of client change (Box 16.2), can be summarized as two series of dialogues of increasing emotional depth and affiliative responding (Brubacher & Wiebe, 2019; Greenman & Johnson, 2013; Wiebe & Johnson, 2016), bookended with specific disclosures. The initial bookend is a disclosure from the IP, naming the injurious event, and the OP's response to this account. The bookend in closing – after the forgiveness and reconciliation dialogue – is a consolidation of the bond where the IP is invited to risk reaching to request that their attachment needs regarding the injury be met, the OP responds, and the couple is supported to create a new narrative of the event.

Dialogue 1: Assembling Each Partner's Experience of the Injury. The first of the two key dialogues, potentially including many encounters is an assembly of each partner's version of the injurious event. This dialogue is the clients' Steps 3 and 4 of the AIRM. The IP identifies the attachment significance of the event and the OP elaborates on how the event evolved. This entails helping the IP to assemble and express the attachment meaning that is at the core of this injury. For example, "You are the one person I thought would never do this to me! I thought I could always count on you, and suddenly I don't know who you are!" This is followed by helping the OP to absorb that their partner's pain is because of their importance to them, and not because they are a bad person due to their actions.

Emily is finding it takes some careful processing to help the OP remain engaged as they listen to their partner describe the impact of the hurtful event, particularly the pain of having someone they counted on, betray them. She pauses to process and integrate using Move 4, "How is it to hear that your partner's pain deep down is about, 'That is not who I knew you to be. You are the last person I thought would do this!'?"

Following her attempt to process and help the OP to take in, "Your partner's pain is about how important you are to them!" she gathers her courage to ask the difficult yet very important question, "How were you able to do this to your partner?" For example, an IP says, "I feel the stab in my back every day," and Emily asks the OP, "How were you able to stab your beautiful partner in the back?" Evoking and then shaping an encounter with Moves 2 and 3, she helps the OP to expand on *how* the injury happened. The IP needs to hear an emotionally engaged explanation from their partner about *how* they could have hurt them in this way, in order for them to become predictable again. The therapist is seeking a response to "*how* could you do this" rather than "*why* did you do it?" An emotionally engaged response comes from an engaged partner.

The OP in the EFT AIRM training program *at* www.attachmentinjuryrepair.com (Brubacher & Buchanan, 2014) says, "As horrible as it sounds, I think I was trying to hurt her." "It does sound horrible," the therapist replies, validating the anguish in his voice as he looks straight into the eyes of his partner, who flashes a slight smile of recognition, as though to say, "I recognize this guy!" Up until this point, the OP remains a stranger. Only after the OP can engage in owning *how* they were able to create this injury can the IP begin to find them predictable again. As the OP makes sense out of how he could have turned away from his wife to have an affair with her best friend, he is essentially recounting his moves in their cycle: When he would be hurting from a conflict between them, he would not send a clear message to her. He would walk away in anger and then fight back in a spiteful reaction. Openly acknowledging, in tears, "I was trying to hurt you, as horrible as that sounds," he authentically reveals his heartfelt remorse at how horrible he feels that he was actually trying to hurt his wife.

Dialogue 2: The Forgiving Injuries/Rebuilding Trust Conversation. The second key dialogue is the crux of forgiveness and rebuilding trust. This dialogue is the clients' Steps 5 and 6 of the AIRM. The therapist shapes encounters where the IP discloses the impact of the event, with increasing depth of experiencing and vulnerability, processing the anger, sadness, shame, and fears related to the injury. The OP, also with increasing emotional depth and vulnerability, offers an emotionally engaged apology that expresses responsibility, remorse, and attuned empathy for their partner's pain. In this vulnerable reaching and responding process, the hurt is reprocessed, forgiveness occurs, and trust is restored. The crucial healing element is when an IP sees in their partner's face and hears in their partner's voice that the one who has hurt them is actually *feeling their pain*. Also significant for rebuilding trust is the OP's genuine disclosure of remorse, regret, and responsibility for causing this injury.

Contrary to folklore that forgiveness is an inside job, from an attachment perspective, forgiveness and rebuilding trust are a relational process. Both partners are changed as trust is rebuilt. The OP moves from feeling helpless and thinking, "There is simply nothing I can say or do to make up for this," to becoming the one who makes a difference for their partner through their engaged, responsive participation in this healing conversation. The IP moves from feeling hopeless and thinking, "This will always hurt, but I just have to not let it bother me," to discovering that the most important source of comfort is right next to them, helping to heal the injury!

Resolving an Attachment Injury in Stage 2: The AIRM with Eric and Aida

Emily first discovers the defining power that one "long forgotten" pivotal event can have on a relationship in her work with Eric and Aida, a couple in their late forties, who had married as teenagers. They entered therapy with a well-entrenched cycle of Aida pursuing with escalating criticism and hostility and Eric shutting down, going cold, and occasionally firing back in self-defense with vicious comments.

The couple and Emily are pleased with the progress they are making. After taking several months to de-escalate and several more weeks for Eric to fully engage, Eric is taking a more assertive place in the relationship. He is stepping close to Aida, asking for reassurance and comfort in ways he had never done before in his life. When he catches sight of her look that to him signals danger, "as if I'm about to get burned," he pauses now and asks for her patience. He lets her know that look freaks him out and makes him feel like getting out of her way, but that he wants to stay connected. This longing to stay connected is a clear indication that he has engaged, since previously, being close to Aida felt dangerous to him. When he feels twinges of the familiar tingling from his heart to his arm – his typical bodily arousal at signs that Aida may be unhappy or disapproving – he says, "Oh no, it's starting up again. That tingling tells me you're about to judge me and wall me off." They repair the moment and come together.

In the midst of softening toward Eric, Aida expresses her fear that if she reaches to him, he will not be there. Emily senses Aida is the most vulnerable she has ever been, and she invites her to share this fear with Eric. As Aida looks over to Eric, she stops abruptly. Suddenly her face goes blank, she begins to wring her hands, and she looks off into the corner of the room. A long-forgotten AI ghost comes roaring out of the closet!

"No, no, no, no! He wasn't there. The darkest moment (pauses). We were so in love. He was my shining knight!" Her eyes fall to the floor. She wraps her arms around her belly and utters in a shakey voice:

> He's been a good father to Micah for 40 years, but I've never quite trusted he really loves him. I've never got over his suggestion that I have an abortion when I became pregnant. He fell off his pedestal that day. Broke my heart, really. Get rid of *our* baby! How could I? Didn't he care? I've never quite trusted him since. Why, I've almost blamed him for Micah's autism!

Emily feels a chill run through her body and her heart pounds with pain: Pain for the broken trust between them, pain for Aida's privately held grief and fear, and pain for Eric, hearing now for the first time how that one seemingly small moment broke her trust and diminished her view of him; that one moment knocked the knight in shining armor off his horse! Emily experiences first hand this common Stage 2 impasse she has read about, where a couple's initial distress lessened through Stage 1, but an unresolved AI from the past blocked their full repair.

Eric and Aida have come so far in repairing their relationship through de-escalation and withdrawer engagement, but when it comes to the final change event of softening, they are stuck. Aida cannot risk being vulnerable with Eric. The memory of the past event resurfaces and stops her in her tracks. Emily sees Eric's total shock that this forgotten event has resurfaced. She resonates with pain, imagining the difficult moment when the couple discovered they were pregnant before marriage – something totally unacceptable to Aida's religious, immigrant family. The couple obviously needs and is ready for the therapist to follow the AIRM to help them resolve an injurious event that has made its unexpected, paralyzing appearance.

The two key dialogues of the AIRM, described earlier, are a condensed version of the model, to portray a felt sense of the essence of the repair process. To make the more detailed AIRM accessible and updated, I illustrate how Emily facilitates the partners' steps of repair (as delineated in Zuccarini et al., 2013) using the moves of the EFT Tango with Aida and Eric.

Cycle De-escalation Related to the Injury

Move 1 to Help the Injured Partner (IP) Articulate the Injury (AIRM Step 1). Emily supports Aida to repaint the scene, engage with the pain, and put it into words.

Aida: He was my world – my knight in shining armor! I loved the baby from the moment I knew I was pregnant! Yes, I was afraid of my family's outrage and judgment, but I was confident that, with Eric, we could handle anything. But his suggestion of an abortion broke me. It felt as if he turned against me and against the baby!

Emily reflects the scene that Aida draws of Eric as her knight in shining armor, feeling she could get through anything if she had his support. She validates Aida's view that together they could survive her family's harsh disapproval and be a successful, happy, teen-parent family. She heightens Aida's description of Eric as her source of strength, that together they could do anything, and how his suggestion shattered that belief for her.

Move 1 to Help Offending Partner (OP) Respond (AIRM Step 2). Eric interrupts at times to express his utter shock at all this. Emily validates his reactions to this triggering moment of hearing that something he did over 35 years ago is still hurting Aida! She validates his disbelief and action tendencies to dismiss its significance and to explain and defend his behaviors. She acknowledges that his experience of that event is very different from Aida's.

Move 2 to Help IP Add the Attachment Significance (AIRM Step 3). Emily assembles Aida's emotional experience, heightening her description of the attachment significance of the event (Eric's importance to her, rather than his flaw). She helps Aida to integrate the story with her attachment fears and longings. She evokes vulnerable hurt, sadness, longings, and fears underlying her anger.

Aida: Something changed after he suggested I have an abortion and even suggested that we break up! I insisted he not break up with me. We got married, we carried on. We did survive my family's judgment. We stuck together but I pulled away from him to care for the baby and to protect the baby *from him*! I never quite trusted him again. I've never quite felt safe or protected by him anymore. I've had to act strong on my own. Inside, I was feeling lonely and scared, always afraid he'd walk away.

Move 3 to Help IP Deepen and Disclose the Attachment Crux of the Injury (AIRM Step 3). Emily shapes an encounter for Aida to tell Eric about this crushing experience of losing the man she trusted.

Moves 4 and 3 to Help OP Process Attachment Significance and Describe How it Happened (AIRM Step 4). Eric begins to hear Aida's pain, not as a sign that he is inadequate or insensitive, but as a sign of how important he is to her. He begins to become predictable again, by disclosing his experience during those dark moments when he had suggested breaking up and having an abortion.

Emily: (With Move 4) What is it like to see this side of Aida that you haven't seen before? What happens on the inside for you to hear her tell you she was scared and felt alone and lost and needed *you*—that she is still hurting and has never shared this before?

Eric: (Face flooded with anguish.) I hurt. I was so selfish, so young. I just wanted to run! I see now how much I hurt her, how lonely and terrified she felt. I had no idea! She's always been the strong one.

He acknowledges directly to Aida how he feels her pain, her loneliness, and how abandoned she must have felt.

Emily: (Shaping an encounter with Move 3.) Can you help Aida understand *how* you came to make this suggestion to her? (Supporting Eric to elaborate on how this event evolved, becomes a pivotal step in their healing process.)

Eric: I panicked. I felt so helpless and terrified of being a father. No idea of how to protect you or even how to take care of myself. I was terrified of your parents' reaction, and I just wanted to run, it's true! I felt so ashamed of who I was and so afraid of being a father and so afraid I couldn't live up to what you and your mother wanted me to be. I was overwhelmed and didn't know what to do. I wanted the best for you and thought I just couldn't do it!

Emily: (Reflecting and validating, could seem like Move 2 assembly; however, it is also part of Move 3, shaping a message for Eric to share with Aida in his encounter.) You had no idea of how to protect Aida and your baby. Your best attempt to support her was to suggest an abortion and to disappear from her life, yes? You are saying—you really thought mostly about your own needs at the time. Your suggestion to have an abortion and to break up broke her heart and you get that now. It hurts to hear that? (Eric is nodding and sobbing.)

As Eric opens up and discloses what was going on for him 40 years ago, he begins to make perfect sense to Aida and to become predictable. She senses his dependability again.

New Cycles of Emotional Engagement – Forgiveness and Reconciliation

Moves 3 and 4 to Help IP Disclose Deeper, Clearer, Vulnerable Expressions of the Impact of the Injury (AIRM Step 5). Emily helps Aida to distil and express the impact of the event directly to Eric. In so doing, she expands her attachment fears and longings and deepens her previously unexpressed loss and fears regarding the attachment bond. She describes years-old fears that Eric could not be trusted to support her or to love their son and to take a genuine interest in him.

As Emily reflects and validates Aida's experience, she is able to organize it more clearly, and to integrate the story of this pivotal event with her underlying vulnerable emotions. She asks Aida (shaping an encounter) to allow Eric to witness her vulnerability, "Can you tell him—show him— how scared and alone you felt?"

Aida: Until that moment you were still my knight – I thought the world of you, I felt so safe with you. You were my partner, and we were together. At that moment you turned into something else. I thought I had lost you, and I so desperately needed you. I didn't feel strong at all. I felt afraid and alone and I needed you.

Emily tracks and heightens the process of how right now, in this moment, Aida is letting Eric see how very vulnerable she is. She is showing Eric a side of her she never, ever shares with anyone: This frightened, "I can't-do-this-alone" part of herself.

With Move 4, Emily supports Eric to be emotionally engaged and moved by Aida's vulnerable expressions.

Moves 2, 3, and 4 to help OP Engage with Partner's Pain and Respond (AIRM Step 6). Slowly, with Move 2 (empathic reflections, evocative responding and heightening), Emily helps Eric to access his internal experience so that he has the space to actually feel Aida's hurt and feel how her pain impacts him.

Emily: How is it to hear Aida share this heart-breaking event where she totally lost her knight in shining armor and decided never again to trust you? (She then shapes an encounter for Eric to respond to Aida.)

Eric: I see your pain—it hurts me. I hurt to see what I've done to you! You are so beautiful, and I didn't get that I was your knight in shining armor! I felt small, ashamed, and frightened. I didn't think you've ever needed me—not really. I am so, so sorry I hurt you. I never want to hurt you like this! Never want you to feel abandoned or afraid.

With Move 4, Emily processes this engaged, responsive encounter of forgiveness and rebuilding trust. Aida sees Eric's face mirroring her pain. She hears caring and tenderness in his voice. She feels his empathy for her pain and his remorse for abandoning her in this critical moment.

Consolidation of the Restored, Trusting Bond

Moves 3, 4, and 5 to Help Partners Reach, Respond, and Create a New Narrative (AIRM Steps 7 and 8). Emily asks Aida to tell Eric what she needs to feel safe now. Aida risks reaching to Eric, "I need to know you want to support me. Inside I am not as strong as I act. I have this old, old wound and this fear. Whenever you become distant, I still fear that you could just give up on us. I need you to know that when I get demanding, underneath I am afraid and trying to hold on to you. Can you be my knight again and care for me? Can you assure me you will not leave, will not go away, will not shut down and pull away from me? Can you assure me I am precious to you? Precious enough to drive across town in bad weather for my favourite restaurant?" she adds with a subtle smile, recalling their last argument.

Eric replies, "I want more than anything to be that man for you. I want you to feel safe and loved! You are everything to me! I want you to feel completely safe with me. I want to care for you every way I can!"

Eric and Aida are creating a new attachment bond. Their relationship is redefined as one of safety and solid support shared between them.

Summary of the AIRM in EFCT

Repairing shattered attachment bonds and rebuilding trust is an interpersonal process with two series of dialogues. First are the conversations to assemble and stabilize each partner's experience of the injurious event. Second are the forgiveness and rebuilding trust dialogues. In stabilizing a pattern with the broken trust of an AI, it is important to assemble and validate the emotional pain of *both* the IPs and OPs. When REC trauma is also present for one or both partners, attending to minority stress, is heightened in both the stabilizing and forgiving injuries dialogues.

In dialogues to assemble and stabilize each partner's experience of the injury, it becomes clear that both partners are living with grief, fears, anger, and shame. First the couple is helped to stabilize enough that they can slow down and stop the cycles of blame, shame, and defense. The OP engages enough that they can tolerate deeply listening to their partner's pain; the IP stabilizes enough that they can share their pain in increasingly vulnerable, non-blaming ways.

The attachment significance of the injury becomes increasingly clear to both partners, in that the enormity of the shattering event is because of the importance the OP has to the IP. When the OP can hear that the event was so shattering precisely because of their importance, not their flaws, and can engage deeply enough with their own emotional experience to describe something about *how* they were able to take this very hurtful action, they become predictable and safer again. Predictability, a fundamental ingredient of rebuilding trust, stands in contrast to a flimsy apology, taking no responsibility, such as, "It was a stupid mistake. I'm sorry and I won't do it again."

In the forgiveness and rebuilding trust dialogues the IP deepens their vulnerability and articulation of their attachment pain. They move beyond accusations into affiliative sharing conversations where their deepest heartbreak is disclosed to a compassionate, attentive listener who is also the focus of their pain. This is a powerful antidote to shattered trust, heartbreak, and the shame that both IP and OP carry. The IP experiences their partner taking responsibility for the injury and risking to feel and taste *their* pain; what they have been enduring alone. The OP who betrayed their partner and shattered their bond of trust, comes to fully feel and to understand their partner's pain, and their own remorse.

Healing occurs for both partners in this interpersonal process of vulnerably sharing pain and responsively engaging with empathy, responsibility, and remorse. The OP who has also been living with fear and shame and pain has the surprisingly restorative experience of finding that their emotional engagement in owning their responsibility, and perhaps even more challenging, in tasting the pain their partner endured because of what they did, is making a difference for the one they hurt.

Multiple attachment injuries will take longer to resolve, although Johnson (2016a) suggests that the steps of the resolution process probably will not need to be followed for each event. After the corrective emotional bonding experience that reshapes the security of the relationship, partners can integrate the shift across the injuries of their relationship. Partners' entire world becomes safer and more secure.

If an AI emerges in Stage 2 during the engagement change event, and the IP is the withdrawer, the process of AIRM will become the engagement change event (Case example, Brubacher, 2018). A softening change event may still be needed after that. The steps of the AIRM form either the withdrawer engagement, if the withdrawer is the IP or, when the IP is the pursuer, they become a significant softening change event (Johnson, 2016b). Stage 3 will then integrate the newly shaped bond across other pragmatic issues and consolidate the shift into the future of the relationship. See Box 16.4 for a summary of tools provided in this chapter for working with attachment injuries in EFCT, including these variations.

The final conversations of repair include dialogues similar to the reach and response encounters in Stage 2. Repairing an AI is much bigger than cognitive forgiveness and letting go of resentment. Consonant with a softening, it is taking the risk to put oneself in the other's hands and once again experience safety and trust. The IP is invited to ask for what they need now, typically what they needed at the time of injury (such as some form of, "Notice my pain, stop hurting me, and come close to value/comfort me"). The OP is invited to respond. Both partners' resilience is strengthened; trust and dignity are restored for both partners as they co-create and consolidate the antidote to the shattered trust. Together they create a new narrative of their relationship. A newly secure bond of trust and connection strengthens the relationship bond and fortifies renewed positive views of self and other. Chapter 16 Support Material contains a fun poem of the AI resolution process from the perspective of the IP (routledge.com/9781032151335).

Box 16.4   Summary of EFCT Attachment Injury Tools

Resounding echoes of anger, shame, grief and fear can be daunting! EFT therapists frequently fear misstepping. Let these tools boost your confidence.

1. Content and Context are important! Name the moment of injury.

    a. Name the injury as soon as it is apparent.

    b. It is common for therapist and partners to be hesitant about addressing the moment of injury. Explicitly naming is regulating.

2. Set the stage for repair.

    a. Stabilize the cycle blocking repair.

    b. Engage the withdrawer.

Note: Withdrawing or pursuing partners can be injured.

- **When the IP is the more pursuing partner:** Both stabilization and engagement are pre-requisites to repair.
- **When the IP is the withdrawer:** The AIRM will be part of the engagement change event.

3. Shape two dialogue series of the Stage 2 Attachment Injury Resolution Model

    a. *Assemble and stabilize* each partner's experience of the injury, with the IP disclosing the attachment significance of the event and the OP expanding on how the injury happened. (AIRM Steps 3 and 4).

    b. Shape the *forgiving injuries conversation* – the crux of forgiveness and rebuilding trust (AIRM Steps 5 and 6), a bonding event of vulnerable sharing and responsive engagement, empathy, and remorse that rebuilds trust.

Attachment Injuries in EFIT and Resolving Injuries in EFIT with the AIRM

The change process in EFT is common across modalities, so it comes as no surprise that the EFCT model of AI repair is also a useful guide for resolution in EFIT. Individual clients frequently re-call pivotal shattering moments with an attachment figure with the same vividness that partners re-experience an AI long after the event has passed. The events range from childhood memories or recent incidents in romantic, friendship, or familial relationships.

Critical, injurious moments also occur with strangers where there is no one to turn to for protection and safety and those from whom one would expect to receive comfort and caring turn away or take the side of the abuser. REC trauma examples come to mind where police, from whom one should expect protection, become the abusers or take the side of the attackers. (See video of Adam (pseudonym) at www.steppingintoeft.com). Another example is when a neurodiverse or trans student is jeered by peers and a teacher ignores or joins in the verbal persecution.

There are many examples of EFIT clients who continue to be impacted by traumatic events where comfort, safety, and caring were not offered in a time of urgent need. Box 16.5 provides a summary of the AIRM model as a useful guide for resolution and repair in EFIT, with dismissive and abusive others. Caveats and modifications to ensure safety are provided.

Box 16.5 AIRM in EFIT: Resolution Process for Unresolved Issues with an Attachment Figure

Stabilization

1. Client articulates the injurious event to an imaginal other (IO). When the IO is an "offending other," as in trauma resolution, take extreme care to hold the other and not self, responsible; validate choice to block IO from responding; validate needs for permanent distance from abuser.
2. Client is in charge of whether they want to hear back from the IO. If they are agreeable to hearing responses from the IO, they are free to change their mind at any point. The IO may deny, discount, or dismiss client's pain. Negative, discounting responses from an IO elicit more assertion and clarity from client about how bad the injury was.
3. Client integrates story and engages with and expresses the attachment pain, fears, and longings with increasing depth (more core emotion and less reactivity). Shares specifics of how the injury was hurtful.
4. IO may understand/ integrate more of the attachment significance, more of the individual's pain and more of their importance to them. They may find words to describe how they could have taken this injurious action – been so hurtful or nonresponsive.

Forgiveness/Resolution – New Bonding Cycle Created – or Permanent Distance from Imaginal Other Affirmed

5. Client moves to deeper levels of emotional engagement; a more integrated, articulation of attachment pain. In the safety of the therapeutic relationship client can face difficult interpersonal encounters with an I.O. who has wounded them and is able to shape a new experience with a new outcome.
6. IO *may* or *may not* empathically engage, acknowledge responsibility and express empathy, and remorse as in, "I feel your pain." If there is no response or client has requested no response, a corrective emotional experience is nevertheless shaped by the client's new congruent position and coherent expression validating their experience in relation to the IO.

Consolidation

7. Client asks for attachment needs to be met or chooses permanent distance.
8. Imaginal Other may respond. Relationship is redefined as a potential safe haven or detachment is consolidated. New narrative is constructed. Views of self and other shift and are consolidated. Reliable, safe others are distinguished from unsafe other(s).

Adapted from, Makinen and Johnson (2006), Elliott et al. (2004), Johnson and Campbell (2022) and Paivio and Pascual-Leone (2010).

As with couples, the antidote corrective emotional experiences to reprocess these AIs and restructure working models of self, other, and the world, are rooted in responsive engagement, empathy, and remorse from the offending other regarding that trust-shattering moment. When the imaginal, relevant other is not safe or responds negatively, dismissively, or not at all, or the client does not want them to respond, resolution for the client can nevertheless be shaped in a safe way as is shown in the following case example of Sahra with her imaginal abusive ex-partner.

AIRM in EFIT with Sahra and Her Abusive Ex-partner

Sahra describes a growing sense of calm and hopefulness:

> I feel like I am starting to get my sense of self back again, but I still feel like I am grieving somehow. That first imaginal conversation I had with Fahrad (her former abusive partner) left me feeling so much better, but I am not finished with him. I know he is still affecting me, even though it has been so long ago!

Emily hears that there are lingering impacts of the abusive relationship that Sahra has not yet processed. Though her tears come readily at mention of this relationship, the anger and fear of the complex emotion of hurt are more difficult for her to touch.

Sahra: There is a moment that still really haunts me. A big, aggressive event that happened in my living room. He ended up creating a huge, huge hole in my wall, and despite repairing the hole and changing everything about that room to make it a safe place, I still can't walk in that room without seeing – Well, I don't see it, but without knowing it's there.

Emily: You feel the danger each time you walk into the room, yes?

Sahra: Yes, and every time I hear loud noises, I jump. My heart races and horrific moments like that come back and haunt me. It's too hard to revisit what happened and to let myself notice I was in that scene…but I don't want it to keep haunting me.

Emily: It's so hard to revisit that scene (Right.) with yourself in it and notice how terrifying it was (Right.) and the memory continues to haunt you and leaves you feeling unsafe in your own home. Unsafe anywhere you hear loud noises.

Sahra: Right. I don't want to talk about it, but I feel like the only way to move past this would be to share my story. Not that I want to, you know.

Emily: When you think right now about Fahrad and how he hurt you – his violence, what comes up for you?

Sahra: Mm… Anger. I used to cower a lot but right now it's anger, for sure. I do get really angry when I think about what he did to me for no reason. (Pauses.) Well, there's a tiny piece of me that's like, "Maybe it was a little bit my fault." (Voice getting quieter, trembling, then rises again.) Maybe it was my fault for staying with him that long, but I didn't do anything to deserve that violence!

Emily: You went from this, "Uugh, I don't really want talk about this terrifying incident of violence," and then when you said, "Yeah. I am angry," there was a shift in your body (Pause.) and you said, "I didn't deserve that" even as a tiny part of you asks, "Did I?"

Sahra: Yeah. I don't know. I'm not really an angry person, but…

Emily: You were very badly hurt by him, and you have lots of tears and fears and a little bit of anger.

Sahra: Yeah. Yeah, a little bit.

Emily: And it feels safe to feel your own anger at him right in this moment?

Sahra: Yes, it does.

Emily: Just notice that. Just notice that it feels safe to notice that you are angry at him. You've kind of feared your own anger (Right) in the past, but right in this very moment, how is it to notice that you can safely feel angry?

Sahra: Interesting. It's, uh, surprising…. Yeah. I wouldn't expect that to be true, but, yeah, I am angry (Pointing to her chest and making a fist.) and I am surprised I am not going numb like I usually do!

Emily: (Beginning to shape an encounter.) Might you be willing to tell the story of what this was like to an image of Fahrad? You've said you've recounted this story many times to friends and family; but that somehow you feel removed from the story – like a factual recounting, over and over and nothing changes. I'm wondering if you might be willing to tell your story to an image of Fahrad, to experience your voice of anger and pain being addressed directly to an image of him.

Sahra: Yikes! It will not be easy. It's going to be very hard, but that's why I'm here. (Laughs. Suddenly frowns, shaking her head.) I don't think he understood what he put me through.

Emily: Mm-hm.

Sahra: He still doesn't. He still texts me every now and then. It's like, "You clearly don't get what you did," but it is so hard to resist! ARGH!! I'm so embarrassed to admit that lots of times I do text him back. (Hangs her head.)

Emily: He had such a strong impact and you invested so much in this relationship that it's still difficult not to respond, even when you don't want him in your life, yes? (validating)

Sahra: Exactly!

Emily: What comes up just noting that? (Evoking present moment awareness.)

Sahra: He still has such a strong hold on me!

Emily: Yeah.

Sahra: And I hate that, because I'm so jumpy.

Emily: Yeah. Still so jumpy. Still feeling the traumatic impact of his aggression.

Sahra: (Dropping her head, voice inaudible, then mumbling.)…Still fearing something is wrong with me.

Emily: You're getting quiet and kind of disappearing, now, yes, starting to doubt yourself? (Tracking reflection.)

Sahra continues to indicate to Emily that she wants to address an image of Fahrad despite how difficult it is, and Emily titrates the risk – persisting and keeping it safe.

Emily: (Firm, strong voice.) Can you feel that anger in your chest again and hear it in your voice and can you picture yourself saying, "Fahrad, what you did was so wrong, there is no way that was ever okay what you did to me!"? (14-second silence. Sahra begins to cry.) Is it a little too scary?

Sahra: It just takes me a while. (28-second silence.)

Emily: Just notice how much courage what you're doing right now is taking. You're facing, in your imagination, this horrific impact that Fahrad has had on you. Yeah. (40 seconds silence.) What do you feel like doing right now? (Focusing on action tendency to keep Sahra within her window of tolerance without losing emotional engagement.)

Sahra: Running.

Emily: Running. Yeah. Right. Like every fiber in your body says, "Run, don't even speak to him, just get out of the way!" (Heightening awareness of action impulse, to validate and keep emotion alive.)

Sahra: I want to speak to him. It's just so hard.

Emily: Let's honor that, Sahra. Let's notice this is so hard, even in the safety of this room (yeah). It is so hard to picture speaking to him. It doesn't feel safe to do that.

Sahra:	No. I want to, but…. I don't know why it's so hard.
Emily:	You just know it feels really hard. (Yeah) Something says, "Don't say it." Yes?
Sahra:	I'm telling myself to say, "What you did was so hard, so hard for me, so horrible." But picturing myself saying it to him. I don't know (voice breaking) if it literally just feels unsafe or what. I just get so tense.
Emily:	Right. Like you're saying, it doesn't feel like I can do it. My throat closes up. (Proxy voice conjecture.)
Sahra:	Yeah.
Emily:	You can tell *me* it wasn't right, but to actually picture yourself saying that to an image of Fahrad feels… feels dangerous? (conjecture). It doesn't feel like you can do it.
Sahra:	No, not yet. But eventually I will.
Emily:	(Validate; proxy voice conjecture) Yeah. Something says, "Not yet. Not yet. Don't tell him. Not yet. This aggression from Fahrad has knocked me over so badly that I can't even speak to an image of him, not yet.
Sahra:	Right. But I will. Give me time.
Emily:	(20 second pause; then to help Sahra find some words.) What do you want him to know? What feels the most important to start with?
Sahra:	(20-second silence.) Mm… That I didn't deserve that. It shouldn't have happened to me, and I will never go back to him (Tearing up.)
Emily:	"I didn't deserve your violence." (Being specific; heightening with proxy voice repetition) What else did you not deserve?
Sahra:	I didn't deserve the violence. I didn't deserve feeling scared. I didn't deserve his lies or cowering in fear. (Pause.) Just saying this to you makes me feel the fear and the sadness that he caused me. And feeling that intense pain is so hard.
Emily:	It is so hard to revisit that intense pain. (Validating.)
Sahra:	Yeah.
Emily:	Yeah. That intense pain that you survived.
Sahra:	Yeah. That he caused.
Emily:	Yes. He caused that pain. Yes. And it's so hard to revisit that pain. Can you picture Fahrad?
Sahra:	I see him standing there as if he has no clue! (20 second pause.) But I need to know I do not need to hear back from an image of him. I don't want to hear his reaction to what I tell him (Shaking head and waving hand – as though pointing at an image of him; crying.)
Emily:	(Proxy voice conjecture / validation.) That's right. You're saying, "I don't want to hear back from him. He's not a safe guy."
Sahra:	Right (Nodding.)

Emily invites Sahra to notice how Fahrad looks as she prepares to address him. This is her first actual encounter with the imaginal abusive other.

Emily:	Can you picture him there now, at a safe distance from you, and can you tell him, "I am going to say my piece and I do not want to hear back from you. I will tell you how badly you have hurt me – and then I'll tell you to leave!" (Setting boundary for safety.) (30 second silence.)
Sahra:	I'm going to tell you what it was like for me, but you don't get to respond.
Emily:	Wow. How is it to hear yourself say that out loud?
Sahra:	It's very empowering.
Emily:	You can feel the power? You can feel your power? That you're free, when you're ready, to let him know how wrong he was, how bad he was for you and then you will tell him to leave.

Sahra: Yeah. (35-second silence.) (To an imaginal Fahrad.) You hurt me. I didn't deserve that. I didn't deserve the pain. (Emily: Yeah) I didn't deserve the trauma. (Emily: Yeah) I didn't deserve cowering. (Emily: Right!) You scared me.

Emily: Yeah. Yeah. "I didn't deserve it. It was very bad!" (Proxy voice.)

Sahra: I didn't deserve that.

Emily: Yeah. You're telling him right now, all that fear is clutching at your throat, and you're getting the words out. Can you hear that? (Sahra: Yeah) What's it like that you've told him this much? (Move 4.)

Sahra: (Nodding.) Hard but good. (Big sigh!)

Emily: Hard and good. Scary and empowering. Yeah. And you can breathe.

Sahra: Yeah. Yeah. Yeah (Weeping, continuing to speak to imaginal Fahrad.) I don't know why you changed. I tried for so long to get you to be your old self. I just couldn't try anymore.

Emily: (Proxy voice reflection.) I just couldn't try anymore. Right. I reached the end. Too scary, too painful, and I was having no impact. (Move 4.) How is it to tell him, "I tried so long, I just couldn't try anymore?"

Sahra: I needed to tell him that, without him talking back. (Gritting teeth, shaking fist.)

Emily: Yeah (shaking fist, mirroring Sahra's gesture). You are so angry!

Sahra: Yes! He just always talked back…always told me I am wrong.

Emily: So right now, this image didn't speak back, and you're saying, "Finally I told you I'm not wrong. I tried so long to help you, and you're not talking back. I'm telling you, I couldn't help you anymore. (Sahra: Right.)

Emily shapes several more encounters with Moves 3 and 4 where Sahra expresses more core anger to an imaginal Fahrad, naming the crux of his injury, that was worse than any of the physical abuse: His lies about his drinking.

Sahra: (Closing her eyes, addressing her image of Fahrad.) I literally hurt in my heart. (Puts hand on her heart and winces.) You knew I couldn't stand lying, and you lied. I was *not* crazy for leaving. I was so hurt! This wasn't all my fault!

Emily: How is it to tell him this?

Sahra: That was hard to tell him. (She spontaneously closes her eyes and repeats the message.) I wasn't crazy. You hurt me. It wasn't me that caused you to lie – to drink. (Another big sigh.)

Emily: (Move 4.) You are feeling how important it is to send this message again to an imaginal Fahrad, "I wasn't crazy, I was hurt, over and over and over. I wasn't crazy. I was hurting. I needed out of this hurtful place. I needed to leave you, and I did." Yes! Take a moment to soak in how you feel, taking this new position. (Pause.) Is there more you need to tell him?

Sahra: I think that's it. You can go now. (To imaginal Fahrad.) (Sigh, followed by laughter.) What a huge relief. I can let him go now! I'm done with him! Ready to block him totally. No more responding to his texts!

Emily: (Move 5, integrating, summarizing and celebrating.) That's amazing, Sahra, that you feel the clarity and the certainty that, "Hey, I don't need him in my life. I have safe others, but I don't need him (Sahra: Right.) and I'm ready to block him."

Sahra: To just be able to move through that pain feels really good and productive. (Big Sigh!)

Emily: You feel that you moved through the pain.

Sahra: At one point, I actually thought, "I think this is what people feel in the beginning of a heart attack." It physically hurt when I said, "You lied to me, that is the worst, that you lied to me!"

Emily: And what do you feel in your heart now?

Sahra: It's healing. (Smiles, winces, cries; ten-second silence.) It's bittersweet, letting him go.

Emily: You're glad you're letting him go, and it feels bittersweet. (Validating both the relief and the grief of bittersweet.)

Sahra: I hoped so much he'd get back to the kind man he first seemed to be. I invested so much, trying to get him back.

Emily: That is bittersweet.... Letting go of all your hopes and dreams and investments in him. And to be ready to let him go and feel yourself reclaiming your goodness and worth! What a huge step!

Sahra: (Big sigh and a bright smile.) Yes!! So good!

At a follow-up session several months later Sahra confirms that her shifts in sense of self as loveable and competent and of some others as trustworthy and responsive have endured. She describes meeting Fahrad in a local restaurant as a cordial passing, feeling calm and safe, with a sense of personal dignity. See Chapter 16 Support Material for transcript of AI resolution between Sahra and her mother (routledge.com/9781032151335). Additionally, an 11-hour EFIT video series at steppingintoeft.com contains numerous similar corrective emotional experiences with parental and ex-partner attachment injuries, illustrating the AIRM in EFIT.

Helping a client to clearly voice their pain – anger, grief, fear, and shame – in a coherently assembled, emotionally engaged encounter, opens models of self and other for revision and restructuring, regardless of an IO's response. Assertive and vulnerable disclosures to IOs reshape the client's sense of self and other, expanding sense of self and increasing ability to connect with others.

Conclusion

Contrary to many clients' assumptions that the pain of interpersonal injury can be obscured or pushed aside but can never go away, EFT offers an alternative for all modalities of therapy: couple, individual and family. It is possible to transform injured views of self and other and to trust others again. EFT offers a process of interpersonal healing conversations that can reshape internal and interpersonal, emotional worlds.

Part VI
The Next Steps

17 Emotionally Focused Family Therapy (EFFT)

Stepping into EFT with Families

James Furrow and Gail Palmer

A main aim of family therapy is to enable all members to relate together in such a way that each member can find a secure base in his relationships within the family, as occurs in every healthily functioning family. (Bowlby, 1979, p. 176)

Introduction

Emily received a call from Jessica six months after Jessica and Wayne completed couple therapy. The couple had worked hard to resolve parenting differences including how to handle their nine-year-old son Jamal and his growing resistance to family rules and disrespect toward Jessica. Recent incidents at school increased their concern as Jamal was singled out by one of his teachers and labeled a "behavior problem" in a report to the guidance counselor. Jessica began the call, "Emily you were so helpful to us in working together to support Jamal, and Wayne and I wonder if you would meet with Jamal; we believe he could use some additional help and you really understand our family." Emily thanked Jessica for her kind words of appreciation and confidence in her work and shared that she would need to get back to them. She acknowledged that she has more expertise in couple therapy than working with families. To herself, she said, "I know EFT but family therapy? Really? I am not sure I am ready to work with families!"

Emily reached out to her colleague Jill, who saw families as a routine part of her practice and asked if she could discuss Jessica's invitation. Emily's confidence working with EFT grew through her work with couples and individuals, but family therapy seemed like a step beyond. She appreciated John Bowlby's approach to parenting, having read *A Secure Base* (1988) cover to cover as she was anticipating the birth of her first child. After reviewing various Emotionally Focused Family Therapy (EFFT) resources she sat down with Jill for a frank discussion of EFT with families, "I understand that stages of change, tango, and interventions are the same, but how do you work with pursuers and withdrawers and cycles when you have three people in the room much less five?"

Jill appreciated Emily's question and honored her concern for this family and their struggles with their son. She reassured Emily that her Tango skills and understanding of attachment processes would provide important resources if she decided to work with this family and noted that there are some important differences to consider in EFFT. Jill highlighted three unique aspects about attachment in her work with families.

First, Jill explained that family work anticipates the various stressors families face as children's developmental needs change and new resources are required. Situational factors, like recent racialized violence at Jamal's school, can impact the demands for helping families keep their emotional balance as a developmental system. Family assessment needs to account for situational, environmental, and developmental factors in the changes that increase tension and distress in parent and child relationships. Emily wondered how Jamal's experience at school was seen by his parents,

DOI: 10.4324/9781003242673-26

given their own experience of racial stress in the neighborhood. Jill appreciated Emily's attention to the ways that the family's emotional climate could be impacted by its own dynamics but also the emotional demands of their context that they each navigate daily.

Second, Jill shared that family relationship dynamics are shaped by the different roles of parents and children in responding to attachment needs. Relationships between parents and children lack the mutual influence that couples have in their interactions that are focused on intimacy and closeness. Jill explains that in working with families we look for relational blocks in the caregiving response of parents to the attachment bids of children. Parents may be overresponsive or under responsive to a child's needs and the child may either amplify or minimize their attachment signals. Themes of anxiety and avoidance organize these patterns, but parents have a different level of responsibility for responding to a child's attachment needs than partners have in couple relationships. Family relationships as a system have reciprocal influences, however, when it comes to responding to attachment needs, the influences are hierarchical rather than mutual. Emily wonders if Jessica's anxious responding in the couple's relationship influences Jamal and she can see how Wayne's more pragmatic approach to Jamal could also play into the intensity of Jessica and Jamal's conflicts.

Third, Jill highlighted the influences of attachment dynamics across generations. She explained that a parent's caregiving is often shaped by the experiences from their own childhood. Emily recalled Wayne's deference to Jessica in difficult parenting moments and she noted Jill's question about Wayne's experience as a child wondering what his parents were like. When Jill learned that Wayne had been raised without a father and while he had father-figures he often questioned his abilities as a parent, she explained that he was working without a model and it made sense he would doubt his effectiveness as a father. Jill underscored the generational influences of attachment and their profound role in shaping a parent's view of self and their responsiveness to their child's emotional needs. The parent's view of self becomes an important focus in working through the relational blocks that disrupt the caregiving and attachment system.

Emily appreciates having an EFT way of conceptualizing the difficulties that might underlie Jessica and Wayne's concerns with Jamal. Still, she wonders how her EFT work would look different in a family session. Jill shares three key differences she finds in her EFT sessions with families. First, the therapist needs to be flexible. The focus of a session can change session to session and may vary between families. Typically, the process of treatment follows the most distressed dyad, but change can happen quickly in a family session and a therapist must be ready to pivot to address emerging needs and changing dynamics in a family system. Second, EFFT sessions combine a mix of sessions involving the family and different subsystems (e.g., parents and siblings). In EFFT the therapist is working within and between family subsystems as she promotes greater parental availability and then engages child vulnerability. In EFFT the therapist may use the structure of who is invited to a session to manage reactivity, increase safety, or promote vulnerability. As they concluded, Jill shares a third difference:

> Family work can be intense, shifting fast. The attachment and caregiving systems are a poignant part of us as humans and we are working in the emotional channel of a family system helping families to build stronger bonds and deeper confidence in caregiving and care seeking. Belonging leads to becoming. We help families do that in EFFT.

Goal of EFFT

EFFT is a brief process-oriented approach that works experientially to transform a family's negative interaction patterns by restructuring attachment bonds through increasing a parent's responsiveness and engaging a child's attachment needs. The goal of EFT with families is to increase the accessibility, responsiveness, and emotional engagement on the part of the parents to foster a more secure base that children grow, and depart from (Johnson, 2020).

In essence, EFFT is a natural extension of EFT where the focus includes working with the relationships that occur within and between generations. As families grow and change, parenting is a "moving target." Thus, the EFT therapist helps parents gather support in regulating their emotions so they can help their child accomplish the same (Johnson, 2019). In EFFT we are helping family members find their emotional balance together.

Throughout EFFT the therapist is following the EFT process of change and guiding families to new experiences through the moves of the EFT Tango. The process unfolds as the therapist engages the family's struggle by tracking the relational patterns associated with their presenting problem. The therapist tunes into the caregiving intentions of parents and the unspoken or disowned attachment emotions of children. Through the EFT Tango, sessions focus on eliciting these core emotions that inform and confirm key messages about safety and felt security (Bowlby, 1988). The EFT therapist reframes the family's distress in terms of relationship blocks that interrupt effective dependency of children on their caregivers and reduce their resilience as a family unit. Prioritizing parental availability, sessions focus on helping parents work through their blocks to accessibility, responsiveness, and emotional engagement with a child's attachment emotions and needs. As parents become more available and responsive, the therapist turns to work through the blocks that interrupt clear bids for attachment and effective responses to a child's need. Through EFFT new emotional signals inform expectations, shape perceptions, and transform the models of self and others that organize family behaviors in times of uncertainty and threat (Johnson, 2019).

Four Functions of EFFT

Four functions guide the EFT therapist's approach to family problems and relationship distress. As an attachment-based approach EFFT combines a focus on tracking systemic interactions, processing emotional experience, promoting felt security, and shaping new interactions around attuned caregiving and vulnerable care seeking.

Tracking Interactional Patterns

The repetitive experience of negative emotions signals patterns of insecurity in family relationships. Attachment theory provides a lens to for conceptualizing the "unique meaning" of disruptive behaviors between children and their caregivers (Morretti & Holland, 2003). An adolescent's silent protest and cut-off responding to a parent's direction escalates to a heated push and pull interaction that repeated over time compromises attunement and reduces confidence in the relationship. Parental blocks to empathic attunement may result from a lack of caregiver availability, distress between caregivers, marital conflict, distress in a family's context, or threats in the community (e.g., racial discrimination and under-housed). Typically, these patterns impact a family's ability to regulate emotional experience effectively across the family system (Morris et al., 2007) and reinforce patterns of negative affect that become absorbing states locking family members into fixed interactional positions informed by underlying anxious or avoidant self-protective strategies (Johnson, 2020). In EFFT these patterns are the initial focus of treatment as disruptive and dysregulated interactions offer access to emotional logic underlying a family's presenting problem (Furrow et al., 2019).

Processing Emotional Experience

Emotion is central to attachment communication and a key focus in the EFT process of change. Patterns of security and insecurity in family interactions reflect the emotional dance taking place within a family (Johnson, 2019). Attachment communication exists first and foremost at an emotional level because attachment bonds are affectional ties (Johnson, 2020), and focusing on the emotional responses of family members enables parents and children to better access their intentions, desires, and needs.

Consider a mother who can express the sadness she feels over the growing distance in her relationship with her son. Her sadness sends a new signal to her son who expects her to respond with negative feelings about his attention problems. The therapist's presence and focus help the mother shift from her frustration to a previously unacknowledged sadness that is first evident in her eyes. As she reflects on her disappointment at their distance, she is more able to expresses a poignant longing to better support and see her son. Accessing a parent's core attachment emotions primes a parent to offer a more attuned and empathic response. The EFT therapist differentiates more vulnerable core emotions from more reactive emotion by actively accessing, and exploring the underlying emotions associated with attachment needs in the family (Furrow et al., 2019).

Promoting Felt Security

A primary aim of EFFT involves promoting felt security as a family based outcome. The therapist role as a process consultant also functions as an attachment resource or "stronger, wiser other" to the family. Felt security supports clearer attachment communication and promotes emotional balance in family relationships (Johnson, 2019). Change in adult caregivers is more likely when those adults have confidence in the availability of another adult (Kobak & Mandelbaum, 2003). The experience of felt security in a family is seen where family members engage a level of vulnerability and openness that promote confidence in the accessibility, responsiveness and emotional engagement of a caregiver and the engagement of trust of a child reaching for support.

Felt security provides a child a resource of internal confidence in an attachment figure's support in exploration and availability in the face of personal threat and emotional distress (Kobak et al., 2015). Parents as caregivers also turn toward one another for mutual support, just as children turn toward parents for care contact and comfort. These positive cycles of security define the family as a "safe haven" of comfort and a critical "secure base" resource for facing ordinary stressors and developmental demands. Attachment security promotes adaptive processes essential to a natural system that supports optimal development and environmental mastery for children (Bowlby, 1982; Mikulincer & Shaver, 2015). When bonds are secure, parents are more likely to provide children with a "secure base" to foster exploration promoting the development of a child's potential and uniqueness and a "safe haven" from the uncertainties and difficulties of life. Together the caregiving and attachment system creates a network of security that ensures the flexibility and cohesion necessary to maintain individual growth and meaningful relationships across the lifespan (Byng-Hall, 2001).

Shaping New Interactions

Throughout the EFFT process, the therapist invites family members to turn toward one another and share their here-and-now experience with other family members. These engaged encounters can capture key moments where new experiences are ordered, and underlying attachment themes are explicitly stated. As Johnson (2019) highlights, the sharing of emotional experience creates the opportunity for a new emotional reality to be made explicit, concrete and more coherent offering a different or new level of connection. In the following example, Lauren experiences a new encounter of her mother's vulnerability, although even as an adult child on her own, she felt her mother's anger and constant disapproval.

Through her EFFT sessions, Lauren and her mother began to face the unresolved tension in their relationship linked to Lauren's father's illicit relationships that eventually ended her parent's marriage. As her mother became more aware and responsive to the burden and fears Lauren carried after discovering her father's affair as an adolescent, Lauren risked sharing her fear that holding this secret had made things worse for her mother. She also shared her fear that not having trusted her mother with this information also would have hurt her. As Lauren expressed her guilt and fear she asked her mother to forgive her for not letting her know and seeking her help. Her fears that this would crush her mother and destroy the family kept her quiet but the secret and surrounding guilt had built a wall between them. Lauren's ability to send a clear and coherent message at a vulnerable level opened a door to her mother's comfort and care for a daughter who was alone and afraid, all the while wanting the best for her mother. As a stronger, wiser other in this moment, her mother provided a safe and secure space for her daughter to be seen and to be freed from a burden that was not her own.

Encounters are at the heart of healing families through EFFT as the caregiving and attachment systems are realigned and the underlying needs and felt experience of children are met effectively by an open and engaged parent or caregiver (Furrow et al., 2019). This ultimate change event in EFFT is built upon many engaged encounters that unfold through the EFT process as new levels of awareness and experience are ordered and shared in the present moment. These moments are the building blocks of constructive dependency that promotes a dynamic developmental engine of growth as families *broaden and build* the resources and resilience necessary for a flourishing family life (Johnson, 2019; Mikulincer & Shaver, 2015).

EFFT Process of Change

In EFFT, the therapist follows the EFT process of change from stabilization through restructuring relationships to consolidating around more secure connections with a particular focus on parent and child interactions (Johnson, 2020). In Stage 1, the focus is on stabilizing the reactive distress in the family through ordering experience and identifying relationship blocks that interrupt effective caregiving and care seeking. A pivotal objective in Stage 1 is promoting greater parent openness and availability as this is a marker of de-escalation in the family system. In Stage 2, the focus shifts to engaging a child's attachment-related emotions and supporting their risk and reach for specific attachment needs. The effective response of a caregiver to the needs of her child and the disclosure of the needs by the child is the pivotal change event in Stage 2. In Stage 3, the therapist's focus is on integrating and solidifying the new steps the family has taken into more secure patterns of engagement. The family consolidates their change by forming new narratives for the family and investing in various rituals that symbolize the importance of their bonds and the flexibility needed to support growth.

Throughout Stage 1, the EFT therapist is building and monitoring their alliance with family members as the presenting problem is understood in the context of the family's experience.

The therapist tracks the relational patterns associated with the presenting problem and the emotional dance that organizes individual responses to the distress they share. These reactive responses are indicative of underlying experiences of fear, pain, sadness, and longing. Attention is given to the most distressed dyad and to the relational blocks to caregiving and attachment seeking that reinforce the negativity often felt throughout the family. Focusing on the specific "pain point" in the family enables the therapist to work from the most acute source of insecurity in the family system and initiate a process for working through this primary relational block toward re-engaging family members in new patterns of security. Following the moves of the EFT Tango, the therapist orders and engages these underlying emotional experiences and focuses attention on the core emotions that motivate caregiving responses. As parental blocks to caregiving are worked through parents become more flexible in their roles and more responsive to the needs of their children. As parental availability is highlighted the family's negative interaction cycle is reframed in terms of relational blocks between caregiving and care seeking. The focus on heightening parental caregiving intentions that were made explicit through the process of Stage 1 leads to greater stabilization and de-escalation of family reactivity.

In Stage 2 the focus shifts to engaging a child's attachment-related experiences and needs. The therapist deepens and distills the child's underlying attachment emotion, distilling unmet attachment needs. In tandem with eliciting and deepening attachment-related affect the therapist promotes a parent's acceptance, responsiveness, and emotional engagement with the child's experience. Parents often need support in working toward acceptance of the mistrust and pain of their child as they are impacted by their own experience of fear and shame given the emerging clarity of what their child needed but did not receive. The therapist invites children to share their attachment needs and guides parents in responding effectively to the child's request. New family responses tend to reflect clearer definitions of self, more assertive boundary definitions, and more explicit expectations of the relationships desired in the family (Johnson, 2020).

As Stage 3 unfolds new patterns of security achieved by the family through the preceding stages are consolidated. The therapist guides the family through revisiting unresolved problems with new relational resources. More secure family interactions demonstrate greater flexibility in responding to developmental demands and are more effective in problem solving (Johnson et al., 1998). In Step 9 the therapist encourages the family to make meaning of the changes that have taken place in their family. New rituals of connection are explored to increase openness and emotional engagement, greater positive affect, and appreciation for their stronger ties as a family.

Working through Relational Blocks in EFFT

The therapist in EFFT relies on the EFT Tango moves and micro interventions, just as an EFT therapist would in working with an individual or couple. As Bowlby (1979) noted the family therapist provides families the opportunity to have conversations that they are not able to have on their own. In EFT we provide families with a sound and secure space to have these conversations in a safe, open, and vulnerable way. The Tango guides the session process through present awareness and deeper experience, which can then be shared with another. These encounters create new opportunities for self-understanding and a new awareness of others. Parents and children are better able to reach their core emotions that are too often disowned or otherwise unspoken in a family's negative pattern. When these experiences are given voice, engaged, and received, they bring a felt understanding that begins a shift in the family's struggle for meaning and connection. A safer space emerges where a child and parent for that matter can see and be seen.

The EFT Tango in EFFT

The emotion work of EFT is put in motion with the five moves of the EFT Tango. For Johnson (2019) these moves capture the focus and shifts a therapist makes in working toward a corrective emotional experience with each move following a particular rhythm and progression. In EFFT the therapist follows these moves in working through the "here-and-now" relational blocks found in distressed family interactions and engaging caregiving responses and attachment bids. These five moves include:

1. **Mirroring the Present Process** brings the therapist focus to an in-session moment of emotional significance. Consider the therapist who tracks a parent's reactive judgment in response to her

daughter's insolent dismissal of a mother's advice. "Right here, right now is where things get difficult between the two of you. Her indifference is maddening especially in the face of how much you have done to try to make things different for her, yes? And your mom's anger is what you have come to expect so it makes sense to keep her worries at a distance." In mirroring the present process focus is placed on the emotional experience of a family member as the impact of a relational interaction is felt. Family blocks to caregiving and care seeking often organize the family's pattern and their efforts to manage its impact in session and the therapist focuses on these moments to access a family's emotional process.

2. **Affect Assembly and Deepening** is at the heart of working through relational blocks in family interactions. Here the therapist accesses the elements of emotion that begin to emerge when focusing on present experience and uses evocative responses to explore the cue/or trigger, perceptions, bodily experiences, meanings, and actions tendencies associated with specific experiences, as she works toward deepening the mother's felt experience.

"Can we stay here a moment? I am wondering about that harsh tone that comes up in these moments when your daughter pulls away, the one you regret later, the angry tone that you say pushes her away. Right, because this tone is much louder than you intend and different from the concern you feel on the inside..." The therapist reflects the cue (i.e., daughter's rejecting mother's advice), and mother's angry defense when her care is rejected. "So, on the inside the voice is quiet, more unsure, more afraid at the distance growing between you. Can we listen to that part of you that fears this distance, this fear of losing touch with your daughter who means so much to you? The therapist engages the mother's frustration exploring and expanding the concern the mother feels when her influence loses its' impact, and she feels more desperate and afraid.

3. **Choreographing Engaged Encounters** follows the deepening and affect assembly as the EFT therapist engages the emotional experience that has been given voice. In EFT emotion is both a target but also an agent of change. In Move 3 the therapist may ask a family member to turn toward another to share a more vulnerable emotional experience. "Can you share this with your daughter? How scary this distance is for you as her mother, because you're afraid the concern and care you have for her won't reach her and she will alone in this struggle?" The therapist now invites the mother to share about the distance she fears and the care she feels for her daughter. This engages the mother's felt experience, enabling her to speak out of her heart-felt concern for her daughter.

4. **Processing the Encounter** follows the disclosure of emotional responses in EFT. The therapist explores the impact of sharing and receiving emotional experiences. The therapist reflects and validates the experiences of risking and reaching to another in the family as attachment-related emotions and needs are shared. The therapist will often acknowledge the caregiving intentions of a parent's vulnerability keeping the focus on the parent's role as caregiver to make clear the purpose of this disclosure. "What this like for you to share this heartfelt concern that your daughter may be alone not really knowing your care?" The therapist also explores the experience of the daughter who may still be in a reactive less receptive position. "It's not that big of a deal, she gets angry all the time it seems. I know she cares but sometimes it would be nice if she acted like it." The therapist would "catch the bullet" of the daughter's harsh response. "Yes, it's kind of like you are always ready for her anger and disappointment so when she goes softer and shows her care, it's surprising, you are not sure what to do with it, right?" The therapist safety provides a validating and accepting response for the daughter, giving space for her to begin to take in a new emotional encounter with her mother.

5. **Integrating and Validating** focuses on the therapist's efforts to make meaning from the experiences just shared by family members. New connections and insights are fostered between

family members and emphasis is placed on new opportunities and engagement. For example, the therapist may acknowledge that the mother's care for her daughter, while not a surprise to the daughter, is felt differently when there is a clear signal of her vulnerability. "Mother, you took a risk to show your care and concern and daughter, and daughter you noticed this was different, different than your mother's anger, which so often shuts down your ability to hear anything other than her disapproval." The therapist response organizes the encounter highlighting the mother's core emotions and validating the daughter's caution and her general understanding that her mother cares.

Micro Interventions Used in the EFT Tango

Throughout EFFT, the therapist uses micro-interventions to move through the five EFT Tango moves to achieve two primary EFT goals. The first goal includes eliciting, ordering, and organizing emotional experience. The therapist uses reflection, validation, empathic conjecture, and evocative questions to access and process the emotional responses associated with stuck family patterns or emerging vulnerabilities. The second goal of forming new interactional patterns is organized around positive cycles of attuned caregiving and attachment security. Encounters are used to engage primary emotional experience leading to the sharing of attachment-related emotions and needs. EFFT differs from EFT with couples in recognizing the hierarchical role of a parent and the primacy of parental caregiving in response to attachment needs expressed by a child. The EFFT therapist uses heightening interventions and encounters to choreograph change events that foster parental responsiveness and accessibility to a child's vulnerability.

Case Example

Jill shared the following case example with Emily to help her see the flow of EFFT through the process of change. Emily follows the challenges that a single parent father of two teenage sons faces, navigating a sea of loss and uncertainty. Jill encourages Emily to give attention to the changing emotional climate of the family and its impact on parent and child behaviors. The family includes Davit (55) who works as a government consultant, and parent of two teenage. boys, Bill (15) and James (13). As the sole parent Davit came to family therapy knowing he needed help in parenting his boys, especially with Bill's misbehavior increasing. Traumatic loss was also a key part of this family's story. Davit had three adult sons from his first marriage, and he stoically reported one of these sons, Matthew, died within the past year of suicide. Additionally, Davit's second wife, Marie, mother of Bill and James, also died by suicide when the boys were four and two years of age. The following summary of the family's EFFT journey begins with a session with Davit, the father, and Bill and James, his two youngest sons.

EFFT Focus: Alliance and Assessment

Jill shares that Davit, Bill and James were invited to the first session. Bill told his father that he was not going to participate or answer any questions. Davit responded by threatening him with a loss of privileges if he failed to attend and did not try. Emily laughed, nervously, "This is like the partner who drags the other into my office under threat of leaving." "Exactly!" Jill noted, "Similar challenge in alliance building, just a different kind of relationship."

Jill describes how she is working with this family to establish an alliance with each family member by making space and honoring each person's perspective. The therapist invites all perspectives, empathizing with each family member and holding differences that may be contradictory and conflictual. The session begins as the therapist asks Davit and his sons for a word or two that describes what it's like to be them in the family. These individual words or phrases provide insight into everyone's felt sense of family life and begin to show their relationship to one another.

James pipes in quickly. "Loving." He likes to get along with everyone in the family and feels close to his dad and brother. Davit smiles at James's response and launches into a long story about family values and how they are disappearing in today's fast-paced world. The therapist refocuses Davit, and his spits out his word, "frustration" revealing his distress and sense of helplessness at raising to teenage boys on his own. The therapist validates his exasperation and normalizes the demands of being their sole parent complimenting his persistence and care for his boys. Bill reluctantly joins in, "Fine" and looks away saying to therapist and his father, "That's all you're going to get from me." The therapist acknowledges his sharing and honors his participation while also wondering about his need to avoid the family spotlight. The therapist thanks the family for their different words and then begins to use these words as an entry point to the family pattern. The therapist asks evocative questions like, "What's that like for you when dad says 'frustrated'?" "What happens to you when James chooses 'loving' or Bill says 'fine'?" In doing so, the therapist creates a visual representation of how the family members interact with each other. Their reactive behaviors are made explicit, and the triggers for the patterned reactions are identified. Tracking the pattern shifts the focus from a "problem child" to the relationship interactions where the heat of the distress lies.

Jill explains to Emily that the in this initial session the therapist sidesteps the family's critical and blaming behaviors by focusing on relationship patterns. She tracks the negative pattern that erupts between family members and tunes into the emotional climate of the family. In her assessment she seeks to identify the most distressed dyad in the family unit. For Davit and his boys, the session begins to highlight how this family does not talk about the recent loss of Matthew, their son and brother. When asked about this loss, Davit shares glibly, "It's tough but I think we have done our best to just move on."

Emily asks about getting an attachment history and wondering about the rest of the EFFT assessment phase. Jill shares that the EFFT assessment phase includes separate conversations with the different subsystems in the family. The parent session provides the therapist more opportunity to strengthen her alliance giving space to Davit's parenting concerns. Davit focuses mostly on his frustration with Bill, describing his difficulty in a dry, logical, analytical manner. He highlights both boy's accomplishments and moves through his concerns in a pragmatic and goal-oriented manner. Davit's dedication and care show through in his energy and efforts to fix what he sees as the Bill's problem, given the school's concerns that Bill's grades were falling, and he was often missing from class. His teacher described him as "checked out" like he didn't seem to care.

Behind Davit's business-like approach to parenting, lay a growing uncertainty about his own ability to handle Bill's behavior and a deepening worry that his influence in Bill's life was diminishing. In session the therapist conjectures about how frightening this might be for any parent, which Davit dismisses, stating he wasn't afraid, just frustrated. The therapist validates Davit's reactive emotion and explores the support available to him. Davit acknowledges that he was on his own mostly and that his patterns of coping were primarily solitary. This included scouring the internet for parenting advice and, on occasion, taking psychedelic drugs to take off the edge of the stress. The therapist honors his strategies as "best attempts to cope with the enormity of his losses" and congratulates him for moving out of his comfort zone by reaching out for therapy.

Davit's parenting values were shaped by his Eastern European culture and the immigration struggles of his family as first generation Canadian. He was a trained litigator, and often approached family problems with an attorney mindset, organizing around managing potential risks. More vulnerable emotions were foreign to Davit and the attachment messages he received in his immigrant family of origin were shaped by his dominant and aggressive father and a passive, often distant mother. Vulnerability was seen as weakness and being strong and resilient under difficult circumstances was expected. Davit's self-sufficiency and limited access to his internal emotional world require that his therapist offer consistent acceptance, relentless empathy, alongside persistent, gentle leadership. These self-protective strategies highlighted the need for the therapist to be a source of secure attachment.

The sibling session provides an opportunity to assess the emotional support and active reliance between the two brothers. Bill and James initially presented as the ideal children, as both denied any problems in the family and seemed eager to please their father. A similar compliance was also present in their interactions with the therapist. The boy's active efforts to avoid conflict and please also functioned to protect their father from further pain and to keep their own needs hidden in a system that is overwhelmed and under supportive. The sons' coping strategies reinforce the family message that they have somehow "moved on" from the tragic death of their brother.

Stage 1: Processing a Parental Block

Jill explains to Emily that a key focus in Stage 1 is working through the parent's side of a family's relationship block. This begins with the most distressed dyad in the family system. Exploring the parent's caregiving block the therapist prioritizes highlighting moments of parental reactivity in session and links a parent's actions to specific cues. These triggers may include nonverbal responses or child behaviors that trigger a parent's reactive response. Care is given to validate these reactions in light of the parent's experience, attachment history, and family's relationship history. The therapist tunes into to core emotions related to the parent's caregiving efforts and parental intentions are reframed as parental efforts to "show care" for the child. As these caregiving intentions and underlying emotions are made explicit, the therapist promotes increasing openness and availability by engaging the expression of attachment and caregiving emotions.

Davit and Bill's relationship is identified as the most distressed dyad in the family and treatment focuses on how father and son manage this distress. The therapist focuses on a specific moment of conflict that ensued when Bill asked for a cell phone and Davit agreed to his request, with the condition that Bill improve his schoolwork and attendance. This interaction set in place a demand-placate pattern where father asserts a clear expectation and son feigns compliance only to be discovered later, which then triggers father to erupt into rageful attempts to control.

In EFFT, the therapist looks beyond the content of the argument giving attention to the emotional experience that plays out in a conflict. The therapist uses an attachment frame to makes sense of reactive responses, also validating and regulating the immediate struggle of the moment. Jill summarizes the therapist's work using the EFT Tango to describe how the therapist in Move 1 tracks the pattern between father and son, focusing on the danger cue of Bill lying (e.g., telling his father what he wants to hear) and the sequence unfolds as dad becomes angry and grounds his son in an attempt to control son's behavior. The more Davit exerts pressure, the more silent Bill becomes, the more withdrawn and distant the Bill is, the more Davit controls, with escalating behavior on both sides. The therapist uses evocative questions and responses inviting exploration of attachment significant emotions. The message from father to son is, "Your reward is based on your success," and the emotional music of mistrust plays underneath as, "I don't really trust you." The therapist conjectures the attachment messages behind the 15-year-old's cell phone request, "It's like you hope your father can see that your time with friends really matters. If, you miss out you will be left out, forgotten by your friends and school is hard enough without your best buds?" For Bill already feeling on the outside, not having a phone in his neighborhood would mean social isolation and rejection by his peers. Davit's frustration escalates to an "all or nothing" response, which is indicative of his relationship block that is expressed in his pragmatic rule-oriented approach to parenting.

Emily wonders how the therapist might move to assemble and deepen Davit's core emotions underlying his rigid parenting block. Jill shared the following session example highlighting how the therapist works from validating Davit's frustration to accessing his underlying fear. Jill describes how the dance of Davit's demands and Bill's lying and placation culminates in Davit's exasperation and bitter disappointment:

> Bill says his homework is done. It's not! He says he's all caught up on assignments. He's not! He plays me for a fool, and I have no idea what's going on inside his mind. At times I don't even know who my son is and what is going to happen to him.

The therapist picks up this emotional handle, "not knowing your son's future" and validates "how difficult it is not to know or see where your son is headed, especially when, as his father, you are working so hard to be the best father you can be." The emotional handle provides a present moment experience that is accessed and explored. In a Tango Move 2, Davit identifies his emotional response as frustration, driven by his felt helplessness in relationship to Bill. When this helplessness takes over his whole body goes hot and tense and he becomes utterly overwhelmed, which is unacceptable for him as a parent. The therapist validates Davit's helplessness as an intolerable emotion and his need to exert control as a natural and understandable response to the trauma that robbed him of agency and left him bereft. As the therapist holds and validates Davit, he is able to slow down the moment and reflect more deeply on his own experience. This experience takes Davit to the loss of his older son Matthew.

Therapist:	I am noticing as I am saying this, you look away, and go silent. I am wondering what it is like, when I say, your frustration makes sense. Davit, you go silent. I am wondering what's happening?
Davit:	(Long pause.) I am thinking of my last conversation with Matt. He said he was afraid, and I told him to just go for it.
Therapist:	(Soft and slow.) Oh that is so hard, so heavy.
Davit:	(Voice changes and goes up.) Look, it was all about the internet with Matthew – I think there were people coaching him, convincing him. Trolls, looking to prey on the vulnerable.
Therapist:	That's terrible to think that the internet exposed Matthew to danger that stole him from you! WOW, that is so hard (refocusing back to present process). It makes so much sense then when it comes to Bill, this isn't really about a cell phone for you. This is about saving your son. It is so hard to really see him when Bill is struggling. You have a whole alarm system going off and screaming, "Protect, protect!"
Davit:	(Exits.) Well it is also about being able to manage a phone and not let it become a problem or worse, an addiction. That's all I hear about from Bill, always about the phone, and meanwhile his performance at school is pretty marginal.
Therapist:	Yes, of course you want Bill to be successful with school, but when he asks for a cell phone, this is bigger than Bill or school, this is danger, danger, you need to protect your son, and then it isn't just about school or a cell phone it's about trying to keep him alive. I can see that, Davit. I know how much you care and want to be the best dad you can be.
Davit:	(Makes a joke.) Well, I do screw up on occasion.
Therapist:	(Smiling.) Like we all do. (Refocusing.) Davit, I can appreciate how hard this is to talk about, but you are here, talking about your relationship with Bill and how things

	get stuck. Your nervous system is on high alert, it couldn't help but be, that is what trauma does to us, it keeps us on guard, ready for the next shoe to drop. So, when you see Bill turning away, staying silent, and seemingly only wanting to chat with his friends on social media, this is dangerous, yes?
Davit:	It scares me half to death.
Therapist:	Right, it is terrifying. You feel like you are losing him, and that feeling is unbearable, so you work harder, you double up your efforts to contact him, put on more controls.
Davit:	And he moves further away.
Therapist:	Right, right. It is so good that you can see this, you can see where your fear takes you. I am wondering if Bill knows that underneath the rules and expectations is the terror that something terrible will happen to him?
Davit:	No, we just argue and then go our separate ways.
Therapist:	Can you look at your son right now and let him know that underneath the anger and the punishments, that you are afraid. This is all about how much he matters to you, it leads you to extremes because of the terror you feel?
Davit:	(Joking.) Hey Bill, what about those Blue Jays?
Therapist:	(Refocus, using proxy voice.) I am so afraid of something bad may happen to you
Davit:	(To Bill.) She's right. I am afraid. It's hard to talk about because I want to be strong and in charge as your father.
Therapist:	And my fear leads me.......
Davit:	To not trust you, to overreact. (Pauses in silence.) I am sorry that I lose it with you and treat you like a six-year-old.
Therapist:	That is so good that you can be that straight with Bill. What's it like to say that to him?
Davit:	Part of me is cringing, and just wanting this session to end but the other part knows I got to get a grip.
Therapist:	Actually, I see you being very courageous and brave right now. It's hard for all of us to be vulnerable but the message you are sending to Bill is that he is important, he does matter, and sometimes your fear makes it hard to see him.
Davit:	(Joking.) If you say so.
Therapist:	This is brand new, Davit, you were never taught this. It's hard being a parent sometimes, but you have never given up and keep trying. It just says to me how much you care.
Davit:	I want to do this differently than my father, I don't want Bill to be afraid of me. In my darkest moments, I know that Matthew kind of fell through the cracks with me. (Softly.) So I am adamant that I am not going to let happen with Bill.
Therapist:	(Softly.) Of course Davit, you love Bill with all your heart, and you want to have a different kind of relationship with your son, which is what you are doing right now. (Pause.) What's that like for you, Bill, to see your dad open up?
Bill:	He doesn't need to worry. I am fine.
Therapist:	I see you trying to reassure your dad right now, of course, you care about him and his feelings. But your dad is saying that you matter to him, that his fear blinds him sometimes, and leads him to get angry and try to control you. What's that like?
Bill:	(With flat affect.) Well I can see that human side of him. It's like there is another side of him than just the angry person.

Jill explains that her clear focus is on the caregiving system and on connecting Davit's reactive anger and control to the vulnerability he experiences when he fears his son may be "falling through the cracks." Emily responds, "It makes so much sense that Davit's fears carry the weight of that traumatic loss into his growing fears that he is losing his ability to protect his son." "Exactly," Jill responds. She continues:

> Yes, you can see how the therapist organizes the father's fear in terms of his caregiving intent and invites the father to emotionally engage with his son. When the father's concern and care is made explicit, his reactive anger is given new understanding.

In EFFT a critical shift occurs in Stage 1 when the father is better able to see his son, an important step toward this dad "knowing where his son is" and greater parental availability.

Stage 2: Processing a Child Block

The therapist, in Stage 2 of EFFT, turns attention to the blocks to child vulnerability and processing unsuccessful attachment bids with a parent. Again, the focus remains on the most distressed dyad as the therapist works through the relational block and now has the added resource of a parent's availability. Emily wonders how this shift in focus differs from the previous work on parental blocks. Jill explains that in Stage 2 the therapist attends to the child's protective responses by accepting and attuning to their experience as a parent initiates interest and care for the child's needs. As expected, these new moves by the parent may trigger the child's anger, mistrust, and other forms of protection rooted in disappointment and uncertainty, given the parent's previous lack of availability. The therapist validates and works through the child's ambivalence anchoring into the underlying vulnerability of their attachment needs. Throughout the process, the therapist repeats and reinforces the parent's newfound accessibility, responsiveness, and emotional engagement. Stage 2 concludes with the child's reach with their attachment needs and the parent's effective response. This completes the resolution of the relational block and sets the relationship on a course toward greater felt security.

Jill returns to the case example as the focus shifts to Davit taking new steps to engage Bill following his clear intention to respond to his son needs. In a Stage 2 session, Davit explicitly reaches for his son, expressing his desire to change their relationship and make more of an effort to listen to him. He says that he understands why Bill would run for cover and stay withdrawn when he loses it. Bill appreciates his dad's attempts to understand him and agrees he had most of it right, but was reluctant to engage his father's initiative, instead minimizing his own needs. Davit's availability triggers Bill's mistrust and he keeps his father at a distance, by placating and trying to please him.

Emily wonders how the enduring impact of loss impacts Bill's coping and need to minimize his own needs. Jill shares that Davit is on high alert wanting to protect his son, and Bill is caught between his grief over his brother's death and his own needs to be seen and affirmed for who he is – separate from his deceased sibling. He carries an added burden of survival guilt, expressed as, "My dad is still hurting, and I don't want to put more on him." Bill questions whether he is worthy of his dad's attention and love in the midst of this terrible loss. Jill conjectures that another layer of Bill's struggle to be vulnerable is the loss of his mother at a very young age, which he expresses when he wonders if he did something wrong to have his mother "choose" to leave him. This compounds his own negative view of self, "Is there is something wrong with me?" and his negative view of others, "There is no one really here for me." Bill's pleasing and placating behaviors function as attempts to assuage his own guilt and take care of his father's grief. Jill and Emily review the following transcript that captures the therapist shoring up Davit's emotional accessibility and invitation to Bill to begin to risk sharing his needs.

Therapist:	So, I am wondering now, Davit as you look at your son, and you see him participating in this session with you, what do you see in him, what would you like to say to him?
Davit:	(Confused.) I am not sure what you mean.
Therapist:	Well, it's like what you said earlier, Bill has grown from a boy to a young man, and all of this has happened in the face of huge challenges as a family, so much loss, and Bill is here, with you, as a 15-year-old, in therapy, talking about your relationship, what is that like to see that in your son?
Davit:	It makes me very proud of him. I would never have done that with my father.
Therapist:	Can you tell him?
Davit:	You are smart, funny and I can see how strong you are. On one hand though that makes me worry, because I don't want you to soldier on, but maybe those are my fears.
Therapist:	It sounds like you can see his strengths and that makes you proud and you also want him to know he can turn to you. He can depend on you. What's that like to hear that, Bill?
Bill:	It makes me feel like I need to work harder to really make you feel proud.
Therapist:	Right, it's like it is really hard to hear that your dad might be proud of you, it's almost like you don't deserve that – you need to work harder, Ohhh, that is tough. When he says he is proud, that hits you. Can you help me, what happens when you hear that? I can see your body kind of stiffen. It's like you need to push that away.
Bill:	I have done nothing for him to be proud of.
Therapist:	That's really hard. How can he really see me, and if he really sees me, he wouldn't be proud of me at all. It makes so much sense how you would need to stay hidden then because if your dad really, really saw you, what would happen?
Bill:	He would be disappointed.
Therapist:	Ahhh, yes, he would be disappointed that would be so painful, so, so, painful, we all need to be good in our parent's eyes and you work so hard to not disappoint him.
Davit:	This isn't about disappointing me.
Therapist:	Can I pause you here Davit? Your son is opening up. Bill is showing you his pain, his fear rather than suppressing. He is letting you see. Can you just stay with him, he is doing what you asked. He is leaning on you and showing his fears?
Davit:	Yes, Bill, I don't want you to have my bad habits and do want you to be able to share what scares you. I love you son.
Therapist:	Can you look at your dad, Bill? Can you see that he is reaching for you, that he wants to know you, all of you? (Bill makes eye contact) You have been alone for a very long time, you can't share everything with your 15-year-old friends, they don't get it. And you need to look after your younger brother because he isn't able to stick up for himself. But when you say, hey dad, this is what is important to me, it's like it doesn't matter, you don't matter and that takes you to a very dark place, like I am just a disappointment, I don't deserve your attention.
BILL:	I don't want anyone feeling sorry for me.
Therapist:	Sure, because that just feels like pity, like there is something wrong with you. So, when your dad says to you right here, right now, that he wants you to lean on him, good, bad, and ugly, and know that he loves you, can you see his face? Do you believe him?
Bill:	Not sure.
Therapist:	Yes, that is hard to believe, your dad has been lost in his own pain and fears and he now sees this gets in the way of seeing clearly. Right now, you are not saying what

your dad wants to hear, but you are being exactly you. You fear you are a disappointment. You don't deserve for your dad to be proud of you, and it is hard to imagine you can feel safe enough to be yourself and for your dad to love you for who you are. That makes total sense. Bill, you are being so brave in just sharing this. Davit, what's that like, when Bill is expressing his uncertainty and his fears to you right now?

Davit: It's good. I get it. Thank you for letting me know.

In this moment of effective caregiving, Bill receives the message that he is not alone, his emotions make sense, and together, dad and son will endure and survive. The therapist continues to tune into the attachment music, with Davit and Bill, turning up the volume, so that Bill can gradually expresses his fears and confusion about his mother's and Matthew's deaths. Davit sees and embraces his son.

Bill's ability to confide and reach for his father's support and care is the antidote for Davit's fear that somehow "I will lose my son." It is also the antidote for Bill's belief that he must perform to be loved, "because I can't really count on others to be there for me." The relationship block is removed. As fears are shared and care is received, a father and son build a more secure base for facing the future tougher. There is also now an opportunity to work with other dyads including Davit's relationship with Matthew's older brothers from Davit's first marriage.

Stage 3: Consolidation

There is now stabilization within the family, and the interactional patterns are restructured in the direction of attachment security. Davit's older sons notice the ease in family gatherings as they see their father more open and relaxed. "He is more at ease with himself and more open." Davit says that he had a "two-year speed bump" where he was not himself. He now has access to his grief and his thoughts reflect on Matthew most days. He is breaking though his isolation, making friends with an older neighborhood woman whom he seeks out regularly. Bill is now 16 and is not the perfect child. Davit reports a recent incident when Bill was caught sneaking in a female friend to the house late at night. Davit did not explode but instead recounted the story with humor and a lightness of being. "I guess this is just normal. We had a serious talk but my relationship with my son is not threatened. We are ok. I guess he has some growing up to do, well both of us do."

The power of traumatic loss can order reality in such a way that those things that are most precious also become fragile. Jill's case example illustrates the power of families to find relationship of resilience when they can turn toward an attachment figure who offers a safe haven in the storms of life and extends a secure base that enables growth and exploration. In EFFT we recognize that the path toward becoming begins with belonging and that life will bring "speed bumps" along the way that can cause a parent or child to lose their emotional balance and react and respond to their uncertainty in ways that only reinforce their dilemma they are trying to solve. As father turns to therapist and son to father the process of regaining attachment security begins with acceptance of one's need for others in the best of times and even more in life's darker more uncertain moments.

Conclusion

Emily thanks Jill for sharing this case and declares, "I'm ready to invite Jessica and Wayne and their son for EFFT now. Walking me through this EFFT case so clearly is giving courage and clarity about the process!" Their discussion then turns to Jamal and his parents, as Emily ponders where the family feels the most distress and how she can work with the family to see their pattern as the problem and EFFT as a resource for working through the understandable relational blocks for the parent's obvious care and concern. For Emily, tuning into the parent's caregiving intention, validating their reactive responses, and accessing their felt concern for Jamal all make sense in ordering the family's experience and moving the family toward greater accessibility, responsiveness, and emotional engagement. Jill expresses confidence in what Emily has to offer the family, encouraging her to lean in with confidence given the ways Jessica and Wayne have grown in their ability to support and rely on one another. Emily smiles in response, concluding:

> As with all of EFT, I can trust the process! As I engage with my clients in this model, I will learn more, and reach the point of integrating a newly structured attachment bond across previous seemingly insurmountable obstacles.

18 Future Steps

You and EFT

> We need a map to guide us on our journey to love – starting with the place where we know what we mean when we speak of love. (bell hooks, 2001, p. 14)

Looking back on the journey you have traveled with Emily and envisioning future steps that you and EFT will take are the themes of this concluding chapter. You have an opportunity to review the key ingredients of change that are summarized in the EAR of attunement in EFT and to receive encouragement and tools for your continuing journey of becoming an EFT therapist. Clients are your greatest teachers and a collegial community can be your greatest source of encouragement. Consonant with the humanistic model of EFT is a focus on strengths, growth, community, and new possibilities. I recap how EFT defines love and provides us with a map for what bell hooks, a Black, feminist writer, calls our *journey to love*. This voyage to love takes us to a place of secure attachment bonds, emotional flexibility and resilience, safe and secure connections with others, a humble willingness to become more culturally sensitive and trauma-informed, and an expanded sense of self as worthy and competent.

The journey to love also takes us to a place of belonging and acceptance for the difficult days that we do not feel competent or even worthy as a therapist. There will be days when you are practicing this gold-standard, empirically validated model of EFT, and you wonder, "What is wrong with me? If I have this great model, how can I be facing these therapeutic ruptures, barriers, and self-doubts?" The journey to love is every bit as important for you, in your moments of discouragement as an EFT therapist, as it is for your clients. Find a companion to ground you and care for you, and to remind you that in attachment, in love, you do not need to be perfect; you need to be present and to notice that you belong. "To ward off life-threatening despair," writes hooks, "more and more individuals are turning toward a love ethic" (hooks, 2001, p. 94). This love ethic – emotional interconnectedness in a climate of trust, care, respect, and kindness – can definitely ward of the despair and shame that are triggered on difficult therapy days.

Furthermore, beginning EFT therapists do well to focus themselves, as they do their work with clients, "on growth through new experience, and new ways of processing that experience, rather than on the correction of inherent deficits or deficiencies" (Johnson, 2020, p. 42). One of the kindest, strongest, and most secure foundations for this growth process can be found in the international community of fellow EFT therapists and in a local consultation/support group. "An empathic way of being can be learned," wrote Rogers (1980, p. 150), and ongoing inter-collegial support from your EFT colleagues ensures that an empathic EFT manner can be integrated into your way of being. The journey of *becoming an EFT therapist* is an ongoing expedition, with endless learning and discoveries, and no destination of perfection. The exciting voyage is sure to last for as long as you are practicing EFT. *Workouts for Stepping into EFT* is designed expressly as an engaging resource

DOI: 10.4324/9781003242673-27

to strengthen and fine tune your EFT muscles and to do so in a way that is validating and built on the ethic of love and interconnectedness.

Seasons have come and gone since Emily first stepped enthusiastically into EFT. Despite challenges and setbacks, she is finding that her clients and the model itself continue to be an inspiration and source of meaning. Emily is increasingly confident in the EFT journey to love. She savors the dramatic shift away from trying to fix clients' presenting problems to taking a more empathic, collaborative stance as a process consultant, helping her clients restructure their negative patterns of interaction into increasingly secure bonds. She is experiencing decreased attachment anxiety and increased compassion for herself and others in her world, unexpected, but not uncommon benefits of EFT training (Montagno et al., 2011; Rodríguez-González et al., 2019). Her confidence and competence in EFCT and EFIT are definitely expanding. After consulting with her colleague, Jill, about working with families (Chapter 17), and hearing from clients who want her to help them with family tensions, Emily feels ready to add the modality of emotionally focused family therapy (EFFT) to her practice.

As you travel through your own steps of learning EFT, hopefully, Emily's integration of the model will encourage you to develop your style of EFT, one step at a time. The process of integrating a new paradigm can be overwhelming, but resources such as this book, its accompanying website (www.steppingintoeft.com) with many EFCT and EFIT training videos, and its companion book, *Workouts for Stepping into Emotionally Focused Therapy: Exercises to Strengthen Your Practice* will carry you far along the journey of EFT fitness, confidence, and self-acceptance. Drawing on these resources, and others found at www.iceeft.com, and an EFT community of support, you are ensured of an inspiring experience with increasing moments of creative competency.

The science and the art of EFT are inextricably combined with attunement to contextual impacts and deep listening to contextual stories and experiences of race, ethnicity, and culture (REC). Practicing EFT across cultures calls upon therapists to be grounded in the model with openness and humility to discover how the model works for a particular client in their context. The EFT therapist is a process consultant collaborating with clients who are the experts on their experience; thus it is well-suited to being a cross-culturally relevant model, respecting different cultural styles of emotional expression. To continue to grow in your competency as an EFT therapist, you are challenged to embrace learning more about diverse experiences of culture, power, and privilege and to continually expand your cultural humility before assuming you can fully understand others' nuanced experience and the impacts of their contexts.

The EFT Pearls of Great Value

"Pearls form as a result of an irritant becoming trapped in the soft tissue of a living creature as this creature attempts to grasp the nutrients needed to sustain life. One way of dealing with the irritant can result in something precious and beautiful" (Johnson, 2010, p. 133). Focusing on Johnson's imagery of the formation of pearls serves to review the key ingredients of change in EFT, as conveyed in the EAR of attunement. It can also encourage therapists in what is sure to seem, at times, a much slower process than they would like – that of becoming an EFT therapist. The image of forming pearls "reflects one of the basic truths about adult love, the need for human connection. Loss of safe emotional connections is a powerful irritant" (Johnson, 2010, p. 133) that leads to relationship and emotional distress! EFT offers a structured guide to restructure distress into effective dependence where partners and individual clients can respond to disconnection in a way that ensures a relationship will become a secure bond and an individual client will discover an expanded sense of self in secure connections with others. This discovery of belonging, that brings to life a new view of self and other, is clearly a pearl of great value.

Effective dependence, or secure belonging, is undeniably one of the most treasured pearls of human existence. Therapists stepping into EFT are likely to discover common challenges and powerful irritants that can form into what Johnson identifies as the three pearls of wisdom at the heart of EFT. Johnson (2010) consolidates the key EFT resources as three valuable pearls, emotion, attachment, and enactments/encounters, all of which support a therapist to remain focused upon engaging with present-moment emotional experience. Although the pearls can be described separately, in practice they are inseparable – effectively dependent upon, and supportive of, one another. Their interdependence reflects a similar interdependence of the elements of the EAR of attunement (Box 3.1; follow emotion, attune to attachment; reshape strategies).

The EAR of attunement keeps *context* in the forefront of emotion, attachment, and the reshaping that is created through interpersonal encounters. Context, like the air we breathe, is everywhere, and each of these pearls, is uniquely, contextually formed.

Pearl One: Emotion

EFT therapists follow emotion because emotion is the heart of change. In intimate relationships it is the most powerful force: A hand can calm jittery neurons in the brain (Johnson et al., 2013), and perceived disconnection can trigger primal panic (Johnson, 2010). Staying with present-moment emotional experience and working with the moment-to-moment unfolding process of emotion, is a central tenet of EFT. Unfolding a client's emotional reality goes beyond naming an emotion. It involves assembling emotion as an active perception-appraisal-motivational process (Chapter 6), expanding and making explicit emotional experience, which has been only implicit (Stern, 2004) or on the leading edge of conscious awareness (Rice, 1974), while exploring the contextual experience of that emotion. Unfolding a client's emotional reality progresses from identifying the different elements of emotion, accessing a felt sense of the emotion, attuning to the cultural and contextual impacts of emotional experience and expression, finding words for emerging emotional experience, and finally, using the newly experienced emotion to create new interactions.

As you treasure this pearl, ask yourself:

Do I recognize subtle verbal and non-verbal markers of emotional experience? How comfortable am I with attuning and getting a felt sense of client's experience? What may interfere with my comfort or discomfort around emotion? Do I know how to assemble the process of emotion, starting with what triggers it? Am I comfortable lingering in emotional experience, assembling and deepening the distilled core, once it is coherent?

Consider how you can expand your competence in working with emotion by remembering to open the four doorways into emotional experience and to follow the verbal and non-verbal markers of emotional and cultural handles. Continue to be aware of your limitations and your need for contextual curiosity and sensitivity to fully attune to clients with different positions of power and privilege from your own. Always attend to you own felt sense of emotional experience while attuning to others.

Pearl Two: Attachment

EFT therapists frame relational-emotional distress as understandable reactions to core attachment fears of abandonment and rejection, including contextual threats of exclusion and survival dangers. As process consultants, EFT therapists are always looking through an attachment lens, to sense explicitly how moment-to-moment experience is illuminated by/filled with survival responses when attachment needs for safety and connection are threatened and REC contextual danger cues are presented. (See Chapter 5 for attachment themes.)

Wearing a solidly dark purple turtleneck sweater to my son's glow-in-the-dark bowling, I was shocked when I looked at my sweater to see not a solidly dark sweater, but instead one covered with white polka dots. Every textured nodule in the wool was accentuated, illuminated as a white dot, glowing in the dark. With continued practice, an EFT therapist finds that attachment themes – needs for safe connection – illuminate the relational landscape like the textured wool glowing in the dark. The drama of self-protective reactions to attachment threats and contextual dangers, such as minority stressors, and the accompanying attachment fears, longings, needs, and resilience become increasingly clear in a culturally sensitive, therapeutic relationship.

You can train yourself to be continually on the lookout for attachment dramas, in and outside of therapy. For example, attend to attachment emotions and cultural danger cues in the supermarket, in films, in the news, and in the relational ruptures and repairs you observe and experience on a daily basis.

Seek opportunities to use the classic attachment reframes: Criticism as a fight for connection, frantic demands as a search to find an emotionally absent other, and increasing volume as a desperate plea for a response; disappearance as hiding in fear of disappointing an exquisitely important other, down-regulating as a survival response to avoid getting hurt, and a lack of response as freezing in fear of fighting back and jeopardizing an entire relationship. Tuning into the attachment survival threat that a client may be managing helps substantially to avert reacting judgmentally to clients. All strategies for engagement (hyperactivating, deactivating, or swinging between the two) have their usefulness, in context.

As you treasure this pearl of attachment, notice how your growing understanding of attachment protest and separation-distress responses helps you form an alliance with two partners at loggerheads with one another, or in tension with you, given the intersectionalities of power and privilege between you. Continually fine-tune your visual and auditory sensitivities to recognize variations of the human cry for belonging in your individual clients. Ground yourself to be continually open to being informed about subtle acts of exclusion you may have committed, ready to respond with gratitude for being told if you have hurt someone and kindness and compassion to listen to how your response may have threatened their sense of safety (Chapter 7; Jana & Baran 2020).

Pearl Three: Reshaping through Encounters

The third pearl is creating therapeutic encounters that reshape clients' relational and inner worlds. Acknowledging minority stressors, and cultural differences in emotion, EFT therapists recognize that change events shaped through interpersonal dialogues (encounters/enactments) can create islands of safety in a world that remains unsafe for some. Deliberately shaped therapeutic encounters, function to shape partners' and individual clients' reaching and responding in new ways. This pearl actively integrates the first pearl of present-moment processing of emotion in all its contextual richness with the second pearl of processing experience within the attachment, relational, systemic context. It also unites the two features shown to contribute to change in EFT: Depth of emotional experiencing and affiliative interactions. Using newly assembled key emotional experience to "prime new responses … in therapeutic enactments [aka encounters] is the heart of change in EFT" (Johnson, 2020, p. 18).

Therapists new to EFT are well aware of the prominent Stage 2 encounters of expressing distilled attachment fears and reaching to ask to have attachment needs met. However, encounters, shaped in a culturally attuned manner, are a standard part of EFT sessions. Beginning EFT therapists benefit from practicing shaping "smaller scale" encounters in each session. The moves of the EFT tango provide a tool kit for shaping change by choreographing encounters. After tracking processes within and between with Move 1 and assembling and deepening emotion with Move 2, the stage is set for a Move 3 encounter where the therapist shapes and directs an engaged disclosure, keeping the client focused and the emotion alive. With Move 4, the therapist mines the moment of this intimate sharing, processing the impact on the discloser as well as the one who receives the message. Depending on the therapeutic modality, the receiver of the disclosure may be personally present or in imagination. While summarizing and heightening the new moves and new moment of interpersonal contact, with Move 5, the therapist validates that clients are truly competent to shape and restructure their emotional and relational lives, moment-to-moment, as they just did.

Culturally sensitive forms of encounters may look different from white middle-class hetero clients, and yet are profoundly effective. For example, Liu describes her flexibility in working with a Chinese man, in his 70s who had never called his wife by her name. Although he tried, he could not utter any words to his wife at Liu's prompting. Instead, while he struggled to speak, his wife reached out to comfort him and assure him he didn't need to speak. Lui immediately used Move 4 to validate and heighten his wife's care for him and processed that experience with each of them. This culturally sensitive creativity with shaping and processing an encounter created a significant corrective emotional experience that reshaped their interactions. "We may not always be able to ask our clients to articulate their feelings and needs in ways that we assume they should," says Liu (Dockett, 2022, p. 28). Respect for different ways of expressing affection and different gender expectations means being flexible about how to reshape connection.

You can begin to integrate EFT into your therapy style, simply by moving through these moves in each session. Furthermore, you can capitalize on the final celebratory Move 5 of summarizing and integrating clients' progress by also celebrating and summarizing your own progress as an EFT therapist. Commend yourself for beginning to attune and move with clients through the EFT steps of change. Acknowledge how you have already expanded how you look at couples, individuals, and families and consider how this is shifting your work with them. Be continually open to enhance the relevance and sensitivity in your EFT practice across REC differences. Focus upon your own emotions and bodily felt sense as you stretch your capacity to increase engagement with clients' internal experience and interpersonal patterns. Validate that, indeed, you are competent to shape loving relationships moment by moment. Seed hope with a picture of the safety and trust you are building with your clients: Picture yourself trusting the process and the ambiguities of your work.

Stepping into Community

One of the key elements of being an effective process consultant is that while engaging with, and reshaping, present-moment process, the consultant simultaneously attends with empathic attunement to their clients and to their own inner felt sense. The potential weight of this personal demand is lessened when a therapist is securely grounded in a community of colleagues. Being surrounded by the compassion, nurturance, and collective knowledge of colleagues can offer therapists a secure base for exploring their own style of becoming an EFT therapist. There are various options to choose from to plan your journey into the culturally sensitive art and science of EFT. Your exploration will be enriched by the company of fellow travelers. You will travel more safely and more happily, together. A community will enhance your theoretical and practical learning as well as provide needed emotional support. Local and international communities of EFT colleagues can be located at www.iceeft.com

International Community

By becoming an EFT therapist, you are joining a movement dedicated to shaping secure connections worldwide. You are embarking on a safe adventure in a vibrant model with like-minded therapists worldwide, dedicated to making a difference and healing the grief of broken attachments and exclusion. Formal training in EFT begins with a four-day introduction offered across the globe in any one of the three modalities: EFCT, EFIT or EFFT. After the introductory training, therapists are eligible to join an online international community that has over 8,000 members from nearly 80 countries – the International Centre for Excellence in EFT. This community provides a listserv of rich dialogue, video and reading resources, and a quarterly newsletter of practical support that validate the complexities and delights of learning this deceptively simple model. Training and resources for therapists are available at www.iceeft.com as well as at www.carolinaeft.com. The international community provides a host of in-person and virtual training opportunities in all modalities of EFT.

Additionally, there are many EFT podcasts, webinars such as www.eftandme.com, and online Facebook groups providing virtual support. "Therapists working with Clients of Color, especially white clinicians, must be professionally trained and racially prepared to deliver racially sensitive, trauma-informed therapy" (Hardy, 2023, p. 28). ICEEFT supports may trainings in culturally sensitive training with Clients of Color, LGBTQ+, and other cultures.

Local Community: Peer Practice Groups

In addition to experiencing oneself as a part of the international community, it will also enhance your capacities to integrate EFT into your way of being and ground you with a sense of belonging and support if you become part of a local or virtual community of fellow therapists. Companions on the journey of learning EFT can provide safe-haven comfort by validating your challenges and self-doubts and create a secure base for exploration.

A helpful next step can be to find a learning partner to embark on the *EFT workouts* in the companion volume to this book. Peer or supervisor-led supervision groups provide opportunities to review each other's video recordings, to discuss common challenges and impasses, to celebrate successes, and to refine personal goal(s) to enhance one's EFT practice. Peer support is indispensable to learning and practicing EFT. Peers are likely to see strengths and contributions easily missed by a struggling therapist. By conveying acceptance and trust, colleagues support and strengthen each other's capacity to remain attuned and curious, both with self and with clients. Having peer support and sharing struggles with one another helps to erase feelings of shame and inadequacy. Peer supervision also nurtures therapist's motivation and hope in the value of pursuing the journey toward the continually expanding competence as an EFT therapist. Experiential learning can be enriched by reviewing each other's videos and practicing the exercises in *Workouts for Stepping into Emotionally Focused Therapy: Exercises to Strengthen Your Practice*. Additionally, an engaging way to enhance your practice and gain empathic understanding and compassion for a challenging client is to engage in a role-play, where you take on the role of that person.

Forming a peer study group, or joining an online supervision group, or an online *EFT Workouts* group are excellent ways to support your learning. The website to accompany this book (www. SteppingintoEFT.com) offers additional resources, such as transcripts and video excerpts of therapy sessions demonstrating EFT's key elements.

Growing by Experiencing the EFT Model

Emily finds the model itself is helping her to ease up on her self-expectations and to trust the role of being a process consultant in clients' lives. She takes encouragement from the realistic perspective offered by Johnson who said, "It does take time and effort to learn. In fact, for myself, after 30 years, I am still learning from every client and couple I see" (2011, p. 428). Emily constantly finds that her clients are her best teachers about attachment dynamics, cultural nuances, learning to work with emotion, and to shape in-session encounters. She learns much from viewing her own recordings and refers frequently to *Workouts for Stepping into EFT: Exercises to Strengthen Your Practice* when she needs encouragement. The flexibility and room for therapist imperfections and client limitations within EFT are additional sources of inspiration.

At times, Emily's clients take a break from therapy for various reasons. Some are financially unable to afford regular therapy and for others travel and work schedules impede regular attendance at therapy. Other times, one partner's ambivalence or reluctance to stay in therapy interrupts therapy progress. Frequently, Emily is encouraged to find that when a couple or individual takes a "break" from therapy for any number of reasons but return months later, the progress essentially continues from where they left off. The problematic pattern might have reappeared with a new vengeance, however, the positive impact and small corrective emotional experiences of early Stage 1 work frequently remain. Similarly, individual clients who return to therapy after a break, despite new life crisis and existential challenges, seem to retain earlier therapeutic gains and corrective emotional experiences endure, as powerful resources. I trust that you too will grow your EFT competence and confidence as you experience it together with your clients and your colleagues.

As another way to immerse yourself in the model, you might consider leading a group based on Johnson's (2008) book for relationship enhancement, *Hold Me* Tight®: *Conversations for Connection*. The *Hold Me Tight Facilitator's Guide* will be a great resource. Other group programs with leaders' guides include, Created for Connection for Christian couples, Healing Hearts Together for cardiac patients and their partners, Hold Me Tight®/Let Me Go for families with teens, and Hold Me Tight®/Let Me Be Me for families with adult children. Your grasp of EFT will also be enhanced by reflecting on your personal experience as you read Johnson's books for the public: *Hold Me Tight*; *Love Sense;* and the *Hold Me Tight Workbook,* as well as exploring the *Hold Me Tight Online* a program for clients to participate in, at their own pace, from home.

The Next Steps for EFT and You

The future of EFT will undoubtedly include expansion in EFIT and EFFT training, publications, and research. Although the EFIT research has not yet been published at the time of this printing, it is likely to refine and validate the effectiveness of EFIT. Data is being gathered and analyzed and, as Mikulincer and Shaver (2023a) predict, "Based on Johnson's previous development and evaluation of EFT for couples, we are optimistic about her new approach, EFIT, becoming another successful form of attachment-based individual psychotherapy" (p. 176). Publications and research are also likely to remain strong in EFCT with separate training tracks emerging for training and certification in the three modalities: EFCT, EFIT, and EFFT.

Adult attachment theory is being extended beyond the traditional romantic dyads, as discussed in Chapter 5, to include "the advantages of an expanded and diverse attachment network...We can move from the classical version of attachment theory, which focuses exclusively on close dyadic relationships, to an expanded version of the theory that includes multiple sources of security" (Mikulincer & Shaver, 2023b, p. 50). Different attachment figures can include romantic partners, consensual nonmonogamous relationships, friends, families, working groups, sociopolitical groups, religious groups, and spiritual figures. The trend to extend both attachment theory and applications of EFT is sure to expand in the next decade. The theoretical growth in attachment theory is already being mirrored in expanded applications of EFT, in fields such as medicine (Rhodius, 2023; the *palliative paradox*), organizational management, education, and therapy with consensual nonmonogamous relationships (Edwards et al., 2023; Kolmes & Witherspoon, 2017).

One great hope for a next step in EFT in the next decade is that it will become increasingly clear how EFT can have a healing impact on the racial trauma of colonialism and slavery and become a beacon in the search for reparations to indigenous peoples and people of color. It has been suggested (Hawkins, 2022) that the EFT model of attachment injury resolution is relevant for healing impacts of racial trauma and intergenerational, ongoing, repetitive injuries done to marginalized groups by dominant groups in society. EFT therapists and scholars have great opportunities to explore how to extend the AIRM to embrace working with the impacts of minority stress experienced by all racial, ethnic, and culturally marginalized groups.

Given its worldwide popularity and its malleability to adapt to other cultures, EFT will continue to be influenced by the traditions of collectivist cultures. Polychroni and Liu, two ICEEFT-certified EFT trainers, describe from the perspectives of Greek and Chinese cultures, respectively, the differently nuanced traditions and notions of what love is and how emotions are expressed (Dockett, 2022). Collectivist cultures where EFT is already thriving include Uganda, Greece, China, and indigenous groups in New Zealand. While the growth of EFT in these and many other collectivist cultures is expected to continue thriving, it is anticipated that it will also serve to enlighten those steeped in the individualism of the Western world. It will influence EFT practitioners to be flexible, attuned, and respectful, putting client needs, not therapist values, in the forefront, being able to reframe, for example, what appears as gender inequality as a loving reach to extend support. Polychroni and Liu's "respect and sensitivity to the client and the culture create a path not to subvert tradition, nor to dismantle old ways of creating strong healthy relationships, but to enhance ways already working" (Dockett, 2022, p. 32). We have only begun to touch the tip of the iceberg of how collectivist cultures that value interdependence and caring and respect for others can influence the development and practice of EFT.

There are many doors to open in terms of diversity in EFT. EFT is expanding to explicitly address working with African Americans (Guillory, 2022; Nightingale et al., 2019), the LGBTQ+ populations (Allan & Westhaver, 2018; Edwards et al., 2023), Chinese clients (Liu & Wittenborn, 2011; Wong, et al., 2017) and cultural diversity more broadly (Allan et al., 2022). EFCT is likely to continue to build on its current integration of treating sexual response (Johnson & Zuccarini, 2010, 2011; Johnson et al., 2018), working with violence (Slootmaeckers & Migerode, 2018, 2020), and compulsive behaviors and addictive processes (Fletcher & MacIntosh, 2018; Love et al., 2016). Literature, research, and training on how all modalities of EFT can effectively serve a diversity of cultural, racial, ethnic, gender, sexual, spiritual, religious orientations, neurodiverse clients and differing family structures is sure to expand. The most current source for literature on these topics can be found at www.iceeft.com. Your growth as an EFT therapist can also include broadening your use of this model across your work with a diversity of clients and a range of presenting problems and diagnoses with couples, individuals, and families.

Hopefully, along with Emily, you will continue to step more fully into EFCT and EFIT with renewed sensitivity to contextual elements and with a keen openness to integrate what the burgeoning research shows. I expect you will be excited to integrate findings from new EFIT publications, showing how EFIT works with depression, anxiety, and trauma-related symptoms. The more you engage with clients in moment-to-moment attunement, forming alliances, identifying and stabilizing problematic patterns, and restructuring bonds and strategies for engaging with self, others and life, the more your clients will become your teachers, and the stronger will be your EFT foundation and confidence. From this foundation, I am optimistic that you will be ready to broaden your work to include families, inspired by Furrow and Palmer's chapter, which builds beautifully upon the EFT foundation you have built along with Emily. You will, no doubt, be motivated by new

EFFT research such as Quinn et al. (2023) which shows a clear path of specific therapist behaviors to create *successful caregiver openness events* – a key finding for EFFT.

The attachment bond is at the core of our existence as individuals, as a society, and as a worldwide community. We now know how to shape the dance called lasting love and togetherness (Johnson & Tronick, 2016), and how to extend this beyond couple relationships (Mikulincer & Shaver, 2023b). Hopefully we will continue building a better world with the power of EFT. The potent model has impacted millions of lives worldwide and is currently being taught in over 40 countries, with professional and self-help EFT literature translated into more than 30 languages. There is every reason to expect that it will continue to flourish, in particular because of its unique capacity to define what we mean when we speak of love and to offer a map of the journey out of trauma and distress toward love. EFT continues to draw therapists encouraged to have a map to reshape attachment/love relationships. The journey to help clients shape new worlds of emotional flexibility and resilience with strategies for engaging that characterize safe and secure relationships with others and within self is a thrilling one for therapists to travel with their clients.

In the preface, I expressed my hope that reading this book would enrich your therapy practice one step at a time, by integrating EFT into your way of being. Throughout the book, I have held EFCT in one hand and EFIT in the other as we followed Emily's journey to learn these modalities. I have shown you how the EFT process that creates change through corrective emotional experiences in couples also shapes change for individuals. Then, in Chapter 17, Furrow and Palmer conveyed Emily's continued search to discover how to add EFFT to her practice. They showed Emily and you the similarities and unique nuances of EFFT, particularly in helping parents to become accessible to their children's vulnerability and the unidirectional dynamic of caregiving.

Before closing, I leave you with an EFCT haiku (Brubacher, 2012) that I wrote during my early years of training therapists in EFT and a visual of a *broaden-and-build* cycle, relevant to EFIT. The haiku portrays the attachment, relational beginnings of EFT and the human need for a secure interpersonal bond. The visual (Figure 18.1) represents the power of belonging – how a safe haven/ secure base is a survival need and a source of comfort and growth for everyone. This is also known as the *secure-base script* (Mikulincer & Shaver, 2023a).

EFCT Haiku

Stage 1
Savor, linger, breathe
Every layer of the dance
Chaos becomes calm

Stage 2
Deepen, taste, disclose
Raw spots that our dance evokes
Healed by your embrace

Stage 3
THEN we danced in fear
NOW to songs of needing you
And finding you near.

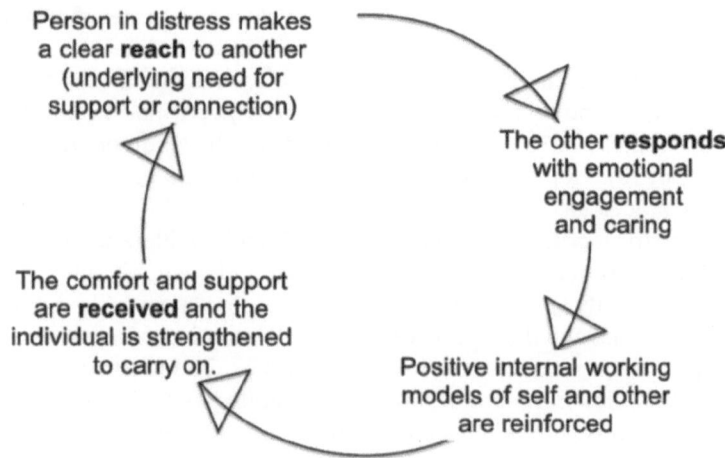

Figure 18.1 EFIT Broaden-and-Build Cycle.

This is an exciting time for attachment theory and EFT as both extend beyond classical attachment theory. I hope you are as motivated as Emily to accelerate your exploration of EFT's art and science of creating secure bonds with a culturally sensitive, attachment-informed orientation. Mikulincer and Shaver suggest that "Bowlby's eclectic approach to theory construction, his theory's insights into intimate relationships, and attachment researchers' diligence in testing his ideas portend an exciting future for attachment-related psychotherapies" (2023a, p. 176). You've picked trustworthy companions and a winning route for your journey. Go for it!

References

Ainsworth, M. D. S. (1967). *Infancy in Uganda: Infant care and the growth of love.* Johns Hopkins Press.

Ainsworth, M. S., Blehar, M. C., Waters, E., & Wall, S. (1978). *Patterns of attachment: A psychological study of the strange situation.* Lawrence Erlbaum.

Ainsworth, M. S., & Bowlby, J. (1991). An ethological approach to personality development. *American Psychologist, 46,* 331–341.

Alcoholics Anonymous: The big book (2001). (4th ed.). Alcoholics Anonymous World Services Inc.

Alder, M. C., Dyer, W. J., Sandberg, J. G., Davis, S. Y., & Holt-Lunstad, J. (2019). Emotionally-focused therapy and treatment as usual comparison groups in decreasing depression: A clinical pilot study. *The American Journal of Family Therapy, 46*(5), 541–555. https://doi.org/10.1080/01926187.2019.1572478

Alexander, B. K. (2022). A final conversation with addiction professionals. *Addiction Research & Theory.* https://doi.org/10.1080/16066359.2022.2144262

Allan, R., Edwards, C., & Lee, N. (2022). Cultural adaptations of emotionally focused therapy. *Journal of Couple & Relationship Therapy.* Advance online publication. https://doi.org/10.1080/15332691.2022.2052391

Allan, R., & Westhaver, A. (2018). Attachment theory and gay male relationships: A scoping review. *Journal of GLBT Family Studies, 14*(4), 295–316.

American Psychiatric Association. (2022). *Diagnostic and statistical manual of mental disorders 2022-2023* (5th ed.). DSM-5-TR™.

American Society for Addiction Medicine. (2019). Retrieved from: https://www.asam.org/quality-care/definition-of-addiction

Amodeo, J. (2015, August 9). Is unconditional love possible? *Psychology Today.* Retrieved from: https://www.psychologytoday.com/ca/blog/intimacy-path-toward-spirituality/201508/is-unconditional-love-possible

Angelou, M. (1987). *The mask.* [Video]. YouTube. Retrieved from: https://www.youtube.com/watch?v=nNCVw0TmJjI

Arnold, K. (2014). Behind the mirror: Reflective listening and its tain in the work of Carl Rogers. *The Humanistic Psychologist, 42,* 354–369.

Arnold, M. B. (1960). *Emotion and personality.* Columbia Press.

Asiimwe, R., Lesch, E., Karume, M., & Blow, A. J. (2021). Expanding our international reach: Trends in the development of systemic family therapy training and implementation in Africa. *Journal of Marital and Family Therapy, 47,* 815–830.

Barlow, D. H. (2002). *Anxiety and its disorders: The nature and treatment of anxiety and panic* (2nd ed.). Guilford Press.

Barlow, D. H., Farchione, T. J., Sauer-Zavala, S., Latin, H. M., Ellard, K. K., Bullis, J. R., Bentley, K. H., Boettcher, H. T., & Casiello-Robbins, C. (2018). *Unified protocol for transdiagnostic treatment of emotional disorders: Therapist's guide* (2nd ed.). Oxford.

Barlow, D. H., Sauer-Zavala, S., Carl, J. R., Bullis, J. R., Ellard, K. K. (2014). The nature, diagnosis, and treatment of neuroticism: Back to the future. *Clinical Psychological Science, 2*(3), 344–365.

Barrett-Lennard, G. (2013). *The relationship paradigm: Human being beyond individualism.* Palgrave Macmillan.

Barrett, L. F. (2017). *How emotions are made: The secret life of the brain*. Houghton Mifflin Harcourt.

Bartholomew, K. (1990). Avoidance of intimacy: An attachment perspective. *Journal of Social and Personal Relationships, 7*, 147–178.

Beasley, C. C., & Ager, R. (2019). Emotionally focused couples therapy: A systematic review of its effectiveness over the past 19 years. *Journal of Evidence-Based Social Work, 16*(2), 144–159. https://doi.org/10.10 80/23761407.2018.1563013

Beckes, L., & Coan, J. A. (2011). Social baseline theory: The role of social proximity in emotion and economy of action. *Social and Personality Psychology Compass, 5*(12), 976–988.

Berscheid, E. (1999). The greening of relationship science. *American Psychologist, 54*(4), 260–266.

Bertalanffy, L. (1968). *General system theory: Foundations, development, applications*. George Braziller.

Bird, J. (2019). *Sorted: Growing up, coming out, and finding my place: A transgender memoir*. Tiller Press.

Birnbaum, G. E. (2023). The enticement of feeling understood, validated, and cared for: How does perceiving a partner as responsive affect the sexual arena? *Current Opinion in Psychology, 52*. https://doi.org/10.1016/j.copsyc.2023.101594

Blow, A. J., Sprenkle, D. H., & Davis, S. D. (2007). Is who delivers the treatment more important than the treatment itself? The role of the therapist in common factors. *Journal of Marital and Family Therapy, 33*(3), 298–317.

Bograd, M., & Mederos, F. (1999). Battering and couples therapy: Universal screening and selection of treatment modality. *Journal of Marital and Family Therapy, 25*(3), 291–312.

Bordin, E. S. (1979). The generalizability of the psychoanalytic concept of the working alliance. *Psychotherapy: Theory, Research and Practice, 16*, 252–260. https://doi.org/10.1037/h0085885

Bowlby, J. (1944). Forty-four juvenile thieves: Their characters and home-life. *International Journal of Psychoanalysis, 25*, 19–52.

Bowlby, J. (1958). The nature of the child's tie to his mother. *International Journal of Psychoanalysis, 39*, 1–23.

Bowlby, J. (1973). *Attachment and loss: Vol. 2. Separation: Anxiety and anger*. Basic Books.

Bowlby, J. (1979). *The making and breaking of affectional bonds*. Tavistock.

Bowlby, J. (1980). *Attachment and loss: Vol. 3. Loss, sadness and depression*. Basic Books.

Bowlby, J. (1982). *Attachment and loss: Vol. 1. Attachment* (2nd ed.). Basic Books.

Bowlby, J. (1988). *A secure base*. Basic Books.

Bradley, B., & Furrow, J. J. (2004). Toward a mini-theory of the blamer softening event: Tracking the moment-by-moment process. *Journal of Marital and Family Therapy, 30*(2), 233–246.

Bradley, B., & Furrow, J. J. (2007). Inside blamer softening: Maps and missteps. *Journal of Systemic Therapies, 26*(4), 25–43.

Bradley, B., & Furrow, J. J. (2010). *Conquering the nemesis: Blamer softening from A-to-Z*. [Paper presentation]. International Centre for Excellence in Emotionally Focused Therapy Summit, San Diego, California.

Bretherton, I. (1992). The origins of attachment theory: John Bowlby and Mary Ainsworth. *Developmental Psychology, 28*, 759–775.

Brill, S., & Kenny, L. (2016). *Transgender teen: A handbook for parents and professionals supporting transgender and non-binary teens*. Cleis Press.

Brubacher, L. (2018). Attachment injury resolution model in emotionally focused therapy. In J. Lebow, A. Chambers, & D. Breunlin (Eds.), *Encyclopedia of couple and family therapy*. Springer Science and Business Media. http://doi.org/10.1007/978-3-319-15877-8_903-1

Brubacher, L. L. (2012). An EFT haiku. *The EFT Community News, 12*, 14.

Brubacher, L. L. (2017). Emotionally focused individual therapy: An attachment-based experiential/systemic perspective. *Person-Centered and Experiential Psychotherapies, 16*(1), 50–57.

Brubacher, L. L. (2020). The EAR of EFIT: Attuned empathic listening. *The EFT Community News, 44*, 5–7.

Brubacher, L. L. (2022). SHAPE emotionally engaged interpersonal encounters. *The EFT Community News, 52*, 6–9.

Brubacher, L. L., & Buchanan, L. (2014). *Emotionally focused therapy attachment Injury Reduction Model (AIRM) Training Program* [Interactive Video Training Program]. Retrieved from www.attachmentinjuryrepair.com

Brubacher, L. L., & Johnson, S. M. (2017). Romantic love as an attachment process: Shaping secure bonds. In J. Fitzgerald (Ed.), *Foundations for couples' therapy: Research for the real world* (pp. 8–19). Routledge.

Brubacher, L. L., & Lee, A. C. (2014). Emotion is more than feeling: The elements of emotion in action. *The EFT Community News, 15*, 11–13.

Brubacher, L. L., & Liu, T. (2023). Emotionally focused couple therapy online: Handholding from a distance. In A. Rolnick, H. Weinberg, & A. Leighton (Eds.), *Theory and practice of online therapy* (pp. 205–216). Routledge.

Brubacher, L. L., & Wiebe, S. A. (2019). Process-research to practice in emotionally focused couple therapy: A map for reflective practice. *Journal of Family Psychotherapy, 30*(4), 292–313. https://doi.org/10.1080/08975353.2019.1679608

Burgess Moser, M., Johnson, S. M., Dalgleish, T. L., Lafontaine, M. F., Wiebe, S. A., & Tasca, G. A. (2015). Changes in relationship-specific attachment in emotionally focused couple therapy. *Journal of Marital and Family Therapy, 42*(2), 231–245.

Burke, M. A., & Embrich, D. G. (2008). Colorism. *International Encyclopedia of the Social Sciences, 2*, 17–18. Thomas Gale.

Burton, L. M., Bonilla-Silva, E., Ray, V., Buckelew, R., & Hordge, E. (2010). Critical race theories, colorism, and the decade's research on families of color. *Journal of Marriage and Family, 72*(3), 440–459.

Byng-Hall, J. (2001). Attachment as a base for family and couple therapy. *Child Psychology & Psychiatry Review, 6*, 31–36.

Cashwell, C. S., Giordano, A. L., King, K., Lankford, C., & Henson, R. K. (2017). Emotion regulation and sex addiction among college students. *International Journal of Mental Health & Addiction, 15*, 16–27.

Cassidy, J., & Shaver, P. R. (Eds.). (2016). *Handbook of attachment: Theory, research, and clinical applications* (3rd ed.). Guilford Press.

Causadias, J. M., Morris, K. S., Cárcamo, R. A., Neville, H. A., Nóblega, M., Salinas-Quiroz, F., & Silva, J. R. (2021). Attachment research and anti-racism: Learning from Black and Brown scholars. *Attachment & Human Development*. https://doi.org/10.1080/14616734.2021.1976936

Chan, C. D., & Howard, L. C. (2020). When queerness meets intersectional thinking: Revolutionizing parallels, histories, and contestations. *Journal of Homosexuality, 67*(3), 346–366. https://doi.org/10.1080/00918369.2018.1530882

Comas-Días, L., Hall, G. N., & Neville, H. A. (2019). Racial trauma: Theory, research, and healing: Introduction to the special issue. *American Psychologist, 74*(1), 1–5. http://dx.doi.org/10.1037/amp0000442

Coan, J. A. (2016). Towards a neuroscience of attachment. In J. Cassidy & P. R. Shaver (Eds.), *Handbook of attachment: Theory, research, and clinical applications* (3rd ed., pp. 242–269). Guilford Press.

Coan, J. A., & Maresh, E. L. (2014). Social baseline theory and the social regulation of emotion. In J. J. Gross (Ed.), *Handbook of emotion regulation* (2nd ed., pp. 221–236). Guilford Press.

Coan. J. A., & Sbarra, D. A. (2015). Social baseline theory: The social regulation of risk and effort. *Current Opinion in Psychology, 1*, 87–91.

Coan, J. A., Schaefer, H. S., & Davidson, R. S. (2006). Lending a hand: Social regulation of the neural response to threat. *Psychological Science, 17*, 1032–1039.

Conrad, C. A. (2015). The evolution of an emotionally focused therapist: A mixed-methods research study. *EFT Community News, 16*, 6–7.

Conradi, H. J., Dingemanse, P., Noordhof, A., Finkenauer, C., & Kamphuis, J. H. (2017). Effectiveness of the 'Hold Me Tight' relationship enhancement program in a self-referred and a clinician-referred sample: An emotionally focused couples therapy-based approach. *Family Process, 57*(3), 613–628.

Crenshaw, K., Gotanda, N., Peller, G., & Thomas, K. (1995). *Critical race theory: The key writings that formed the movement.* The New Press.

Dalgleish, T., Johnson, S. M., Burgess Moser, M., Wiebe, S. A., & Tasca, G. (2015). Predicting key change events in emotionally focused couple therapy. *Journal of Marital and Family Therapy, 41*(3), 260–275.

Damasio, A. R. (1999). *The feeling of what happens: Body and emotion in the making of consciousness.* Harcourt.

Davis, D. E., DeBlaere, C., Hook, J. N., Choe, E., Worthington, E. L., Owen, J., Rivera, D. P., Van Tongeren, D. R., & Placers, V. (2018). The multicultural orientation framework: A narrative review. *Psychotherapy, 55*(1), 89–100.

Day-Vines, N. L., Ammah, B. B., Steen, S., & Arnold, K. M. (2018). Getting comfortable with discomfort: Preparing counselor trainees to broach racial, ethnic, and cultural factors with clients during counseling. *International Journal of Advanced Counselling, 40*, 89–104.

Day-Vines, N. L., Cluxton-Keller, F., Agorsor, C., Gubara, S., & Otabil, N. A. A. (2020). The multidimensional model of broaching behavior. *Journal of Counseling & Development, 98*, 107–118.

Degruy, J. (2017). *Post traumatic slave syndrome: America's legacy of enduring injury and healing.* Uptone.

Dockett, L. (2022). Couples therapy around the world: Putting EFT to work in two cultures. *Psychotherapy Networker*, 26–33.

Edwards, C., Allan, R., Marzo, N. Wynfield, T., & Hicks, R. (2023). The use of emotionally focused therapy with polyamorous relationships. *Family Process*, 1–15. Advance online publication. https://doi.org/10.1111/famp.12934

Ehrenwald, L. (Ed.). (1976). *The history of psychotherapy: From healing magic to encounter.* Jason Aronson.

Ein-Dor, T., & Doran, G. (2015). Psychopathology and attachment. In J. A. Simpson & W. S. Rholes (Eds.), *Attachment theory and research: New directions and emerging themes* (pp. 346–373). Guilford.

Eisenberger, N. I. (2016). Social pain and social pleasure: Two overlooked but fundamental mammalian emotions? In L. F. Barret, M. Lewis, & J. Haviland-Jones (Eds.), *The handbook of emotions* (pp. 440–452). Guilford Press.

Ekman, P. (2007). *Emotions revealed: Recognizing faces and feelings to improve communication and emotional life.* St Martin's Griffin.

Elliott, R., Watson, J. C., Goldman, R. N., & Greenberg, L. S. (2004). *Learning emotion-focused therapy: The process experiential approach to change.* American Psychological Association.

Estevez, A., Jauregui, P., Sanchez-Marcos, I., Lopez-Gonzalez, H., & Griffiths, M. D. (2017). Attachment and emotion regulation in substance addictions and behavioral addictions. *Journal of Behavioral Addictions, 6*, 534–544.

Feeney, B. C., & Collins, N. L. (2014). A theoretical perspective on the importance of social connections for thriving. In M. Mikulincer & P. R. Shaver (Eds.), *Mechanisms of social connection: From brain to group* (pp. 291–314). American Psychological Association.

Feeney, B. C., van Fleet, M., & Jakubiak, B. K. (2015). An attachment-theoretical perspective on optimal dependence in close relationships. In J. A. Simpson & W. S. Rholes (Eds.), *Attachment theory and research: New directions and emerging themes* (pp. 195–233). Guilford.

Felitti, V. J., Anda, R. F., Nordenberg, D., Williamson, D. F., Spitz, A. M., Edwards, V., Koss, M. P., & Marks, J. S. (1998). Relationship of childhood abuse and household dysfunction to many of the leading causes of death in adults: The Adverse Childhood Experiences (ACE) Study. *American Journal of Preventive Medicine, 14*(4), 245–258. https://doi.org/10.1016/S0749-3797(98)00017-8

Fern, J. (2020). *Polysecure: Attachment, trauma and consensual nonmonogamy.* Thorntree Press.

Fletcher, K., & MacIntosh, H. (2018). Emotionally focused therapy in the context of addictions: A case study. *The Family Journal: Counseling and Therapy for Couples and Families, 26*(3), 330–340. https://doi.org/10.1177/1066480718795125

Flores, P. J. (2004). *Addiction as an attachment disorder.* Jason Aronson.

Frijda, N. H. (1986). *The emotions.* Cambridge University Press.

Frijda, N. H. (2007). *The laws of emotion.* Lawrence Erlbaum.

Furrow, J. L., & Bradley, B. (2011). Emotionally focused couple therapy: Making the case for effective therapy. In J. L. Furrow, S. M. Johnson, & B. A. Bradley (Eds.), *The emotionally focused casebook: New directions in treating couples* (pp. 3–29). Routledge.

Furrow, J. L., Edwards, S. A., Choi, Y., & Bradley, B. (2012). Therapist presence in emotionally focused couple therapy blamer softening: Promoting change through emotional experience. *Journal of Marital and Family Therapy, 38*(1), 39–49.

Furrow, J. L., Johnson, S. M. with Bradley, B., Brubacher, L. L., Campbell, T. L., Kallos-Lilly, V., Palmer, G., Rheem, K., & Woolley, S. (2022). *Becoming an emotionally focused therapist: The workbook.* Routledge.

Furrow, J. L., Palmer, G., Johnson, S. M., Faller, G., & Palmer-Olsen, L. (2019). *Emotionally focused family therapy: Restoring connection and promoting resilience.* Routledge.

Galán, C. A., Sequeira, S. L., Jamal-Orozco, N., Boness, C. L., Tung, I., Tabachnick, A. R., Novacek, D. M., Kahhale, I., Gonzalez, J. C., Bowdring, M. A., & Bekele, B. M. (2022). Combating the conspiracy of silence: Clinician recommendations for talking about racism-related events with youth of color. *Journal of the American Academy of Child & Adolescent Psychiatry, 61*(5), 586–590.

Ganz, M. B., Rasmussen, H. F., McDougall, T. V., Corner. G. W., Black, T. T., & De Los Santos, H. F. (2022). Emotionally focused couple therapy within VA healthcare: Reductions in relationship distress, PTSD, and depressive symptoms as a function of attachment-based couple treatment. *Couple and Family Psychology: Research and Practice, 11*(1), 15–32.

Gendlin, E. T. (1961). Experiencing: A variable in the process of therapeutic change. *American Journal of Psychotherapy, 15*(2), 233–245. https://doi.org/10.1176/appi.psychotherapy.1961.15.2.233

Gendlin, E. T. (1981). *Focusing* (2nd ed.). Bantam Books.

Gillath, O., & Ai, T. (2021). The dual-function model of attachment priming. In R. A. Thompson, J. A. Simpson, & L. J. Berlin (Eds.), *Attachment: The fundamental questions* (pp. 93–100). Guilford.

Gillath, O., Selchuck, E., & Shaver, P. R. (2008). Moving toward a secure attachment style: Can repeated security priming help? *Social and Personality Compass, 2*(4), 1651–1666.

Giordano, A. L. (2022). *A clinical guide to treating behavioral addictions: Conceptualizations, assessments, and clinical strategies*. Springer.

Glanzer, D. (2014). Edge-sensing as embodiment. *Person-Centered and Experiential Psychotherapies, 13*(1), 57–59.

Gorman, A. (2021). *Call us what we carry*. Viking.

Gottman, J. M. (1991). Predicting the longitudinal course of marriages. *Journal of Marital and Family Therapy, 17*(1), 3–7.

Greenman, P. S., & Johnson, S. M. (2012). United we stand: Emotionally focused therapy for couples in the treatment of posttraumatic stress disorder. *Journal of Clinical Psychology: In Session, 68*(5), 561–569.

Greenman, P. S., & Johnson, S. M. (2013). Process research on emotionally focused therapy (EFT) for couples: Linking theory to practice. *Family Process, 52*, 46–61. https://doi.org/10.1111/famp.12015

Greenman, P. S., & Johnson, S. M. (2022). Emotionally focused therapy: Attachment, connection, and health. *Current Opinion in Psychology, 43*, 146–150.

Greenman, P. S., Young, M., & Johnson, S. (2009). Emotionally focused couple therapy with intercultural couples. In M. Rastogi & V. Thomas (Eds.), *Multicultural couple therapy* (pp. 143–165). Sage.

Griffiths, M. (2005). A 'components' model of addiction within a biopsychosocial framework. *Journal of Substance Use, 10*, 191–197. https://doi.org/10.1080/14659890500114359

Gross, J. J. (2014). Emotion regulation: Conceptual and empirical foundations. In J. J. Gross (Ed.), *Handbook of emotion regulation* (2nd ed., pp. 3–20). Guilford.

Guillory, P. T. (2022). *Emotionally focused therapy with African American couples: Love heals*. Routledge.

Guillory, P. T., Villodas, F., & Berhe, Z. (2022, April 8, 9). Attachment and culture: Deep roots, courageous conversations, and self-reflections. [Online Workshop]. North California Center for EFT.

Halchuk, R. E., Makinen, J. A., & Johnson, S. M. (2010). Resolving attachment injuries in couples using emotionally focused therapy: A three-year follow-up. *Journal of Couple & Relationship Therapy: Innovations in Clinical and Educational Interventions, 9*, 31–47.

Hallendy, N. (2000). *Inuksuit: Silent messengers of the Arctic*. Douglas & McIntyre.

Hannah-Jones, N. (2019). *The 1619 project*. The New York Times.

Hari, J. (2015). *Chasing the scream: The first and last days of the war on drugs*. Bloomsbury.

Hari, J. (2018). *Lost connections: Why you're depressed and how to find hope*. Bloomsbury.

Hardy, K. V. (2016). Toward the development of a multicultural relational perspective in training and supervision. In K. V. Hardy & T. Bobes (Eds.), *Culturally sensitive supervision and training* (pp. 3–10). Routledge. https://doi.org/10.4324/9781315648064

Hardy, K. V. (Ed.). (2022). *The enduring, invisible, and ubiquitous centrality of whiteness*. W. W. Norton.

Hardy, K. V. (2023). *Racial trauma: Clinical strategies and techniques for healing invisible trauma wounds*. W. W. Norton.

Harper, D. (2001–2016). *Online Etymology dictionary*. Retrieved from: www.etymonline.com

Harrell, W. J. Jr. (2010). *We wear the mask: Paul Laurence Dunbar and the politics of representative reality*. The Kent State University Press.

Hatkoff, I., Hatkoff, C., & Kahumbu, P. (2007). *Owen and Mzee: Best friends*. Scholastic.

Hawkley, L. C., Masi, C. M., Berry, J. D., & Cacioppo, J. T. (2006). Loneliness is a unique predictor of age-related differences in systolic blood pressure. *Psychology and Aging, 21*(1), 152–164.

Hawkins, J. (2022, February 13). Using emotionally focused therapy to repair social injuries. YouTube. [Video]. We Heart Therapy. Retrieved from: https://www.youtube.com/watch?v=L25bfDQmsBo

Hazan, C., & Shaver, P. (1987). Romantic love conceptualized as an attachment process. *Journal of Personality and Social Psychology, 52*, 511–524.

Heather, N., Field, M., Moss, A. C., & Satel, S. (Eds.). (2022). *Evaluating the brain disease model of addiction*. Routledge.

Hendricks, M. N. (2007). The role of experiencing in psychotherapy: Attending to the "bodily felt sense" of a problem makes any orientation more effective. *Journal of Contemporary Psychotherapy, 37*(1), 41–46.

Herman, J. L. (1992). *Trauma and recovery*. Basic Books.

Hill Collins, P., & Bilge, S. (2020). *Intersectionality* (2nd ed.). Polity Press.

Hinson, M., & James, T. (2022, October 21, 22). Multi-cultural faux pas: The benefits of being aware of cultural differences. [Workshop]. Online, Carolina Center for Emotionally Focused Therapy.

Hogue, A. Schumm, J. A., MacLean, A., & Bobek, M. (2022). Couple and family therapy for substance use disorders: Evidence-based update 2010–2019. *Journal of Marital and Family Therapy, 48*, 178–203. https://doi.org/10.1111/jmft.12546

hooks, b. (2001). *All about love: New visions*. William Morrow.

Howard, A. (2021, October 29). Interview with Dr. S Johnson on EFIT. UBC Department of Psychiatry.

Jacobson, N. S., & Gottman, J. M. (2007). *When men batter women: New insights into ending abusive relationships*. Simon & Schuster.

Jana, T., & Baran, M. (2020). *Subtle acts of exclusion: How to understand, identify, and stop microaggressions*. Berrett-Koehler.

Johnson, S. M. (1993). Healing broken bonds [DVD]. *International Centre for Excellence in EFT (Producer)*. Retrieved from: www.iceeft.com/index.php/training-dvds

Johnson, S. M. (1998). Listening to the music: Emotion as a natural part of systems theory. *Journal of Systemic Therapies: Special Edition. The Use of Emotions in Couples and Family Therapy, 17*, 1–17.

Johnson, S. M. (2002). *Emotionally focused couple therapy with trauma survivors: Strengthening attachment bonds*. Guilford Press.

Johnson, S. M. (2003). Attachment theory: A guide for couple therapy. In S. M. Johnson & V. Whiffen (Eds.), *Attachment processes in couple and family therapy* (pp. 103–123). Guilford Press.

Johnson, S. M. (2004). *The practice of emotionally focused couple therapy: Creating connection* (2nd ed.). Brunner-Routledge.

Johnson, S. M. (2007). A new era for couple therapy: Theory, research, and practice in concert. *Journal of Systemic Therapies, 26*, 5–16.

Johnson, S. M. (2008). *Hold me tight: Seven conversations for a lifetime of love*. Little Brown.

Johnson, S. M. (2009a). Attachment theory and emotionally focused therapy for individuals and couples. In J. H. Obegi & E. Berant (Eds.), *Attachment theory and research in clinical work with adults* (pp. 410–433). Guilford Press.

Johnson, S. M. (2009b). Extravagant emotion: Understanding and transforming love relationships in emotionally focused therapy. In D. Fosha, D. J. Siegel, & M. F. Solomon (Eds.), *The healing power of emotion: Affective neuroscience, development and clinical practice* (pp. 257–279). W.W. Norton.

Johnson, S. M. (2010). Emotionally focused couple therapy: It's all about emotion and connection. In M. Kerman (Ed.), *Clinical pearls of wisdom: 21 leading therapists offer their key insights* (pp. 133–143). Norton.

Johnson, S. M. (2011). Commentary on the special section on learning emotionally focused couples therapy. *Journal of Marital and Family Therapy, 37*, 247–248.

Johnson, S. M. (2012). EFT and trauma. *Interview*, February 29 (R. Jorgenson, Interviewer). ICEEFT Trainer Talk. Retrieved from: http://connectpro67534013.adobeconnect.com/p63t5nb74ur/-

Johnson, S. M. (2013). *Love sense: The revolutionary new science of romantic relationships*. Little Brown.

Johnson, S. M. (2015). Emotionally focused couple therapy. In A. S. Gurman, J. L. Lebow, & D. K. Snyder (Eds.), *Clinical handbook of couple therapy* (pp. 97–128). Guilford Press.

Johnson, S. M. (2016a). *Attachment and the dance of sex: Integrating couple and sex therapy.* Presented to Psychotherapy Networker Symposium, Washington, DC, 19 March. Retrieved from: www.drsuejohnson. com/attachment-sex/attachment-and-the-dance-of-sex-integrating-couple-and-sex-therapy/#more-1957

Johnson, S. M. (2016b). Emotionally focused therapy: On target couple interventions in the age of attachment (DVD). Retrieved from: www.iceeft.com/index.php/training-dvds

Johnson, S. M. (2016c). *Shaping love: A seminal study [Blog post]*, January. Retrieved from: drsuejohnson. com/science-2/shaping-love-a-seminalstudy/#more-1888

Johnson, S. (2017). An emotionally focused approach to sex therapy. In Z. D. Peterson (Ed.), *The Wiley handbook of sex therapy* (pp. 250–266). John Wiley & Sons.

Johnson, S. M. (August, 2019). *Externships in emotionally focused couple therapy: Participant's manual.* International Centre for Excellence in Emotionally Focused Therapy.

Johnson, S. M. (2019). *Attachment theory in practice: Emotionally focused therapy with individuals, couples, and families.* Guilford Press.

Johnson, S. M. (2020). *The practice of emotionally focused couple therapy: Creating Connection* (3rd ed.). Routledge.

Johnson, S. M. (February, 2021). *Externships in emotionally focused therapy (EFT): Participant's manual.* International Centre for Excellence in Emotionally Focused Therapy.

Johnson, S. M. (2022). *The hold me tight workbook: A couple's guide for a lifetime of love.* Little Brown.

Johnson, S. M., & Brubacher, L. L. (2016). Emotionally focused couple therapy: Empiricism and art. In T. Sexton & J. Lebow (Eds.), *Handbook of family therapy* (pp. 326–348). Routledge.

Johnson, S. M., Burgess Moser, M., Beckes, L., Smith, A., Dalgleish, T., Halchuk, R., Hasselmo, K., Greenman, P. S., Merali, Z., & Coan, J. A. (2013). Soothing the threatened brain: Leveraging contact comfort with emotionally focused therapy. *PLoS ONE, 8*(11), e79314.

Johnson, S. M., & Campbell, T. L. (2022). *A primer for emotionally focused individual therapy: Cultivating fitness and growth in every client.* Routledge.

Johnson, S. M., & Faller, G. (2011). Dancing with the dragon of trauma: EFT with couples who stand in harm's way. In J. L. Furrow, S. M. Johnson, & B. A. Bradley (Eds.), *The emotionally focused casebook: New directions in treating couples* (pp. 165–192). Routledge.

Johnson, S. M., & Greenberg, L. S. (1985). Differential effects of experiential and problem-solving interventions in resolving marital conflict. *Journal of Consulting and Clinical Psychology, 53*(2), 175–184.

Johnson, S. M., & Greenberg, L. S. (1988). Relating process to outcome in marital therapy. *Journal of Marital and Family Therapy, 14*(2), 175–183.

Johnson, S. M., Hunsley, J., Greenberg, L., & Schindler, D. (1999). Emotionally focused couples therapy: Status & challenges. *Clinical Psychology: Science & Practice, 6*, 67–79.

Johnson, S. M., Lafontaine, M-F., & Dalgleish, T. L. (2015). Attachment: A guide to a new era of couple interventions. In J. A. Simpson & W. S. Rholes (Eds.), *Attachment theory and research: New directions and emerging themes* (pp. 393–421). Guilford Press.

Johnson, S. M., Maddeaux, C., & Blouin, J. (1998). Emotionally focused family therapy for bulimia: Changing attachment patterns. *Psychotherapy, 25*, 238–247.

Johnson, S. M., Makinen, J. A., & Milliken, J. W. (2001). Attachment injuries in couple relationships: A new perspective on impasses in couples therapy. *Journal of Marital and Family Therapy, 27*(2), 145–155.

Johnson, S. M., & Sanderfer, K. (2016). *Created for connection: The "Hold Me Tight" guide for Christian couples.* Little Brown.

Johnson, S. M., Simakhodskaya, Z., & Moran, M. (2018). Addressing issues of sexuality in couples therapy: Emotionally focused therapy meets sex therapy. *Current Sexual Health Report, 10*, 65–71. https://doi. org/10.1007/s11930-018-0146-5

Johnson, S. M., & Talitman, E. (1997). Predictors of success in emotionally focused marital therapy. *Journal of Marital & Family Therapy, 23*, 135–152.

Johnson, S. M., & Tronick, E. (2016). *Love sense: From infant to adult (Video).* Retrieved from: www.youtube.com/watch?v=OyCHT9AbDY

Johnson, S. M., & Zuccarini, D. (2010). Integrating sex and attachment in emotionally focused couple therapy. *Journal of Marital and Family Therapy, 36*(4), 431–445.

Johnson, S. M., & Zuccarini, D. (2011). EFT for sexual issues: An integrated model of couple and sex therapy. In J. L. Furrow, S. M. Johnson, & B. A. Bradley (Eds.), *The emotionally focused casebook: New directions in treating couples* (pp. 219–246). Routledge.

Jones, T. D. W. (2016). Location of self in training and supervision. In K. V. Hardy & T. Bobes (Eds.), *Culturally sensitive supervision and training* (pp. 16–14). Routledge. https://doi.org/10.4324/9781315648064

Jordan, J. V. (2008). Recent developments in relational-cultural theory. *Women & Therapy, 31*(2/3/4), 1–4.

Jordan, J. V. (2018). *Relational–cultural therapy* (2nd ed.). American Psychological Association. https://doi-org.libproxy.uncg.edu/10.1037/0000063-000

Josephson, G. J. (2003). Using an attachment-based intervention with same-sex couples. In S. M. Johnson & V. E. Whiffen (Eds.), *Attachment processes in couple and family therapy* (pp. 300–317). Guilford Press.

Kailanko, S., Wiebe, S. A., Tasca, G. A., & Laitila, A. A. (2021a). Impact of repeating somatic cues on the depth of experiencing for withdrawers and pursuers in emotionally focused couple therapy. *Journal of Marital and Family Therapy, 48*(3), 677–692.

Kailanko, S., Wiebe, S. A., Tasca, G. A., Laitila, A. A., & Allan, R. (2021b). Somatic experience of emotion in emotionally focused couple therapy: Experienced trainer therapists' views and experiences. *Journal of Marital and Family Therapy, 48*(3), 693–708.

Kailanko, S., Wiebe, S. A., Tasca, G. A., & Laitila, A. A. (2022). Somatic interventions and depth of experiencing in emotionally focused couple therapy. *International Journal of Systemic Therapy, 33*(2), 109–128.

Karen, R. (1994). *Becoming attached: First relationships and how they shape our capacity to love.* Oxford University Press.

Karantzas, G. C., Simpson, J. A., & Pizzarini, B. (2022). The loss of humanness in close relationships: An interpersonal model of dehumanization. *Current Opinion in Psychology, 46*, 1–5.

Katehakis, A. (2016). *Sex addiction as affect dysregulation: A neurobiologically informed holistic treatment.* W. W. Norton & Company.

Keller, H. (2021). *Attachment theory: Fact or fancy?* In R. A. Thompson, R. A. Simpson, & L. J. Berlin (Eds.), *Attachment: The fundamental questions* (pp. 229–236). Guilford.

Keller, H. (2022). *The myth of attachment theory: A critical understanding for multicultural societies.* Routledge.

Kelly, R. M., Hastings, J. and West, R. (2022). How an addiction ontology can unify competing conceptualizations of addiction. In N. Heather, M. Field, A. C. Moss & S. Satel (Eds.), *Evaluating the brain disease model of addiction* (pp. 484–496). Routledge.

Kennedy, N. W., Johnson, S. M., Wiebe, S. A., & Tasca, G. A. (2018). Conversations for connection: An outcome assessment of the hold-me-tight relationship-education program for couples, and recommendations for improving future research methodology in relationship education. *Journal of Marital and Family Therapy, 45*(3), 432–446.

Klein, M. H., Mathieu, P. L., Gendlin, E. T., & Kiesler, D. J. (1969). *The experiencing scale. A research and training manual (Vol. I).* Wisconsin Psychiatric Institute.

Klein, M. H., Mathieu-Coughlan, P., & Kiesler, D. J. (1986). The experiencing scales. In L. S. Greenberg & W. M. Pinsof (Eds.), *The psychotherapeutic process: A research handbook* (pp. 21–71). Guilford.

Kobak, R., & Mandelbaum, T. (2003). Caring for the caregiver: An attachment approach to assessment and treatment of child problems. In S. Johnson & V. Whiffen (Eds.), *Attachment processes in couple and family therapy* (pp. 144–164). Guilford.

Kobak, R., Zajac, K., Herres, J., & Krauthamer Ewing, E. S. (2015). Attachment based treatments for adolescents: The secure cycle as a framework for assessment, treatment and evaluation. *Attachment & Human Development, 17*, 220–239.

Knudson-Martin, C., Wells, M. A., & Samman, S. K. (Eds.). (2015). *Socio-emotional relationship therapy: Bridging emotion, societal context, and couple interaction.* Springer.

Kolmes, K., & Witherspoon, R. J. (2017). Therapy with a consensually nonmonogamous couple. *Journal of Clinical Psychology, 73*, 954–964.

Koren, R., Woolley, S. R., Danis, I., & Török, S. (2022). Training therapists in emotionally focused therapy: A longitudinal and cross-sectional analysis. *Journal of Marital and Family Therapy, 48*, 709–725. https://doi.org/10.1111/jmft.12495

Lafontaine, M-F., Lonergan, M., Brubacher, L., & Johnson, S. (in preparation). Attachment injuries in romantic couples: A qualitative thematic analysis.

Landau-North, M., Johnson, S. M., & Dalgleish, T. L. (2011). Emotionally focused couple therapy and addiction. In J. L. Furrow, S. M. Johnson, & B. A. Bradley (Eds.), *The emotionally focused casebook: New directions in treating couples* (pp. 193–218). Routledge.

Ledoux, J. (1996). *The emotional brain: The mysterious underpinnings of emotional life*. Simon & Schuster.

Lee, N. A., Spengler, P. M., Mitchell, A. M., Spengler, E. S., & Spiker, D. A. (2017). Facilitating withdrawer re-engagement in emotionally focused couple therapy: A modified task analysis. *Couple and Family Psychology: Research and Practice, 6*(3), 205–225. http://doi.org/10.1037/cfp00 00084

Lewis, T., Amini, F., & Lannon, R. (2000). *A general theory of love*. Random House.

Lietaer, G., Rombauts, J., & van Balen, R. (1990). *Client-centered and experiential psychotherapy in the nineties*. Leuven University Press.

Liu, T., & Wittenborn, A. (2011). Emotionally focused therapy with culturally diverse couples. In J. L. Furrow, S. M. Johnson, & B. A. Bradley (Eds.), *The emotionally focused casebook: New directions in treating couples* (pp. 295–316). Routledge.

Love, H. A., Moore, R. M., & Stanish, N. A. (2016). Emotionally focused therapy for couples recovering from sexual addiction. *Sexual and Relationship Therapy, 31*(2), 176–189.

Magnavita, J. J., & Anchin, J. C. (2014). *Unifying psychotherapy: Principles, methods, and evidence from clinical science*. Springer.

Makinen, J. A., & Johnson, S. (2006). Resolving attachment injuries in couples using EFT: Steps toward forgiveness and reconciliation. *Journal of Consulting and Clinical Psychology, 74*, 1055–1064.

Mandela, N. (1995). *Long walk to freedom: The autobiography of Nelson Mandela*. Little Brown.

Martin, D. (2016). *Counseling and therapy skills* (4th ed.). Waveland Press.

Maté, G. (2010). *In the realm of hungry ghosts*. North Atlantic Books.

McGoldrick, M., & Hardy, K. V. (Eds.). (2019). *Re-visioning family therapy: Addressing diversity in clinical practice*. Guilford.

Menakem, R. (2017). *My grandmother's hands: Racialized trauma and the pathway to mending our hearts and bodies*. Central Recovery Press.

Mesman, J. (2021). Attachment theory's universality claims: Asking different questions. In R. A. Thompson, J. A. Simpson, & L. J. Berlin (Eds.), *Attachment: The fundamental questions* (pp. 245–251). Guilford.

Mesman, J., van IJzendoorn, M. H., & Sagi-Schwartz, A. (2016). Cross-cultural patterns of attachment: Universal and contextual dimensions. In J. Cassidy & P. R. Shaver (Eds.), *Handbook of attachment: Theory, research, and clinical applications* (3rd ed., pp. 852–877). Guilford Press.

Mikulincer, M., & Shaver, P. R. (2015). Boosting attachment security in adulthood: The "broaden-and-build" effects of security-enhancing mental representations and interpersonal contexts. In J. A. Simpson & W. S. Rholes (Eds.), *Attachment theory and research: New directions and emerging themes* (pp. 124–144). Guilford Press.

Mikulincer, M., & Shaver, P. R. (2016). *Attachment in adulthood: Structure, dynamics, and change* (2nd ed.). Guilford Press.

Mikulincer, M., & Shaver, P. R. (2019). Attachment orientations and emotion regulation. *Current Opinion in Psychology, 25*, 6–10.

Mikulincer, M., & Shaver, P. R. (2021). Enhancing the "broaden-and build" cycle of attachment security as a means of overcoming prejudice, discrimination, and racism. *Attachment & Human Development*. http://doi.org/10.1080/14616734.2021.1976921

Mikulincer, M., & Shaver, P. R. (2023a). *Attachment theory applied: Fostering personal Growth through healthy relationships*. Guilford.

Mikulincer, M., & Shaver, P. R. (2023b). *Attachment theory expanded: Security dynamics in individuals, dyads, groups, and societies*. Guilford.

Minuchin, S., & Fishman, H. C. (1981). *Family therapy techniques*. Harvard University Press.

Montagno, M., Svatovic, M., & Levenson, H. (2011). Short-term and long-term effects of training in emotionally focused couple therapy: Professional and personal aspects. *Journal of Marital and Family Therapy, 37*(4), 380–392.

Morgis, B., Ewing, E., Liu, T., Slaughter-Acey, J., Fisher, K., & Jampol, R. (2019). A hold me tight workshop for couple attachment and sexual intimacy. *Contemporary Family Therapy, 41*(4), 368–383.

Morretti, M. M., & Holland, R. (2003). The journey of adolescence: Transitions in self within the context of attachment relationships. In S. Johnson & V. Whiffen (Eds.), *Attachment processes in couple and family therapy* (pp. 234–257). Guilford.

Morris, A. S., Silk, J. S., Steinberg, L., Myers, S. S., & Robinson, L. R. (2007). The role of the family context in the development of emotion regulation. *Social Development, 16*(2), 361–388.

Moors, A. C., Ryan, W., & Chopik, W. J. (2019). Multiple loves: The effects of attachment with multiple concurrent romantic partners on relational functioning. *Personality and Individual Differences, 147*, 102–110. https://doi.org/10.1016/j.paid.2019.04.023

Morrison, T. (1992). *Playing in the dark: Whiteness and the literary imagination*. Vintage.

Myung, H. S., Furrow, J. L., & Lee, N. A. (2022). Understanding the emotional landscape in the withdrawer re-engagement and blamer softening EFCT change events. *Journal of Marital and Family Therapy, 48*(3), 758-776. https://doi.org/10.1111/jmft.12583

Nightingale, M. A. (2021). Emotionally focused therapy with African American couples: An exploratory acceptability and feasibility study (Publication No. 28547842) [Doctoral dissertation, Drexel University]. ProQuest Dissertations and Theses Global.

Nightingale, M., Awosan, C. I., & Stavrianopoulos, K. (2019). Emotionally focused therapy: A culturally sensitive approach for African American heterosexual couples. *Journal of Family Psychotherapy, 30*(3), 221–244.

Ogner, R. (2015). *Re: Growing in our craft decades in and on.* [ICEEFT members' electronic mailing list: therapists@list.efters.com], 14 August.

Oluo, I. (2019). *So you want to talk about race*. Hachette.

Paivio, S. C., & Pascual-Leone, A. (2010). *Emotion-focused therapy for complex trauma: An integrative approach*. American Psychological Association.

Panksepp, J. (2003). Feeling the pain of social loss. *Science, 302*(5643), 237–239.

Panksepp, J., Solms, M., Schläpfer, T. E., & Volker, A. (2014). Primary-process separation-distress (panic/grief) and reward eagerness (seeking) processes in the ancestral genesis of depressive affect and addictions. In M. Mikulincer & P. R. Shaver (Eds.), *Mechanisms of social connection: From brain to group* (pp. 33–53). American Psychological Association.

Pascual-Leone, A., & Yeryomenko, N. (2017). The client "experiencing" scale as a predictor of treatment outcomes: A meta-analysis on psychotherapy process. *Psychotherapy Research, 27*(6), 653–665. http://doi.org/10.1080/10503307.2016.1152409

Perls, F. S. (1969). *Gestalt therapy verbatim*. Real People.

PettyJohn, M. E., Tseng, C-F., & Blow, A. J. (2020). Therapeutic utility of discussing therapist/client intersectionality in treatment: When and how? *Family Process, 59*(2), 313–327. http://doi.org/10.1111/famp.12471

Pinel, J. P. (2015). *Introduction to biopsychology* (9th ed.). Pearson Higher Education.

Porges, S. W. (2011). *The polyvagal theory: Neuro-physiological foundations of emotions, attachment, communication, self-regulation*. Norton.

Porges, S. W. (2015). Making the world safe for our children: Down-regulating defence and up-regulating social engagement to 'optimise' the human experience. *Children Australia, 40*, 114–123.

Porges, S. W. (2016). The polyvagal theory, vocal prosody, neuro-exercises and the face-heart connection. [Webinar]. Talk Time Featuring Dr. Stephen Porges. Retrieved from: https://drrebeccajorgensen.com/talk-time-stephen-porges/

Quinn, B., Davis, S., Greaves, B., Furrow, J., Palmer-Olsen, L., & Woolley, S. (2023). Caregiver openness in emotionally focused family therapy: A critical shift. *Family Process*, 1–19. Advance online publication.

Rheem, K. (2012). Helping a combat vet face his vulnerability: Connecting with the shut-down client. *Psychotherapy Networker, 36*(3). Retrieved from: www.psychotherapynetworker.org

Rhodius, C. (2023). How attachment transformed my palliative practice: Discovering the palliative paradox. *Attachment, 17*(1), 58–68.

Rice, L. N. (1974). The evocative function of the therapist. In D. A. Wexler & L. N. Rice (Eds.), *Innovations in client-centered therapy* (pp. 289–311). Wiley.

Rice, L. N., & Kerr, G. P. (1986). Measures of client and therapist vocal quality. In L. S. Greenberg & W. M. Pinsof (Eds.), *The psycho therapeutic process: A research handbook* (pp. 73–105). Guilford.

Rice, L. N., Koke, C. J., Greenberg, L. S., & Wagstaff, A. (1979). *Manual for client vocal quality*. York University Counselling and Development Centre.

Robertson, J. (1952). *A two-year-old goes to hospital (DVD)*. Retrieved from: https://www.youtube.com/watch?v=s14Q-_Bxc_U

Rodríguez-González, M., Schweer-Collins, M., Greenman, P. G., Lafontaine, M.-F., Fatás, M., & Sandberg, J. G. (2019). Short-term and long-term effects of training in EFT: A multi-national study in Spanish-speaking countries. *Journal of Marital and Family Therapy, 46*(2), 304–320.

Rogers, C. (1957). The necessary and sufficient conditions of therapeutic personality change. *Journal of Consulting Psychology, 21*(2), 95–103.

Rogers, C. R. (1961). *On becoming a person*. Constable.

Rogers, C. R. (1975). Empathic: An unappreciated way of being. *Counseling Psychologist, 5*(2), 2–10.

Rogers, C. R. (1980). *A way of being*. Houghton Mifflin.

Sandberg, J. G., & Knestel, A. (2011). The experience of learning emotionally focused couples therapy. *Journal of Marital and Family Therapy, 37*(4), 398–410.

Seiff-Haron, J. M., & Calamur, N. (2022, July 14, 20, 26). Navigating the rapids: Power, culture, and difference in EFT. [Workshop]. Alliant International University, online.

Sexton, T., Coop Gordon, K., Gurman, A., Lebow, J., Holtzworth-Munroe, A., & Johnson, S. (2011). Guidelines for classifying evidence-based treatments in couple and family therapy. *Family Process, 50*, 377–392.

Shaver, P. R., & Mikulincer, M. (2006). A behavioral systems approach to romantic love relationships: Attachment, caregiving, and sex. In R. J. Sternberg & K. Weiss (Eds.), *The new psychology of love* (2nd ed., pp. 35–64). Yale University Press.

Shaver, P. R., & Mikulincer, M. (2014). Attachment bonds in romantic relationships. In M. Mikulincer & P. R. Shaver (Eds.), *From brain to group* (pp. 273–290). American Psychological Association.

Shaver, P. R., Mikulincer, M., Gross, J. T., Stern, J. A., & Cassidy, J. (2016). A lifespan perspective on attachment and care for others: Empathy, altruism, and prosocial behavior. In J. Cassidy & P. R. Shaver (Eds.), *Handbook of attachment: Theory, research, and clinical applications* (3rd ed., pp. 878–916.). Guilford Press.

Shore, A. N. (2014). Introduction. In J. J. Magnavita & J. C. Anchin (Eds.), *Unifying psychotherapy: Principles, methods, and evidence from clinical science* (pp. xxi–xxxiv). Springer.

Siegel, D. J. (2009). Emotion as integration: A possible answer to the question, what is emotion? In D. Fosha, D. J. Siegel, & M. F. Solomon (Eds.), *The healing power of emotion: Affective neuroscience, development & clinical practice* (pp. 145–171). W. W. Norton.

Siegel, D. J. (2010). *The mindful therapist: A clinician's guide to mindsight and neural integration*. Norton.

Siegel, D. J. (2012). *The developing mind: How relationships and the brain interact to shape who we are* (2nd ed.). Guilford.

Simons, S.-A., (Host). (2020, June 1). *To be in a rage almost all the time* [Audio Podcast]. NPR. Retrieved from: https://www.npr.org/2020/06/01/867153918/-to-be-in-a-rage-almost-all-the-time

Simpson, J., & Karantzas, G. C. (2019). Editorial overview: Attachment in adulthood: A dynamic field with a rich past and a bright future. *Current Opinion in Psychology, 25*, 177–181.

Simpson, J., & Rholes, W. (1994). Stress and secure base relationships in adulthood. In K. Bartholomew & D. Perlman (Eds.), *Attachment processes in adulthood* (pp. 181–204). Jessica Kingsley.

Simpson, J., & Rholes, W. (2015). *Attachment theory and research: New directions and emerging themes*. Guilford Press.

Slootmaeckers, J., & Migerode, L. (2018). Fighting for connection: Patterns of intimate partner violence. *Journal of Couple & Relationship Therapy: Innovations in Clinical and Educational Interventions, 17*(4), 294–312.

Slootmaeckers, J., & Migerode, L. (2020). EFT and intimate partner violence: A roadmap to de-escalating violent patterns. *Family Process, 59*(2), 328–345.

Smith, W. A., Hung, M., & Franklin, J. D. (2011). Racial battle fatigue and the miseducation of Black men: Racial microaggressions, societal problems, and environmental stress. *Journal of Negro Education, 80*(1), 63–82.

Snyder, D. K., Castellani, A. M., & Whisman, M. A. (2006). Current status and future directions in couple therapy. *Annual Review of Psychology, 57*, 317–344.

Spengler, P. M., Lee, N. A., Wiebe, S. A., & Wittenborn, A. K. (2022). A comprehensive meta-analysis on the efficacy of emotionally focused couple therapy. *Couple and Family Psychology: Research and Practice*. Advance online publication.

Sroufe, L. A. (1996). *Emotional development: The organization of emotional life in the early years.* Cambridge University Press. https://doi.org/10.1017/CBO9780511527661

Stern, D. N. (2004). *The present moment in psychotherapy and everyday life.* Norton.

Szalavitz, M. (2021). *Undoing drugs: The untold story of harm reduction and the future of addiction.* Hachette Go.

Thompson, A., & Samoilow, D. (2022). Stepping into the EFT Tango. *The EFT Community News, 53,* 2–4.

Thompson, R. A., Simpson, R. A., & Berlin, L. J. (2021). *Attachment: The fundamental questions.* Guilford.

Tilley, D., & Palmer, G. (2013). Enactments in emotionally focused couple therapy: Shaping moments of contact and change. *Journal of Marital and Family Therapy, 39*(3), 299–313.

Trimane, R. (2022, June). Cultural competency and trauma-informed care for working with trans and trans BIPOC clients: Create a welcoming and gender-affirming safe and trusting environment. [online conference session]. LGBTQIA2S+ Summit: Breaking Down the Barriers to Inclusive Mental Health Care and Connection, PESI, Inc.

Tronick, E. Z. (1989). Emotion and emotional communication in infants. *American Psychologist, 44,* 112–119.

Tronick, E. Z. (2007). *The neurobehavioral and social-emotional development of infants and children.* W. W. Norton.

Vangelisti, A. L. (2009). *Feeling hurt in close relationships.* Cambridge University Press.

Wagamese, R. (2012). *Indian horse.* Douglas & McIntyre.

Walant, K. B. (1995). *Creating the capacity for attachment: Treating addictions and the alienated self.* Jason Aronson.

West, C. (1993/2017). *Race matters.* Beacon Press.

Wiebe, S. A., & Johnson, S. M. (2016). A review of the research in emotionally focused therapy for couples. *Family Process, 55*(3), 390–407.

Wiebe, S. A., Elliott, C., Johnson, S. M., Burgess Moser, M., Dalgleish, T. L., LaFontaine, M-F., & Tasca, G. A. (2019). Attachment change in emotionally focused couple therapy and sexual satisfaction outcomes in a two-year follow-up study. *Journal of Couple and Relationship Therapy, 18*(1), 1–21. http://doi.org/10.1080/15332691.2018.1481799

Wiebe, S. A., Johnson S. M., Allan, R., Campbell, L., Greenman, P., Fairweather, D., Ismail, M., & Tasca, G. (in preparation). A randomized controlled trial of emotionally focused individual therapy for depression and anxiety.

Wiebe, S. A., Johnson, S. M., Burgess Moser, T., Dalgleish, T. L., & Tasca, G. A. (2017). Predicting follow-up outcomes in emotionally focused couple therapy: The role of change in trust, relationship-specific attachment, and emotional engagement. *Journal of Marital and Family Therapy, 43*(2), 213–226.

Wiebe, S. A., Johnson, S. M., Lafontaine, M.-F., Burgess Moser, T., Dalgleish, T. L., & Tasca, G. A. (2017). Two-year follow-up outcomes in emotionally focused couple therapy: An investigation of relationship satisfaction and attachment trajectories. *Journal of Marital and Family Therapy, 43*(2), 227–244.

Williams, M. T. (2020). *Managing microaggressions: Addressing everyday racism in therapeutic spaces.* Oxford.

Williams, M. T., Malcoun, E., Sawyer, B. A., Davis, D. M., Nouri, L. B., & Bruce, S. L. (2014). Cultural adaptations of prolonged exposure therapy for treatment and prevention of posttraumatic stress disorder in African Americans. *Behavioral Sciences, 4,* 102–124. http://doi.org/10.3390/bs4020102

Wittenborn, A. K., Liu, T., Ridenour, T. A., Lachmar, E. M., Rouleau, E., & Seedall, R. B. (2019). Randomized controlled trial of emotionally focused couple therapy compared to treatment as usual for depression: Outcomes and mechanisms of change. *Journal of Marital and Family Therapy, 45,* 395–409.

Wong, T. Y., Greenman, P. S., & Beaudoin, V. (2017). '*Hold Me Tight*': The generalizability of an attachment-based group intervention to Chinese Canadian couples. *Journal of Couple & Relationship Therapy — Innovations in Clinical and Educational Interventions, 17*(1), 42–60.

Yoshino, K. (2007). Covering: *The hidden assault of our civil rights.* Random House.

Zuccarini, D., & Karos, L. (2011). Emotionally focused therapy for gay and lesbian couples: Strong identities, strong bonds. In J. L. Furrow, S. M. Johnson, & B. A. Bradley (Eds.), *The emotionally focused casebook: New directions in treating couples* (pp. 317–342). Routledge.

Zuccarini, D. J., Johnson, S. M., Dalgleish, T. L., & Makinen, J. A. (2013). Forgiveness and reconciliation in emotionally focused therapy for couples: The client change process and therapist interventions. *Journal of Marital & Family Therapy, 39,* 148–162.

Index

Note: **Bold** page numbers refer to tables and *italic* page numbers refer to figures.